Handbook of Lung Cancer and Other Thoracic Malignancies

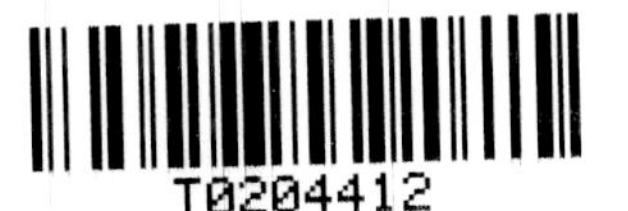

Handbook of Lung Cancer and Other Thoracic Malignancies

Editors

Gregory P. Kalemkerian, MD
Professor, Co-Director of Thoracic Oncology
Division of Hematology/Oncology
Department of Internal Medicine
University of Michigan
Ann Arbor, Michigan

Jessica S. Donington, MD
Associate Professor
Cardiothoracic Surgery
NYU Medical Center
New York, New York

Elizabeth M. Gore, MD
Professor, Department of Radiation Oncology
Medical College of Wisconsin
Milwaukee, Wisconsin

Suresh S. Ramalingam, MD
Professor of Hematology and Medical Oncology
Director, Division of Medical Oncology
Assistant Dean for Cancer Research
Emory University School of Medicine;
Deputy Director, Winship Cancer Institute
Atlanta, Georgia

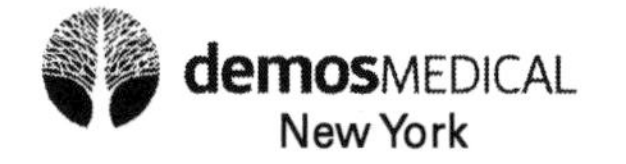

New York

Visit our website at www.demosmedical.com

ISBN: 9781620700969
e-book ISBN: 9781617052729

Acquisitions Editor: David D'Addona
Compositor: diacriTech

Medicine is an ever-changing science. Research and clinical experience are continually expanding our knowledge, in particular our understanding of proper treatment and drug therapy. The authors, editors, and publisher have made every effort to ensure that all information in this book is in accordance with the state of knowledge at the time of production of the book. Nevertheless, the authors, editors, and publisher are not responsible for errors or omissions or for any consequences from application of the information in this book and make no warranty, expressed or implied, with respect to the contents of the publication. Every reader should examine carefully the package inserts accompanying each drug and should carefully check whether the dosage schedules mentioned therein or the contraindications stated by the manufacturer differ from the statements made in this book. Such examination is particularly important with drugs that are either rarely used or have been newly released on the market.

Library of Congress Cataloging-in-Publication Data

Names: Kalemkerian, Gregory, editor. | Donington, Jessica, editor. | Gore, Elizabeth (Professor), editor. | Ramalingam, Suresh, editor.
Title: Handbook of lung cancer and other thoracic malignancies / editors, Gregory P. Kalemkerian, MD, Professor, Co-Director of Thoracic Oncology, Division of Hematology/Oncology, Department of Internal Medicine, University of Michigan, Ann Arbor, Michigan, Jessica S. Donington, MD, Associate Professor, Cardiothoracic Surgery, NYU Medical Center, New York, New York, Elizabeth M. Gore, MD, Professor, Department of Radiation Oncology, Medical College of Wisconsin, Milwaukee, Wisconsin, Suresh S. Ramalingam, MD, Professor of Hematology and Medical Oncology, Director, Division of Medical Oncology, Assistant Dean for Cancer Research, Emory University School of Medicine, Deputy Director, Winship Cancer Institute, Atlanta, Georgia.
Description: New York : Demos Medical, [2017] | Includes bibliographical references and index.
Identifiers: LCCN 2016039960 | ISBN 9781620700969
Subjects: LCSH: Lungs—Cancer.
Classification: LCC RC280.L8 H342 2017 | DDC 616.99/424—dc23 LC record available at https://lccn.loc.gov/2016039960

Printed in the United States of America by McNaughton & Gunn.
16 17 18 19 20 / 5 4 3 2 1

"We collectively dedicate this book to the many patients who have taught us so much over the years about strength, determination and perseverance."

"To my wife Mary and my boys Peter and John for all their patience and support"

—Gregory P. Kalemkerian, MD

"For Pamela Steiner, my mother, friend, and role model."

—Jessica S. Donington, MD

"To my husband Stuart Wong and my children Allie, Stuart, Hank, and Russell for their endless support."

—Elizabeth M. Gore, MD

"To my parents R. Sakkaraiappan and S. Saraswathi, for their support and personal sacrifices, that made my journey possible"

—Suresh S. Ramalingam, MD

Contents

Contributors

Joseph A. Bovi, MD
Associate Professor of Radiation Oncology
Department of Radiation Oncology
Medical College of Wisconsin
Froedtert Memorial Lutheran Hospital
Milwaukee, Wisconsin

Bryan M. Burt, MD
Assistant Professor of Surgery
Division of General Thoracic Surgery
Baylor College of Medicine
Houston, Texas

Jessica S. Donington, MD
Associate Professor
Cardiothoracic Surgery
NYU Medical Center
New York, New York

Vinicius Ernani, MD
Assistant Professor of Medicine
University of Nebraska Medical Center
Omaha, Nebraska

Shirish M. Gadgeel, MD
Professor
Department of Oncology
Karmanos Cancer Institute
Wayne State University School of Medicine
Detroit, Michigan

Michael F. Gensheimer, MD
Instructor of Radiation Oncology
Department of Radiation Oncology
Stanford Cancer Institute
Stanford University School of Medicine
Stanford, California

Elizabeth M. Gore, MD
Professor
Department of Radiation Oncology
Medical College of Wisconsin
Milwaukee, Wisconsin

Raffit Hassan, MD
Senior Investigator
Thoracic and GI Oncology Branch
Center for Cancer Research
National Cancer Institute
National Institutes of Health
Bethesda, Maryland

James A. Hayman, MD
Professor
Department of Radiation Oncology
University of Michigan
Ann Arbor, Michigan

Cheryl Ho, MD, FRCPC
Clinical Associate Professor
British Columbia Cancer Agency
Division of Medical Oncology
University of British Columbia
Vancouver, British Columbia, Canada

James Jett, MD
Professor of Medicine
Division of Oncology
Department of Medicine
National Jewish Health
Denver, Colorado

Gregory P. Kalemkerian, MD
Professor, Co-Director of Thoracic Oncology
Division of Hematology/Oncology
Department of Internal Medicine
University of Michigan
Ann Arbor, Michigan

Vaishnavi Kundel, MD
Postdoctoral Fellow
Department of Medicine
Division of Pulmonary, Critical Care, and Sleep Medicine
Icahn School of Medicine at Mount Sinai
New York, New York

Janessa Laskin, MD, FRCPC
Clinical Associate Professor
British Columbia Cancer Agency
Division of Medical Oncology
University of British Columbia
Vancouver, British Columbia, Canada

Jean Lee, MD
Assistant Professor
Department of Medicine
Division of Hematology and Oncology
NYU School of Medicine
New York, New York

Steven E. Lommatzsch, MD
Assistant Professor of Medicine
Division of Pulmonary and Critical Care Medicine
Department of Medicine
National Jewish Health
Denver, Colorado

Billy W. Loo Jr., MD, PhD
Associate Professor of Radiation Oncology
Department of Radiation Oncology
Stanford Cancer Institute
Stanford University School of Medicine
Stanford, California

Smitha P. Menon, MD
Assistant Professor
Department of Hematology/Oncology
Medical College of Wisconsin
Milwaukee, Wisconsin

Taofeek K. Owonikoko, MD, PhD
Associate Professor
Co-Director, Thoracic Oncology Program
Department of Hematology and Medical Oncology
Winship Cancer Institute
Emory University School of Medicine
Atlanta, Georgia

Sukhmani K. Padda, MD
Assistant Professor of Medicine
Department of Medicine
Division of Oncology
Stanford Cancer Institute
Stanford University School of Medicine
Stanford, California

Edwin R. Parra, MD, PhD
Postdoctoral Fellow
Department of Translational Molecular Pathology
The University of Texas, MD Anderson Cancer Center
Houston, Texas

Charles A. Powell, MD
Janice and Coleman Rabin Professor of Medicine and Chief
Division of Pulmonary, Critical Care, and Sleep Medicine
Icahn School of Medicine at Mount Sinai
New York, New York

Suresh S. Ramalingam, MD
Professor of Hematology and Medical Oncology
Director, Division of Medical Oncology
Assistant Dean for Cancer Research
Emory University School of Medicine;
Deputy Director, Winship Cancer Institute
Atlanta, Georgia

Bryan J. Schneider, MD
Associate Professor of Medicine
Department of Internal Medicine
Division of Hematology/Oncology
University of Michigan
Ann Arbor, Michigan

Ann G. Schwartz, PhD, MPH
Deputy Center Director
Department of Oncology
Karmanos Cancer Institute
Wayne State University School of Medicine
Detroit, Michigan

Conor E. Steuer, MD
Assistant Professor of Hematology and Medical Oncology
Winship Cancer Institute
Emory University School of Medicine
Atlanta, Georgia

Anish Thomas, MD, MBBS
Staff Clinician
Thoracic and GI Oncology Branch
Center for Cancer Research
National Cancer Institute
National Institutes of Health
Bethesda, Maryland

Susan Urba, MD
Professor of Internal Medicine
Division of Hematology/Oncology
University of Michigan Comprehensive Cancer Center
Ann Arbor, Michigan

Heather A. Wakelee, MD
Associate Professor of Medicine
Department of Medicine
Division of Oncology
Stanford Cancer Institute
Stanford University School of Medicine
Stanford, California

Ying Wang, MD
Medical Oncology Fellow
British Columbia Cancer Agency
Division of Medical Oncology
University of British Columbia
Vancouver, British Columbia, Canada

Ignacio I. Wistuba, MD
Professor and Chair
Department of Translational Molecular Pathology
The University of Texas, MD Anderson Cancer Center
Houston, Texas

Preface

"How do I care for this patient sitting in front of me?" This is the question that drove the development of the *Handbook of Lung Cancer and Other Thoracic Malignancies*. Until recently, the answer to this question was relatively straightforward for patients with lung cancer. However, over the past few years, we have witnessed a quantum leap of new knowledge and novel therapeutic options that have positioned lung cancer at the forefront of the personalized medicine revolution in oncology. In just the past two years, the U.S. Food and Drug Administration has granted eight new approvals for drugs used to treat lung cancer.

The management of people with lung cancer now requires the understanding and utilization of numerous multidisciplinary modalities, including minimally invasive surgical procedures, adjuvant chemotherapy, stereotactic radiotherapy, radiofrequency ablation, combined-modality therapy, maintenance therapy, targeted systemic therapy guided by molecular diagnostic testing, immunotherapy, and site-directed treatment of oligometastatic disease. This plethora of therapeutic options not only provides our patients with an increased potential for cure and improved quality-of-life, but also makes it increasingly more difficult for busy practitioners to keep up with the essential knowledge required to provide state-of-the-art care. In addition, health care providers are now facing increasing demands on their time from electronic medical record keeping, interactions with third-party payers, regulatory oversight by health care institutions, and the maintenance of professional competency. Driven by these concerns, we endeavored to create a practical guide to the management of lung cancer and other thoracic malignancies for practicing oncologists, trainees, and other health care providers.

While other textbooks might offer comprehensive data on various aspects of lung cancer, our objective was to provide a concise and practical resource to assist in real-time, clinical decision making. The chapters have been written by highly respected leaders in thoracic oncology, based not only on their research expertise, but also on their extensive experience in patient care. The text is organized by treatment-based themes and is supplemented with tables, graphics, and key points that highlight the most relevant data that drive management decisions for both common and uncommon clinical scenarios. The format is succinct and readable, with multiple subheadings and bulleted points emphasizing overall treatment guidelines and more nuanced applications of therapy for individual patient subgroups. Our goal is that the entire health care team and their patients will benefit from the evidence-based, practical discussions of management paradigms presented in this concise volume.

Finally, we acknowledge the time and effort of all the authors who contributed outstanding chapters for this handbook, and thank David D'Addona and Norman Graubart at Demos Medical Publishing for believing in this project and bringing our concept to fruition.

Gregory P. Kalemkerian, MD
Jessica S. Donington, MD
Elizabeth M. Gore, MD
Suresh S. Ramalingam, MD

Handbook of Lung Cancer and Other Thoracic Malignancies

Epidemiology and Etiology of Lung Cancer 1

Ann G. Schwartz

INCIDENCE AND MORTALITY

In 2015, lung cancer was the second most common cancer diagnosed in both men and women in the United States, accounting for 14% of all new cancer diagnoses among men and 13% among women. However, lung cancer continues to be the leading cause of cancer-related mortality, accounting for 28% of cancer deaths in men and 26% in women. In 2015, there were 221,000 new diagnoses and 158,000 deaths due to lung cancer in the United States (1). The median age at diagnosis is 70 years, with little difference by sex. In men, incidence and mortality rates increased steadily until the early 1980s and early 1990s, respectively, following a decline in cigarette smoking. In women, incidence and mortality rates did not decrease until the mid-2000s. Average annual age-adjusted incidence rates (2008–2012) are 70.1 per 100,000 men (down by ~30% from peak rates) and 50.2 per 100,000 women (down by ~5% from peak rates); the respective mortality rates are 59.8/100,000 and 37.8/100,000 in men and women (2).

In the United States, incidence and mortality rates vary by race/ethnicity (Figure 1.1). The highest incidence rates are seen in African Americans (67.0 per 100,000), followed by whites (60.2 per 100,000). African Americans also have a median age at diagnosis that is 4 to 5 years younger than that among whites. Incidence rates among Asian/Pacific Islanders (37.1 per 100,000), American Indians/Alaska Natives (39.9 per 100,000), and Hispanics (30.4 per 100,000) are substantially lower. Globally, lung cancer was responsible for approximately 1.6 million deaths in 2012, making it the leading cause of death due to cancer worldwide (3). Mortality varies with smoking prevalence, with the highest mortality rates in Central and Eastern Europe and Eastern Asia in men and in North America and Northern Europe in women.

SURVIVAL

The 5-year survival rate after a lung cancer diagnosis in the United States was 19.7% for patients diagnosed in 2005 to 2011 (2). While still relatively low, the 5-year survival rate has risen from

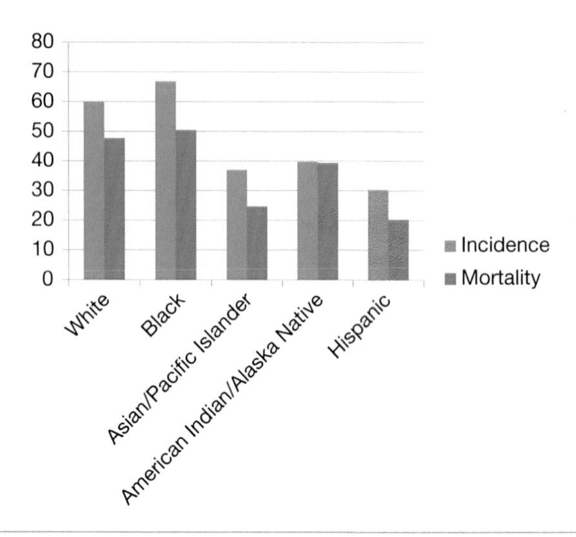

Figure 1.1 Lung Cancer Incidence and Mortality Rates per 100,000 From 2008–2012 by Race/Ethnicity
Source: From Ref. (2). Howlander N, Krapcho M, Garshell J, et al. (eds). *SEER Cancer Statistics Review, 1975-2012*. Bethesda, MD: National Cancer Institute; 2015.

12.2% for those diagnosed in 1975 to 1977. Women continue to have higher 5-year survival rates than men (21.2% vs. 15.8%). These poor survival rates reflect the high frequency of late-stage disease at diagnosis, with 57% of lung cancer patients in 2005 to 2011 diagnosed at distant stage with only a 4.2% 5-year survival rate. For the 16% of patients diagnosed with localized disease, the 5-year survival rate was 54.8%. Figure 1.2 illustrates the disparity in survival by race/ethnicity. The 5-year survival rate is highest among Asians (21.2%), followed by whites (20.0%), Hispanics (19.1%), Pacific Islanders (17.5%), African Americans (16.6%), and American Indians/Alaska Natives (14.5%). So, while lung cancer is one of the few cancers for which the major etiologic factor, cigarette smoking, is well known, these statistics reflect the lack of substantial progress that has been made in smoking prevention and cessation, early diagnosis, and treatment.

RISK FACTORS FOR LUNG CANCER

The risk factors for lung cancer are summarized in Table 1.1.

Tobacco and Inhaled Smoke Exposures

Smoking Prevalence

In 2012, 18.1% of U.S. adults aged 18 years or older were current smokers, with 7.0% of current smokers smoking ≥30 cigarettes

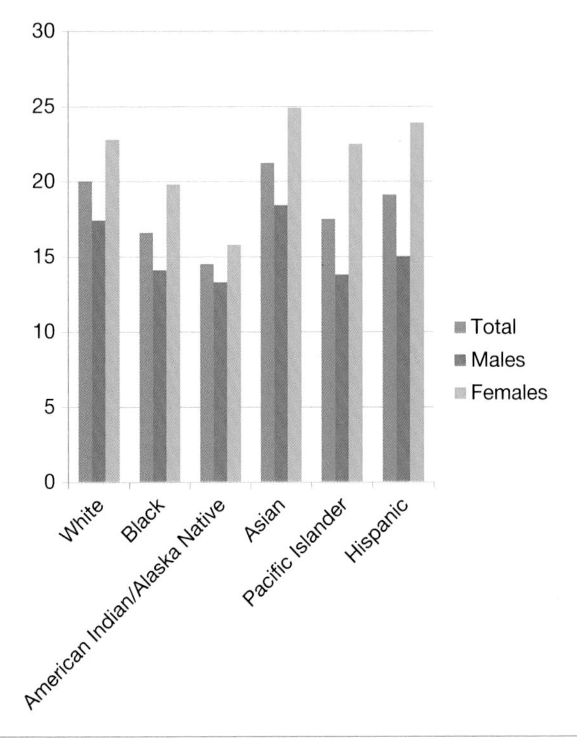

Figure 1.2 Five-Year Lung Cancer-Specific Survival Rates by Race/Ethnicity
Source: From Ref. (2). Howlander N, Krapcho M, Garshell J, et al (eds). *SEER Cancer Statistics Review, 1975-2012*. Bethesda, MD: National Cancer Institute; 2015.

per day (4). Mean cigarettes smoked per day was 14.6. Current smoking is more prevalent among men than women (20.5% vs. 15.8%). The prevalence of cigarette smoking varies by race/ethnicity, with rates among whites being 19.7%, African Americans 18.1%, American Indian/Alaska Natives 21.8%, Hispanics 12.5%, and Asians 10.7%. Both current smokers and former smokers continue to be at increased risk of lung cancer.

Smoking and Lung Cancer Incidence

The association between cigarette smoking and lung cancer is well known, with a landmark report on smoking and health released by the Surgeon General of the U.S. Public Health Service in 1964. At the time of this report, the risk for lung cancer in smoking men was estimated to be approximately 10-fold higher than in never-smoking men, with lower risk among women. Risk was shown to increase with greater amount smoked and decline with cessation of

Table 1.1 Risk factors for lung cancer

Risk factor	Estimate of risk (odds ratio or relative risk)		Comments	Reference
Cigarette smoking (cigarettes/day)	Men	Women	NIH-AARP Diet and Health Study	5
1–10	17.3	12.2		
11–20	27.9	19.8		
21–40	37.3	28.4		
>40	53.0	44.3		
ETS	1.2–1.4		Estimates of exposure usually by self-report	9
Cigar and pipe smoking	2.0–5.0		Ever vs. never use	10
Asbestos	Case-Control Studies	Cohort Studies	Meta-analysis	19
>100 airborne fiber-yr/mL of environmental air for >5% of work time	1.7	8.7		
Exposure as earlier + smoking >15 cigarettes per day	2.7	8.9		
Radon	1.10 per 100 Bq/m^3		Residential exposure	20,21
Household coal use	2.0		Meta-analysis	25
Diesel fuel	1.3–1.5		Occupational exposure	29,30
First-degree family history of lung cancer	1.5–2.0		Meta-analysis adjusting for smoking history among relatives	37
COPD	2.0–3.0		Meta-analysis	56,65
TB	1.7		Meta-analysis	76
HIV	1.5–5.0		Review	79

COPD, chronic obstructive pulmonary disease; ETS, environmental tobacco smoke; TB, tuberculosis.

smoking. This report resulted in a steep decline in smoking among men, driving a decline in lung cancer incidence beginning in the mid-1980s. A somewhat slower decline in cigarette use has been reported among women, with incidence rates beginning to decline in the mid-2000s. The incidence rates for lung cancer reflect the change in the use of tobacco, with women now smoking at rates comparable to men and both sexes starting in their teens.

The National Institutes of Health-American Association of Retired Persons (NIH-AARP) Diet and Health Study provides some of the most current data on smoking habits with follow-up for lung cancer in a cohort of 186,057 women and 266,074 men born between 1924 and 1945, who were enrolled in 1995 and followed for 11 years (5). Among women, 17% were current smokers and 44% were never smokers; among men, 13% were current smokers and 26% were never smokers, with most beginning to smoke between ages 15 and 19. Lung cancer incidence rates increased with amount smoked, with rates similar in men and women within comparable cigarette per day categories. In women, smoking 1 to 10, 11 to 20, 21 to 40, and greater than 40 cigarettes per day was associated with relative risks of 12.2, 19.8, 28.4, and 44.2, respectively. Among men in the same cigarette per day categories, relative risks were 17.3, 27.9, 37.3, and 53.0, respectively.

African Americans are more likely than other racial/ethnic groups to smoke menthol cigarettes, with one study reporting that 86% of African Americans smoked menthol cigarettes compared to only 23% of whites (6). Smokers of menthol cigarettes in this study, while at increased risk of lung cancer compared with never smokers, had lower rates of lung cancer than smokers of nonmenthol cigarettes. Other tobacco exposures in the form of cigar and pipe use are associated with a two- to fivefold increase in lung cancer risk (7). This risk is lower than that seen for cigarette smoking, since exposures are typically lower and smoke inhalation is not as deep.

Smoking Cessation

Several studies have shown that quitting smoking is associated with a reduction in lung cancer risk that continues to decrease with years since quitting, although risk never reaches the level among never smokers. Studies in the United Kingdom showed that among men who stopped smoking at ages 60, 50, 40, and 30, the cumulative risks of lung cancer by age 75 were 10%, 6%, 3%, and 2%, respectively, compared to a cumulative risk of death from lung cancer of 16% in men who did not quit (8). Using published data, Fry et al. estimated that after quitting it took 7.9 years in women and 10.7 years in men for the excess lung cancer risk to become half that of a continuing smoker (9).

Environmental Tobacco Smoke

More than two decades after the Surgeon General's report linking cigarette smoking to lung cancer, a second report from the Surgeon General detailed the risk associated with second-hand smoke, or environmental tobacco smoke (ETS), in nonsmoking individuals. Several known carcinogens in tobacco smoke are also present in ETS including aromatic amines, polycyclic aromatic hydrocarbons, and tobacco-specific nitrosoamines. ETS is associated with a 20% to 40% increase in lung cancer risk (10). While this is a much more moderate risk of lung cancer than that seen with cigarette smoking, ETS still poses a substantial risk.

Tobacco Alternatives

Alternatives to tobacco use include e-cigarettes, marijuana, and hookah use. E-cigarettes deliver aerosolized nicotine. Their use is not yet regulated by the Food and Drug Administration (FDA), so animal and human safety of e-cigarettes has not been evaluated. Little is known about lung cancer risks associated with e-cigarettes given the recent nature of use. What is known is that e-cigarettes deliver similar levels of nicotine as smoking cigarettes, that is enough to evoke physiologic responses in humans. Nicotine and its metabolites are carcinogenic; they contain potentially toxic aldehydes and reactive oxygen species, and alter cytokine levels in murine models.

Risks of lung cancer associated with marijuana use have been difficult to estimate. There is substantial evidence that habitual use is associated with respiratory symptoms, airflow limitation and airway inflammation, and in murine models, marijuana smoke condensate is associated with alterations in gene expression similar to that seen with tobacco smoke condensate (11). In a Swedish study, use of marijuana more than 50 times in men aged 18 to 20 was associated with a twofold increased risk of lung cancer after adjustment for tobacco use (12). Marijuana use is relatively prevalent, with 23.1% of 10- to 24-year olds in the United States in 2011 reporting use within 30 days of being surveyed (13). With new state laws allowing medical and recreational marijuana use, continued study of the long-term effects of this exposure is needed.

Another practice that is increasing in prevalence is hookah use (waterpipe tobacco smoking). In 2011, 18.5% of 12th grade students in the United States had used a hookah in the past year (14), with rates of use in university students ranging from 22% to 40% (15, 16). Exposure to smoke from a hookah results in mean peak plasma nicotine concentrations similar to those resulting from smoking a cigarette, with a 3.75-fold greater increase in carboxyhemoglobin levels and an inhaled smoke volume over 50-fold greater than that of a cigarette (17). The full effects of alternative inhaled smoke will not be fully realized for many decades.

Environmental Exposures

Asbestos

One of the strongest environmental risk factors for lung cancer is asbestos. Asbestos includes several types of naturally occurring mineral fibers that have been widely used in industry. Use peaked in the 1970s, with a subsequent decline in industrial use in the United States due to bans in certain products by the Consumer Product Safety Commission in 1977 and reductions in Occupational Safety and Health Administration (OSHA) guidelines for permissible exposure limits. Asbestos exposure has been linked to increased lung cancer risk in multiple studies, with latency times of 20 to 40 years. Risk is both dose-dependent and related to the size and composition of the inhaled fibers (18). A synergistic effect on lung cancer risk is seen with cigarette smoking (19).

Radon

Radon was first linked to lung cancer among underground miners with high exposures. Outside of occupational settings, individual exposures can occur when radon appears as a contaminant of indoor air. Residential exposures have been associated with an approximately 10% increase in lung cancer risk per 100 Bq/m^3 increase in measured radon, with a linear dose–response relationship. Synergistic effects with cigarette smoking result in a 25-fold higher risk among smokers than among non-smokers (20,21). It is estimated that 20,000 lung cancers diagnosed annually in the United States are attributable to radon exposure, prompting the Environmental Protection Agency in 2011 to develop plans for increased awareness and risk reduction (22).

Ionizing Radiation

In studies of Hiroshima and Nagasaki atomic bomb survivors, ionizing radiation has been associated with increased lung cancer risk with a linear dose–response relationship (23). Much lower doses of ionizing radiation, such as those received during diagnostic medical procedures, have not generally been associated with increased lung cancer risk. As lung cancer screening with low-dose CT becomes more prevalent, evaluation of associated lung cancer risk trends should be conducted. The risks associated with repeated medical screening and diagnostic procedures should be weighed against the benefits (24).

Air Pollution

Exposure to indoor air pollution from use of coal for cooking and heating, and the heating of cooking oils has been associated with increased lung cancer risk, particularly in studies conducted in China where such exposures are high. Household coal use was evaluated in a meta-analysis of 25 studies, showing an overall two-fold increased risk of lung cancer with exposure (25). In Chinese nonsmoking women, heating cooking oils to high temperatures is also associated with an increased risk of lung cancer (26). Outdoor air pollution in the form of ambient fine particulate matter ($PM_{2.5}$) has been linked to lung cancer mortality, but these associations tend to be weak (27,28).

Occupational exposure to diesel fuel is associated with an approximately 30% increase in lung cancer risk, with a significant dose-response trend (29). The risk of lung cancer is increased about 50% among farmers with diesel exposure related to daily tractor use, with higher risk seen for adenocarcinoma (30). While diesel exhaust contains known carcinogens, more study is needed to understand the risks associated with long-term, low-level exposures. Other exposures associated with increased lung cancer risk include wood dust (31) and low-level environmental exposure to cadmium (32).

Genetic Susceptibility

Familial Risk

A hallmark of genetic susceptibility to cancer is aggregation in families. Studying familial aggregation in lung cancer is challenging given that smoking clusters in families and is such a strong risk factor for the disease. Even with these challenges, there is consistent evidence demonstrating a two- to fourfold increased risk associated with having a first-degree relative with lung cancer after accounting for other risk factors, including smoking amount and duration, with variation in risk estimates by age of lung cancer diagnosis, smoking status, and race (33–36). Meta-analyses demonstrate fairly consistent findings, with an approximately 1.5- to 2-fold increased risk of lung cancer associated with family history (37). Variation in risk estimates are seen by race (1.5 for whites, 2.1 for African Americans) and by age at diagnosis (2.0 for onset <50 years).

The level of risk associated with family history is similar to that seen for breast, colon, and prostate cancer, suggesting an underlying genetic contribution to lung cancer susceptibility. Family studies to identify rare, highly penetrant, inherited mutations have been limited to one study that reported the first evidence of a lung cancer susceptibility locus on chromosome 6q23-25 segregating in high-risk lung cancer families (38). As the number of relatives and generations affected with lung cancer increased, so did the significance of this finding. Most importantly, putative carriers of risk in this locus were at higher risk even if they were never smokers or had light smoking histories, suggesting that any level of tobacco exposure increases risk among those with inherited lung cancer susceptibility. A germline mutation in *PARK2* in this region was linked to lung cancer risk in one family with eight affected members (39). Additional evidence of linkage was found for regions on chromosomes 1q, 8q, 9p, 12q, 5q, 14q, and 16q (38). A two-stage genome-wide association study (GWAS) that focused on variants associated with a family history of lung cancer, identified SNPs on chromosomes 4p15.2 and 10q23.33 (40). GWAS data have also been used to estimate overall heritability and the proportion of heritability associated with smoking. It is estimated that 24% of the heritability of lung cancer is attributable to genetic determinants of smoking (41).

Genome-Wide Association Studies

Beyond rare, highly penetrant inherited mutations contributing to lung cancer risk, there is also evidence for contributions to susceptibility due to more common, low-penetrant genetic alterations identified by GWAS (Table 1.2). Several early GWAS identified a region on chromosome 15q25 that is more common in lung cancer cases than in controls (42–44). A neuronal nicotinic acetylcholine receptor gene cluster comprising *CHRNA3* and *CHRNA5* subunits lies within this region. Genetic variation here is associated with an approximate 30% increased risk of lung cancer among individuals carrying a heterozygous mutation and an 80% increase for those who are homozygous for a mutation. A meta-analysis of smokers with or without lung cancer and/or chronic obstructive pulmonary disease (COPD) reported that multiple loci within this region are associated with cigarettes smoked per day and at least one locus is associated with lung cancer independent of amount smoked (45).

Additional regions of interest have been identified on chromosomes 6p21 and 5p15 (42–44). A large meta-analysis of 14,900 lung cancer cases and 29,485 controls of European ancestry from 16 GWAS validated associations between lung cancer risk and genetic variation at 5p15, 6p21, and 15q25 (46). Imputation has been used to expand the data available from GWAS, resulting in the identification and validation of associations between squamous cell carcinoma of the lung and rare variants of *BRCA2*-K3326X (odds ratio [OR] 2.5, $P = 4.7 \times 10–20$) and *CHEK2*-I157T (OR 0.38, $P = 1.27 \times 10–13$) (47).

Table 1.2 Genome-wide association study results in lung cancer

Chromosomal loci	Candidate genes	Populations	Reference
3q28	*P63*	European ancestry (adenocarcinoma) Chinese Japanese Never-smoking Asian women	47 50 52 53
5p15	*TERT, CLPTM1L*	European ancestry African American Chinese Japanese Never-smoking Asian women	42–44,46 49 50 52 53
6p21	*BAT3, MSH5*	European ancestry African American Japanese Never-smoking Asian women	42–44,46 49 52 53
13q12-13	*BRCA2 MIPEP-TNFRSF19*	European ancestry (squamous cell carcinoma) Chinese	47 50
15q25	*CHRNA3/5*	European ancestry African American	42–46 48,49
22q12	*CHEK2 MTMR3*	European ancestry (squamous cell carcinoma) Chinese	47 50

The largest GWAS have included only individuals of European ancestry. The varied genetic architecture and smoking histories of different race/ethnic groups make GWAS in other populations necessary for the eventual identification of lung cancer susceptibility genes. The findings among whites on 15q25, 5p15, and 6p21 have been replicated in African Americans (48, 49). In the Han Chinese population, GWAS identified lung cancer risk associations on 5p15, 3q28, 13q12, and 22q12 (50), and 10p14, 5q32, and

20q13 (51). In the Japanese population, the findings on 5p15, 3q28, and 6p21 were also replicated (52).

GWAS in never smokers has been limited. In never-smoking Asian women, the 6p21, 5p15, and 3q28 findings were replicated and regions on 10q25 and 6q22 were also identified as being associated with lung cancer (53). A large GWAS in never smokers of European ancestry is underway. These studies, across multiple populations and exposure groups, have the potential to uncover mechanisms of carcinogenesis and to identify high-risk individuals to target for prevention and screening efforts.

Chronic Obstructive Pulmonary Disease

COPD and Lung Cancer Incidence

Substantial evidence has been published demonstrating a link between COPD and lung cancer. These diseases share a common risk factor, cigarette smoking, but studies also suggest that a history of COPD is related to a two- to threefold increased risk for lung cancer independent of cigarette smoke exposure (54–57). This link between COPD and lung cancer is evident even among never smokers (58). COPD represents a disease with multiple phenotypes, including emphysema and chronic bronchitis, and it is less clear how lung cancer risk varies by COPD phenotype (57,59). Epidemiologic data relying on self-report of COPD show some differences in risk by COPD phenotype. The largest meta-analysis reported that lung cancer was associated with a previous history of COPD (OR 2.2, 95% CI 1.7–3.0), chronic bronchitis (OR 1.5, 95% CI 1.3–1.8), and emphysema (OR 2.0, 95% CI 1.7–2.4) (56).

Clinical studies have used CT evidence of emphysema and/or spirometry-defined measures of airflow obstruction to evaluate subsequent risk of lung cancer, reducing the potential for disease misclassification and recall bias. Increased risk of lung cancer has been associated with decreasing forced expiratory volume in 1 second (FEV_1) even in smokers with only minimal declines in FEV_1 (59). Several studies report a two- to fourfold increased risk of lung cancer in the presence of CT evidence of emphysema, with no or lower risk associated with airflow obstruction (55,60–62). In studies using quantitative image analysis of CTs (qCT), CT measures of emphysema have not been associated with lung cancer independent of other COPD measures (63,64). In a meta-analysis including seven studies, Smith et al. (65) reported a threefold (95% CI 2.71, 4.51) increased risk of lung cancer associated with visually detected emphysema, but a nonsignificant 1.16-fold (95% CI 0.48, 2.81) increased risk of lung cancer with qCT-defined emphysema. These studies demonstrate the need to consistently define COPD to better understand the relationship between COPD and lung cancer.

COPD and Genetic Risk

Candidate gene studies in COPD and lung cancer have identified common and shared genetic variation in inflammation, extracellular matrix proteolysis, and oxidative stress pathways (66,67), including SNPs in epoxide hydrolase 1 (*EPHX1*), matrix metalloproteinases, and interleukin 1β (*IL1B*) (68–70). Inflammatory pathway gene SNPs in *IL7R*, *IL15*, *TNF*, *TNFRSF10A*, *IL1RN*, and *IL1A* have been associated with lung cancer risk differentially by self-reported history of COPD (71). SNPs in *IL1A* have also been reported to be more strongly associated with lung cancer risk in those with emphysema (69). Genetic variation on 15q25.1, as reported from GWAS in lung cancer, has been reported in GWAS for COPD-related phenotypes as well (45,72–74). Limited studies have specifically evaluated a joint lung cancer and COPD phenotype. Summary data show that the 15q25 locus is associated with risk of both diseases, genetic variants on 4q31 and 4q22 are associated with reduced risk of both diseases, loci on 6p21 are most strongly associated with lung cancer risk in smokers with COPD, and variants on 5p15 and 1q23 alter lung cancer risk when COPD is not present (75). It is clear that additional work is needed to untangle the COPD-lung cancer relationship.

Infectious Agents

Tuberculosis

Lung cancer risk has been associated with several infectious diseases, including tuberculosis (TB). In a meta-analysis of 37 case-control studies and four cohort studies, TB was associated with a 70% increased risk of lung cancer (95% CI 1.5–2.0), adjusting for smoking. Similar risk is observed among never smokers and the highest risk is seen within 5 years of a TB diagnosis (76).

Human Papillomavirus

Human papillomavirus (HPV) prevalence in lung tumor tissue ranges from 0% to 100%, with differences by geographic regions, histology subtype of lung cancer, sex, and HPV subtype (77,78), but little is known about HPV-lung cancer risk profiles.

Human Immunodeficiency Virus

HIV infection has been associated with a 1.5- to 5.0-fold increased risk of lung cancer. In a review of 65 studies, lung cancer risk in HIV-positive populations varied by geographic region. Standardized incidence ratios or incidence rate ratios were 1.5 to 3.4 in Europe, 0.7 to 6.9 in the United States, and 5.0 in Africa (79). Lung cancer risk among HIV-infected patients receiving highly active antiretroviral therapy (HAART) is similar to that among patients not receiving HAART (80,81). The cumulative incidence of lung cancer by age 75 is 3.4% among those with HIV and 2.8% among those without HIV (82).

SUMMARY

Lung cancer is the leading cause of cancer-related death globally and, while incidence and mortality rates have declined with decreased smoking rates, the 5-year survival rate continues to be less than 20%. Although the major risk factor for this disease is well known (cigarette smoking), progress in prevention and early diagnosis has been slow. In addition to cigarette smoking, lung cancer has been associated with exposure to asbestos, radon, ionizing radiation, and indoor air pollution. A contribution for genetic susceptibility is well described in both family-based studies and GWAS. Continued exploration of the role of COPD, infections and exposure to smoke from marijuana, hookah, and e-cigarettes, is needed to further define lung cancer risk. Well-defined high-risk groups, based on more than just smoking history, will be needed to best target populations for lung cancer prevention and screening.

KEY POINTS

- Worldwide, lung cancer is the leading cause of cancer-related death.
- In the United States, lung cancer is the second most common cancer diagnosed in both men and women and the leading cause of cancer-related death in both sexes. The 5-year overall survival for patients with lung cancer is less than 20%.
- Approximately 80% of all lung cancers are attributable to cigarette smoking. While smoking prevalence has declined to 18% in the United States, former smokers continue to be at risk for years after smoking cessation.
- Alternatives to cigarette smoking, such as e-cigarettes, hookah use, and marijuana, are on the rise, but their association with lung cancer risk remains unclear.
- Environmental exposure to asbestos, radon, indoor air pollution, and diesel fuel has been associated with an increased risk of lung cancer.
- A first-degree family history of lung cancer is associated with a twofold increased risk of lung cancer.

(*continued*)

(*continued*)

This information should be part of the medical history and contribute to discussions about lung cancer screening.

- Several genetic loci have been associated with small increases in lung cancer risk, but their routine use as predictive markers is not yet warranted.
- COPD is associated with a two- to threefold increased risk of lung cancer. A detailed medical history regarding COPD phenotype would help clinicians offer better recommendations on lung cancer screening.
- A history of infectious diseases, including TB, HPV, and HIV, should be considered when evaluating lung cancer risk and appropriateness of screening.

REFERENCES

1. American Cancer Society. *Cancer Facts & Figures 2015*. Atlanta: American Cancer Society; 2015.
2. Howlander N, Krapcho M, Garshell J, et al. (eds). *SEER Cancer Statistics Review, 1975-2012*. Bethesda, MD: National Cancer Institute; 2015.
3. Islami F, Torre LA, Jemal A. Global trends of lung cancer mortality and smoking prevalence. *Transl Lung Cancer Res*. 2015;4(4):327-338. doi:10.3978/j.issn.2218-6751.2015.08.04. PubMed PMID: 26380174; PubMed Central PMCID: PMC4549470.
4. Agaku IT, King BA, Dube SR, Centers for Disease Control and Prevention. Current cigarette smoking among adults—United States, 2005-2012. *MMWR Morb Mortal Wkly Rep*. 2014;63(2):29-34. PubMed PMID: 24430098.
5. Freedman ND, Abnet CC, Caporaso NE, et al. Impact of changing US cigarette smoking patterns on incident cancer: risks of 20 smoking-related cancers among the women and men of the NIH-AARP cohort. *Int J Epidemiol*. 2015. doi:10.1093/ije/dyv175. PubMed PMID: 26411408.
6. Blot WJ, Cohen SS, Aldrich M, et al. Lung cancer risk among smokers of menthol cigarettes. *J Natl Cancer Inst*. 2011;103(10):810-816. doi:10.1093/jnci/djr102. PubMed PMID: 21436064; PubMed Central PMCID: PMC3096798.
7. McCormack VA, Agudo A, Dahm CC, et al. Cigar and pipe smoking and cancer risk in the European Prospective Investigation into Cancer and Nutrition (EPIC). *Int J Cancer*. 2010;127(10):2402-2411. Epub 2010/02/18. doi: 10.1002/ijc.25252. PubMed PMID: 20162568.
8. Peto R, Darby S, Deo H, et al. Smoking, smoking cessation, and lung cancer in the UK since 1950: combination of national statistics with two case-control studies. *BMJ*. 2000;321(7257):323-329. PubMed PMID: 10926586; PubMed Central PMCID: PMC27446.

9. Fry JS, Lee PN, Forey BA, Coombs KJ. How rapidly does the excess risk of lung cancer decline following quitting smoking? A quantitative review using the negative exponential model. *Regul Toxicol Pharmacol.* 2013;67(1):13-26. doi:10.1016/j.yrtph.2013.06.001. PubMed PMID: 23764305.
10. Zhong L, Goldberg MS, Parent ME, Hanley JA. Exposure to environmental tobacco smoke and the risk of lung cancer: a meta-analysis. *Lung Cancer.* 2000;27(1):3-18. Epub 2000/02/15. PubMed PMID: 10672779.
11. Biehl JR, Burnham EL. Cannabis smoking in 2015: a concern for lung healthŒ *Chest.* 2015;148(3):596-606. doi:10.1378/chest.15-0447. PubMed PMID: 25996274; PubMed Central PMCID: PMC4556119.
12. Callaghan RC, Allebeck P, Sidorchuk A. Marijuana use and risk of lung cancer: a 40-year cohort study. *Cancer Causes Control.* 2013;24(10):1811-1820. doi:10.1007/s10552-013-0259-0. PubMed PMID: 23846283.
13. Eaton DK, Kinchen S, Shanklin S, et al. Youth risk behavior surveillance—United States. *Morb Mortality Wkly Rep.* 2012;61(SS04):1-162.
14. Johnston LD, O'Malley PM, Bachman JG, Schulenberg JE. *Monitoring the Future National Survey Results on Adolescent Drug Use, 1975-2011: Volume I, Secondary School Students.* Ann Arbor, MI: Institute for Social Research; 2010.
15. Heinz AJ, Giedgowd GE, Crane NA, et al. A comprehensive examination of hookah smoking in college students: use patterns and contexts, social norms and attitudes, harm perception, psychological correlates and co-occurring substance use. *Addict Behav.* 2013;38(11):2751-2760. Epub 2013/08/13. doi:10.1016/j.addbeh.2013.07.009. PubMed PMID: 23934006.
16. Holtzman AL, Babinski D, Merlo LJ. Knowledge and attitudes toward hookah usage among university students. *J Am Coll Health.* 2013;61(6):362-370. Epub 2013/08/13. doi:10.1080/07448481.2013.818000. PubMed PMID: 23930750.
17. Cobb CO, Shihadeh A, Weaver MF, Eissenberg T. Waterpipe tobacco smoking and cigarette smoking: a direct comparison of toxicant exposure and subjective effects. *Nicotine Tob Res.* 2011;13(2):78-87. Epub 2010/12/04. doi:10.1093/ntr/ntq212. PubMed PMID: 21127030; PubMed Central PMCID: PMC3107609.
18. McCormack V, Peto J, Byrnes G, et al. Estimating the asbestos-related lung cancer burden from mesothelioma mortality. *Br J Cancer.* 2012;106(3):575-584. Epub 2012/01/12. doi:10.1038/bjc.2011.563. PubMed PMID: 22233924; PubMed Central PMCID: PMC3273352.
19. Ngamwong Y, Tangamornsuksan W, Lohitnavy O, et al. Additive synergism between asbestos and smoking in lung cancer risk: a systematic review and meta-analysis. *PLOS ONE.* 2015;10(8):e0135798. doi:10.1371/journal.pone.0135798. PubMed PMID: 26274395; PubMed Central PMCID: PMC4537132.

20. Darby S, Hill D, Deo H, et al. Residential radon and lung cancer—detailed results of a collaborative analysis of individual data on 7148 persons with lung cancer and 14,208 persons without lung cancer from 13 epidemiologic studies in Europe. *Scand J Work Environ Health*. 2006;32(suppl 1):1-83. Epub 2006/03/17. PubMed PMID: 16538937.
21. Krewski D, Lubin JH, Zielinski JM, et al. A combined analysis of North American case-control studies of residential radon and lung cancer. *J Toxicol Environ Health*. 2006;69(7):533-597. PubMed PMID: 16608828.
22. U.S. Environmental Protection Agency. *Protecting People and Families From Radon: A Federal Action Plan for Saving Lives*; 2011. https://www.epa.gov/sites/production/files/2014-08/documents/Federal_Radon_Action_Plan.pdf
23. Preston DL, Ron E, Tokuoka S, et al. Solid cancer incidence in atomic bomb survivors: 1958-1998. *Radiat Res*. 2007;168(1):1-64. Epub 2007/08/29. doi:10.1667/RR0763.1. PubMed PMID: 17722996.
24. Brenner DJ. Radiation risks potentially associated with low-dose CT screening of adult smokers for lung cancer. *Radiology*. 2004;231(2):440-445. Epub 2004/05/07. doi:10.1148/radiol.2312030880. PubMed PMID: 15128988.
25. Hosgood HD, 3rd, Wei H, Sapkota A, et al. Household coal use and lung cancer: systematic review and meta-analysis of case-control studies, with an emphasis on geographic variation. *Int J Epidemiol*. 2011;40(3):719-728. Epub 2011/02/01. doi:10.1093/ije/dyq259. PubMed PMID: 21278196; PubMed Central PMCID: PMC3147068.
26. Mu L, Liu L, Niu R, et al. Indoor air pollution and risk of lung cancer among Chinese female non-smokers. *Cancer Causes Control*. 2013;24(3):439-450. Epub 2013/01/15. doi:10.1007/s10552-012-0130-8. PubMed PMID: 23314675; PubMed Central PMCID: PMC3574203.
27. Pope CA, 3rd, Burnett RT, Thun MJ, et al. Lung cancer, cardiopulmonary mortality, and long-term exposure to fine particulate air pollution. *JAMA*. 2002;287(9):1132-1141. Epub 2002/03/07. PubMed PMID: 11879110.
28. Turner MC, Krewski D, Pope CA, 3rd, et al. Long-term ambient fine particulate matter air pollution and lung cancer in a large cohort of never-smokers. *Am J Respir Crit Care Med*. 2011;184(12):1374-1381. Epub 2011/10/08. doi:10.1164/rccm.201106-1011OC. PubMed PMID: 21980033.
29. Olsson AC, Gustavsson P, Kromhout H, et al. Exposure to diesel motor exhaust and lung cancer risk in a pooled analysis from case-control studies in Europe and Canada. *Am J Respir Crit Care Med*. 2011;183(7):941-948. Epub 2010/11/03. doi:10.1164/rccm.201006-0940OC. PubMed PMID: 21037020.
30. Tual S, Silverman DT, Koutros S, et al. Use of dieselized farm equipment and incident lung cancer: findings from the agricultural health study cohort. *Environ Health Perspect*. 2015. doi:10.1289/ehp.1409238. PubMed PMID: 26452295.
31. Hancock DG, Langley ME, Chia KL, et al. Wood dust exposure and lung cancer risk: a meta-analysis. *Occup Environ Med*. 2015;72(12):889-898. doi:10.1136/oemed-2014-102722. PubMed PMID: 26403531.

32. Nawrot TS, Martens DS, Hara A, et al. Association of total cancer and lung cancer with environmental exposure to cadmium: the meta-analytical evidence. *Cancer Causes Control*. 2015;26(9):1281-1288. doi:10.1007/s10552-015-0621-5. PubMed PMID: 26109463.
33. Ooi WL, Elston RC, Chen VW, et al. Increased familial risk for lung cancer. *J Natl Cancer Inst*. 1986;76(2):217-222. PubMed PMID: 3456060.
34. Cote ML, Kardia SL, Wenzlaff AS, et al. Risk of lung cancer among white and black relatives of individuals with early-onset lung cancer. *JAMA*. 2005;293(24):3036-3042. PubMed PMID: 15972566.
35. Schwartz AG, Yang P, Swanson GM. Familial risk of lung cancer among nonsmokers and their relatives. *Am J Epidemiol*. 1996;144(6):554-562. PubMed PMID: 8797515.
36. Jonsson S, Thorsteinsdottir U, Gudbjartsson DF, et al. Familial risk of lung carcinoma in the Icelandic population. *JAMA*. 2004;292(24):2977-2983. doi:10.1001/jama.292.24.2977. PubMed PMID: 15613665.
37. Cote ML, Liu M, Bonassi S, et al. Increased risk of lung cancer in individuals with a family history of the disease: a pooled analysis from the International Lung Cancer Consortium. *Eur J Cancer*. 2012;48(13): 1957-1968. Epub 2012/03/23. doi:10.1016/j.ejca.2012.01.038. PubMed PMID: 22436981; PubMed Central PMCID: PMC3445438.
38. Amos CI, Pinney SM, Li Y, et al. A susceptibility locus on chromosome 6q greatly increases lung cancer risk among light and never smokers. *Cancer Res*. 2010;70(6):2359-2367. Epub 2010/03/11. doi:0008-5472. CAN-09-3096 [pii] 10.1158/0008-5472.CAN-09-3096. PubMed PMID: 20215501; PubMed Central PMCID: PMC2855643.
39. Xiong D, Wang Y, Kupert E, et al. A recurrent mutation in PARK2 is associated with familial lung cancer. *Am J Hum Genet*. 2015;96(2):301-308. doi:10.1016/j.ajhg.2014.12.016. PubMed PMID: 25640678; PubMed Central PMCID: PMC4320264.
40. Poirier JG, Brennan P, McKay JD, et al. Informed genome-wide association analysis with family history as a secondary phenotype identifies novel loci of lung cancer. *Genet Epidemiol*. 2015;39(3):197-206. doi:10.1002/gepi.21882. PubMed PMID: 25644374; PubMed Central PMCID: PMC4554719.
41. Sampson JN, Wheeler WA, Yeager M, et al. Analysis of heritability and shared heritability based on genome-wide association studies for thirteen cancer types. *J Natl Cancer Inst*. 2015;107(12). doi:10.1093/jnci/djv279. PubMed PMID: 26464424.
42. Hung RJ, McKay JD, Gaborieau V, et al. A susceptibility locus for lung cancer maps to nicotinic acetylcholine receptor subunit genes on 15q25. *Nature*. 2008;452(7187):633-637. PubMed PMID: 18385738.
43. Thorgeirsson TE, Geller F, Sulem P, et al. A variant associated with nicotine dependence, lung cancer and peripheral arterial disease. *Nature*. 2008;452(7187):638-642. PubMed PMID: 18385739.
44. Amos CI, Wu X, Broderick P, et al. Genome-wide association scan of tag SNPs identifies a susceptibility locus for lung cancer at 15q25.1. *Nature Genet*. 2008;40(5):616-622. PubMed PMID: 18385676.

45. Saccone NL, Culverhouse RC, Schwantes-An TH, et al. Multiple independent loci at chromosome 15q25.1 affect smoking quantity: a meta-analysis and comparison with lung cancer and COPD. *PLOS Genet*. 2010;6(8). Epub 2010/08/12. doi:10.1371/journal.pgen.1001053. PubMed PMID: 20700436; PubMed Central PMCID: PMC2916847.
46. Timofeeva MN, Hung RJ, Rafnar T, et al. Influence of common genetic variation on lung cancer risk: meta-analysis of 14 900 cases and 29 485 controls. *Human Mol Genet*. 2012;21(22):4980-4995. Epub 2012/08/18. doi:10.1093/hmg/dds334. PubMed PMID: 22899653; PubMed Central PMCID: PMC3607485.
47. Wang Y, McKay JD, Rafnar T, et al. Rare variants of large effect in BRCA2 and CHEK2 affect risk of lung cancer. *Nat Genet*. 2014;46(7):736-741. doi:10.1038/ng.3002. PubMed PMID: 24880342; PubMed Central PMCID: PMC4074058.
48. Schwartz AG, Cote ML, Wenzlaff AS, et al. Racial differences in the association between SNPs on 15q25.1, smoking behavior, and risk of non-small cell lung cancer. *J Thorac Oncol*. 2009. Epub 2009/07/31. doi:10.1097/JTO.0b013e3181b244ef. PubMed PMID: 19641473; PubMed Central PMCID: PMC19641473.
49. Walsh KM, Gorlov IP, Hansen HM, et al. Fine-mapping of the 5p15.33, 6p22.1-p21.31, and 15q25.1 regions identifies functional and histology-specific lung cancer susceptibility loci in African-Americans. *Cancer Epidemiol Biomarkers Prev*. 2013;22(2):251-260. Epub 2012/12/12. doi:10.1158/1055-9965.EPI-12-1007-T. PubMed PMID: 23221128; PubMed Central PMCID: PMC3565099.
50. Hu Z, Wu C, Shi Y, et al. A genome-wide association study identifies two new lung cancer susceptibility loci at 13q12.12 and 22q12.2 in Han Chinese. *Nat Genet*. 2011;43(8):792-796. Epub 2011/07/05. doi:10.1038/ng.875. PubMed PMID: 21725308.
51. Dong J, Hu Z, Wu C, et al. Association analyses identify multiple new lung cancer susceptibility loci and their interactions with smoking in the Chinese population. *Nat Genet*. 2012;44(8):895-899. Epub 2012/07/17. doi:10.1038/ng.2351. PubMed PMID: 22797725.
52. Shiraishi K, Kunitoh H, Daigo Y, et al. A genome-wide association study identifies two new susceptibility loci for lung adenocarcinoma in the Japanese population. *Nat Genet*. 2012;44(8):900-903. Epub 2012/07/17. doi:10.1038/ng.2353. PubMed PMID: 22797724.
53. Lan Q, Hsiung CA, Matsuo K, et al. Genome-wide association analysis identifies new lung cancer susceptibility loci in never-smoking women in Asia. *Nat Genet*. 2012;44(12):1330-1335. Epub 2012/11/13. doi:10.1038/ng.2456. PubMed PMID: 23143601.
54. Mannino DM, Aguayo SM, Petty TL, Redd SC. Low lung function and incident lung cancer in the United States: data from the First National Health and Nutrition Examination Survey follow-up. *Arch Intern Med*. 2003;163(12):1475-1480. PubMed PMID: 12824098.
55. Wilson DO, Weissfeld JL, Balkan A, et al. Association of radiographic emphysema and airflow obstruction with lung cancer. *Am J Respir Crit Care Med*. 2008;178(7):738-744. PubMed PMID: 18565949.

56. Brenner DR, McLaughlin JR, Hung RJ. Previous lung diseases and lung cancer risk: a systematic review and meta-analysis. *PLOS ONE*. 2011;6(3):e17479. Epub 2011/04/13. doi:10.1371/journal.pone.0017479. PubMed PMID: 21483846; PubMed Central PMCID: PMC3069026.
57. Schwartz AG, Cote ML, Wenzlaff AS, et al. Chronic obstructive lung diseases and risk of non-small cell lung cancer in women. *J Thorac Oncol*. 2009;4(3):291-299. Epub 2009/02/05. doi:10.1097/JTO.0b013e3181951cd1. PubMed PMID: 19190518; PubMed Central PMCID: PMC2745706.
58. Turner MC, Chen Y, Krewski D, et al. Chronic obstructive pulmonary disease is associated with lung cancer mortality in a prospective study of never smokers. *Am J Respir Crit Care Med*. 2007;176(3):285-290. PubMed PMID: 17478615.
59. Wasswa-Kintu S, Gan WQ, Man SF, et al. Relationship between reduced forced expiratory volume in one second and the risk of lung cancer: a systematic review and meta-analysis. *Thorax*. 2005;60(7):570-575. PubMed PMID: 15994265.
60. de Torres JP, Bastarrika G, Wisnivesky JP, et al. Assessing the relationship between lung cancer risk and emphysema detected on low-dose CT of the chest. *Chest*. 2007;132(6):1932-1938. PubMed PMID: 18079226.
61. Ueda K, Jinbo M, Li TS, et al. Computed tomography-diagnosed emphysema, not airway obstruction, is associated with the prognostic outcome of early-stage lung cancer. *Clin Cancer Res*. 2006;12(22):6730-6736. doi:10.1158/1078-0432.CCR-06-1196. PubMed PMID: 17121893.
62. Li Y, Swensen SJ, Karabekmez LG, et al. Effect of emphysema on lung cancer risk in smokers: a computed tomography-based assessment. *Cancer Prev Res (Phila)*. 2011;4(1):43-50. doi:10.1158/1940-6207.CAPR-10-0151. PubMed PMID: 21119049; PubMed Central PMCID: PMC3018159.
63. Maldonado F, Bartholmai BJ, Swensen SJ, et al. Are airflow obstruction and radiographic emphysema risk factors for lung cancer? A nested case-control study using quantitative emphysema analysis. *Chest*. 2010. Epub 2010/03/30. doi:chest.09-2567 [pii] 10.1378/chest.09-2567. PubMed PMID: 20348193.
64. Wilson DO, Leader JK, Fuhrman CR, et al. Quantitative computed tomography analysis, airflow obstruction, and lung cancer in the pittsburgh lung screening study. *J Thorac Oncol*. 2011;6(7):1200-1205. doi:10.1097/JTO.0b013e318219aa93. PubMed PMID: 21610523; PubMed Central PMCID: PMC3157578.
65. Smith BM, Pinto L, Ezer N, et al. Emphysema detected on computed tomography and risk of lung cancer: a systematic review and meta-analysis. *Lung Cancer*. 2012;77(1):58-63. doi:10.1016/j.lungcan.2012.02.019. PubMed PMID: 22437042.
66. Yoshida T, Tuder RM. Pathobiology of cigarette smoke-induced chronic obstructive pulmonary disease. *Physiol Rev*. 2007;87(3):1047-1082. PubMed PMID: 17615396.
67. Macnee W. Pathogenesis of chronic obstructive pulmonary disease. *Clinics Chest Med*. 2007;28(3):479-513, v. PubMed PMID: 17720039.

68. Schwartz AG, Prysak GM, Bock CH, Cote ML. The molecular epidemiology of lung cancer. *Carcinogenesis*. 2006;28(3):507-518. PubMed PMID: 17183062.
69. Engels EA, Wu X, Gu J, et al. Systematic evaluation of genetic variants in the inflammation pathway and risk of lung cancer. *Cancer Res*. 2007;67(13):6520-6527. PubMed PMID: 17596594.
70. Smolonska J, Wijmenga C, Postma DS, Boezen HM. Meta-analyses on suspected chronic obstructive pulmonary disease genes: a summary of 20 years' research. *Am J Respir Crit Care Med*. 2009;180(7):618-631. Epub 2009/07/18. doi: 200905-0722OC [pii] 10.1164/rccm.200905-0722OC. PubMed PMID: 19608716.
71. Van Dyke AL, Cote ML, Wenzlaff AS, et al. Cytokine and cytokine receptor single-nucleotide polymorphisms predict risk for non-small cell lung cancer among women. *Cancer Epidemiol Biomarkers Prev*. 2009;18(6):1829-1840. Epub 2009/06/10. doi: 18/6/1829 [pii] 10.1158/1055-9965.EPI-08-0962. PubMed PMID: 19505916; PubMed Central PMCID: PMC19505916.
72. Pillai SG, Ge D, Zhu G, et al. A genome-wide association study in chronic obstructive pulmonary disease (COPD): identification of two major susceptibility loci. *PLOS Genet*. 2009;5(3):e1000421. PubMed PMID: 19300482.
73. Lambrechts D, Buysschaert I, Zanen P, et al. The 15q24/25 susceptibility variant for lung cancer and chronic obstructive pulmonary disease is associated with emphysema. *Am J Respir Crit Care Med*. 2010;181(5):486-493. Epub 2009/12/17. doi: 200909-1364OC [pii]10.1164/rccm.200909-1364OC. PubMed PMID: 20007924.
74. Wilk JB, Shrine NR, Loehr LR, et al. Genome-wide association studies identify CHRNA5/3 and HTR4 in the development of airflow obstruction. *Am J Respir Crit Care Med*. 2012;186(7):622-632. doi:10.1164/rccm.201202-0366OC. PubMed PMID: 22837378; PubMed Central PMCID: PMC3480517.
75. Young RP, Hopkins RJ, Whittington CF, et al. Individual and cumulative effects of GWAS susceptibility loci in lung cancer: associations after sub-phenotyping for COPD. *PLOS ONE*. 2011;6(2):e16476. Epub 2011/02/10. doi:10.1371/journal.pone.0016476. PubMed PMID: 21304900; PubMed Central PMCID: PMC3033394.
76. Liang HY, Li XL, Yu XS, et al. Facts and fiction of the relationship between preexisting tuberculosis and lung cancer risk: a systematic review. *Int J Cancer*. 2009;125(12):2936-2944. doi:10.1002/ijc.24636. PubMed PMID: 19521963.
77. Srinivasan M, Taioli E, Ragin CC. Human papillomavirus type 16 and 18 in primary lung cancers—a meta-analysis. *Carcinogenesis*. 2009;30(10):1722-1728. doi:10.1093/carcin/bgp177. PubMed PMID: 19620233; PubMed Central PMCID: PMC2764507.
78. Hasegawa Y, Ando M, Kubo A, et al. Human papilloma virus in non-small cell lung cancer in never smokers: a systematic review of the literature. *Lung Cancer*. 2013. doi:10.1016/j.lungcan.2013.10.002. PubMed PMID: 24252423.

79. Hou W, Fu J, Ge Y, et al. Incidence and risk of lung cancer in HIV-infected patients. *J Cancer Res Clin Oncol*. 2013;139(11):1781-1794. doi:10.1007/s00432-013-1477-2. PubMed PMID: 23892408.
80. Clifford GM, Polesel J, Rickenbach M, et al. Cancer risk in the Swiss HIV Cohort Study: associations with immunodeficiency, smoking, and highly active antiretroviral therapy. *J Natl Cancer Inst*. 2005;97(6):425-432. doi:10.1093/jnci/dji072. PubMed PMID: 15770006.
81. Engels EA, Brock MV, Chen J, et al. Elevated incidence of lung cancer among HIV-infected individuals. *J Clin Oncol*. 2006;24(9):1383-1388. doi:10.1200/JCO.2005.03.4413. PubMed PMID: 16549832.
82. Silverberg MJ, Lau B, Achenbach CJ, et al. Cumulative incidence of cancer among persons with HIV in North America: a cohort study. *Ann Intern Med*. 2015;163(7):507-518. doi:10.7326/M14-2768. PubMed PMID: 26436616.

2 Biologic Basis of Lung Cancer

Charles A. Powell and Vaishnavi Kundel

LUNG CARCINOGENESIS

Exposure and Susceptibility

Tobacco smoking is the major cause of lung cancer (1). Individuals with predisposition to nicotine addiction are more prone to continue smoking, and thus, be exposed to high doses of tobacco-associated carcinogens, including the polycyclic aromatic hydrocarbon (PAH) benzo-[a]-pyrene and the key nicotine metabolite nicotine-derived nitrosamine ketone (NNK) (Figure 2.1). These carcinogens can be activated or eliminated through endogenous enzyme systems whose activity is determined by specific genetic polymorphisms. For example, the glutathione-S-transferase (GST) system detoxifies carcinogens by adding a glucuronide metabolite to PAHs. Individuals with a GST-Mu 1 (GSTM1) genotype are deficient in this process, so GSTM1 smokers will have an increased risk of lung cancer. Conversely, the cytochrome P450 system metabolically activates carcinogens, such as PAHs, by adding an epoxide metabolite. Individuals with a P450 CYP1A1 genotype have increased activity of this enzyme, so CYP1A1 smokers have an increased risk for lung cancer. Thus, individual genetic differences can confer susceptibility to lung cancer upon specific carcinogen exposure.

Activated PAHs can covalently bind to DNA to form specific DNA adducts, an early sign of lung carcinogenesis. These adducts can be repaired by endogenous DNA repair enzymes, which have differential activity conferred by genetic variation. If not repaired, damaged DNA can induce cell death. However, if these alterations persist, they can lead to oncogenic, somatic alterations of tumor suppressor genes (e.g., *p53*, *Rb*) or oncogenes (e.g., *KRAS*, *BRAF*), or to DNA instability as indicated by loss of heterozygosity. These alterations are commonly found in the bronchial epithelium of cigarette smokers leading to field carcinogenesis. In some individuals, this process gives rise to a cell that undergoes clonal transformation and develops into a tumor. The full series of events that facilitate cellular transformation remain unclear,

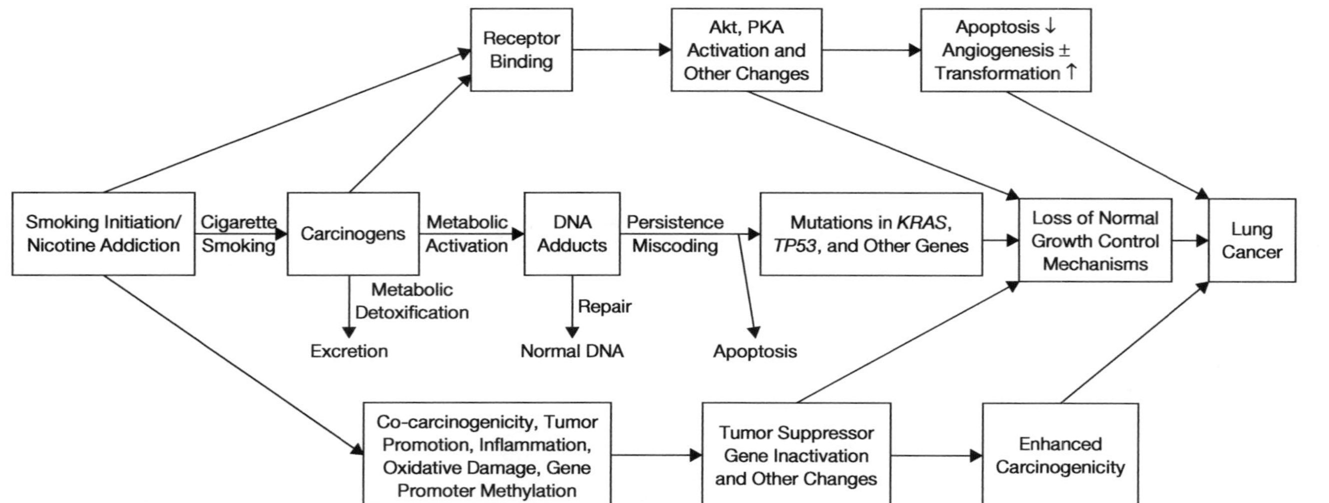

Figure 2.1 Mechanistic Framework for Understanding How Cigarette Smoking Causes Lung Cancer. All Events Can Occur Chronically Since a Smoker Typically Uses Multiple Cigarettes per Day for Many Years

Source: From Ref. (1). Hecht SS. Lung carcinogenesis by tobacco smoke. *Int J Cancer*. 2012;131:2724-2732. Reprinted by permission of John Wiley & Sons, Inc.

but likely includes a stochastic process of mutation accumulation, transformation of key pluripotent cells or stem cells, and cooperation between mutations in epithelial cells and a permissive immune environment that allows the proliferation of cells bearing foreign neoantigens (2).

Field Carcinogenesis

Recent studies of bronchial field carcinogenesis provide insight into the molecular pathogenesis of lung cancer, and may directly impact the care of those at risk for lung cancer by providing novel strategies for early detection and targeted chemoprevention. For example, two multicenter trials (Airway Epithelial Gene Expression in the Diagnosis of Lung Cancer [AEGIS] 1 and 2) demonstrated that a gene expression classifier from normal-appearing bronchial epithelial cells was a sensitive biomarker for diagnosing lung cancer among smokers undergoing bronchoscopy for suspected disease (3). Other studies have identified spatial and temporal variations in cellular alterations within field of cancerization in smokers, including transcriptional dysregulation of *AKT* and *ERK1/2*, epigenetic alterations of micro-RNAs (miRNAs) such as miR4423, and somatic chromosomal alterations. These aberrations can have a significant impact on the entire bronchial epithelial field, including basal cells that may serve as progenitors for lung carcinoma (4).

Lung Development and Carcinogenesis

Many of the interactions that occur between epithelial cells and stromal cells during lung carcinogenesis are similar to those that are essential to normal lung development. The pathways involved in the development and differentiation of the normal lung are also important for tumor initiation, progression, and histologic differentiation. Current paradigms suggest that lung carcinomas arise from pluripotent stem cells and progenitor cells that are capable of differentiation into several histologic cell types. The hypothesis that lung cancer is caused by the aberrant expression of genes involved in lung development is supported by gene expression studies demonstrating similarities between genetic signatures obtained from human lung tumors and those that are characteristically noted during normal lung development (5, 6). These studies show that the molecular profiles of high-grade tumors (e.g., large-cell carcinoma) demonstrate derangements in genes involved in the regulation of both the cell cycle and transcription, resulting in developmental arrest at a stage close to the undifferentiated progenitor cell. However, the molecular signatures of low-grade tumors (e.g., adenocarcinoma) are comprised of genes involved in terminal differentiation pathways. This linkage between poorly differentiated tumors and the molecular parameters of early development suggests that these genetic signatures are important for lung cancer progression and are potential biomarkers of clinical outcome.

MOLECULAR DETERMINANTS OF HISTOLOGIC SUBTYPES

The clinical significance of the developmental regulation of histologic differentiation is highlighted by recent clinical trials showing the differential efficacy of selected lung cancer therapies within specific histological and molecular subtypes. These findings have helped transform the clinical management of non–small-cell lung cancer (NSCLC) from a "one-size-fits-all" approach to a strategy based on personalized medical care (7).

In the most recent World Health Organization (WHO) lung cancer classification scheme, the major subtypes of lung cancer have been reorganized and renamed based upon seminal clinical and biological studies (8). The major changes include grouping all neuroendocrine tumors together, restricting the designation of large-cell carcinoma to tumors that lack differentiation by both morphologic and immunohistochemical criteria, and the adoption of the IASLC/ATS/ERS Lung Adenocarcinoma Classification scheme (9). These modifications are supported by biological studies that demonstrated that specific molecular signatures are associated with clinically relevant histological subtypes (10). This refined histologic classification and routine molecular testing protocols now facilitate the assignment of lung cancer treatment by specific histological and molecular subtypes (Figure 2.2). For example, the chemotherapeutic agent pemetrexed has activity in non-squamous NSCLC, but not squamous cell carcinoma, while necitumumab, an anti-epidermal growth factor receptor (EGFR) monoclonal antibody, may augment the activity of standard chemotherapy in some patients with squamous cell carcinoma, but not non-squamous NSCLC.

For early stage lung adenocarcinoma, the revised classification scheme captures distinct histological and biological subtypes with prognostic significance. For example, tumors with a preinvasive histology, such as adenocarcinoma in situ (AIS) or microinvasive adenocarcinoma (MIA), have 5-year survival rates of 95% to 100% after complete surgical resection. The histologic classification is also supported by the biological data demonstrating unique molecular properties of specific subtypes. Gene expression profiling studies from North America, Asia, and Europe have

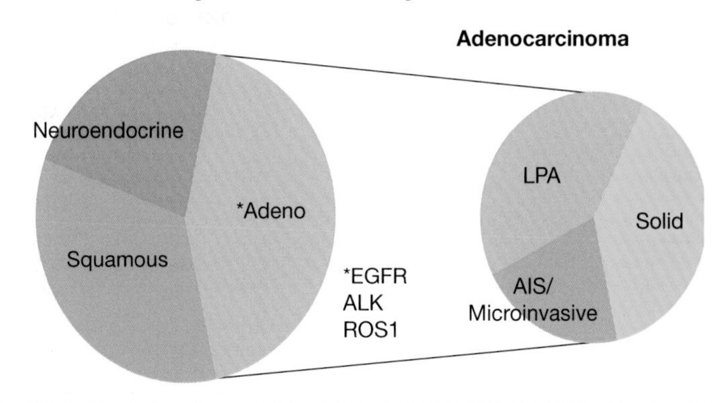

Figure 2.2 Classification of Lung Carcinoma
The major lung cancer histologies are neuroendocrine, squamous cell, and adenocarcinoma. Within adenocarcinoma, the major histological subtypes include the preinvasive adenocarcinoma in situ (AIS), microinvasive adenocarcinoma; lepidic predominant adenocarcinoma (LPA), and solid adenocarcinoma. For patients with advanced adenocarcinoma with actionable molecular alterations in EGFR, ALK, or ROS1, treatment with targeted therapy is recommended.

reproducibly demonstrated that early stage lung adenocarcinomas cluster into three major genomic subgroups that correlate with histology (Figure 2.3) (11). These studies have led to incorporation of these subgroups into the new WHO classification scheme and the revised lung cancer TNM staging system, with annotations for AIS and MIA now included for T1 tumors (12). It will be important to prospectively validate the prognostic accuracy of the revised staging system for preinvasive cancers and to evaluate the clinical significance of specific subtypes of invasive adenocarcinoma. For example, recent studies indicate that the micropapillary and solid variants are associated with a poorer prognosis after resection than other subtypes, such as lepidic-predominant adenocarcinoma.

LUNG CANCER GENETICS

Large-scale efforts to comprehensively evaluate the biology of lung cancer by high-throughput transcriptional analysis, sequencing, and copy number analysis has provided a catalog of genomic alterations that are associated with specific histological subtypes of lung cancer (Table 2.1) (8,13,14). For adenocarcinoma, the most common somatic mutations occur in *KRAS*, *EGFR*, and *P53*, with gene rearrangements of *ALK*, *RET*, and *ROS1*. For squamous cell carcinoma, mutations in *P53* and *PIK3CA* are common, as is

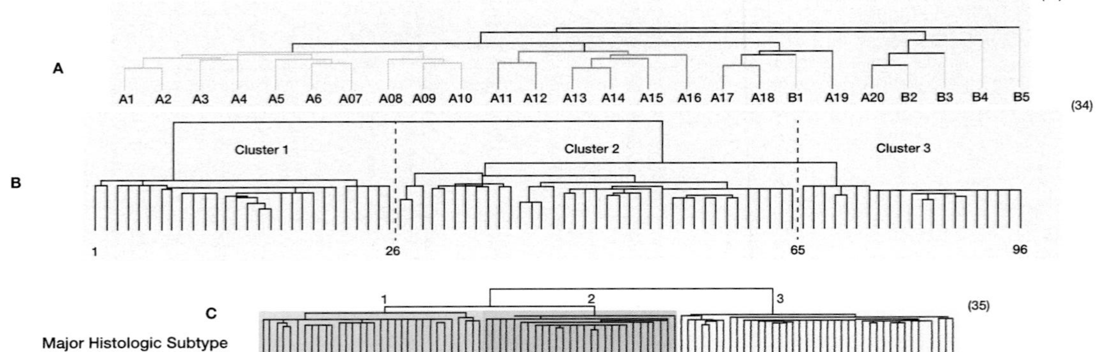

Figure 2.3 Adenocarcinoma Molecular Profiles Correlate With Histological Subtype Class
Independent studies (A–C) with different genomics analysis platforms all show that early-stage lung adenocarcinomas cluster into three major genomic subgroups that correlate with three major adenocarcinoma pathological subtypes (preinvasive adenocarcinoma in-situ and minimally invasive; lepidic predominant adenocarcinoma; solid adenocarcinoma).

Panel A, from Ref. (33), reprinted with permission of the American Thoracic Society, copyright © 2016 American Thoracic Society. Panel B, from Ref. (34), reprinted by permission from Macmillan Publishers Ltd. Panel C, from Ref. (35), reprinted with permission.

Table 2.1 Major genetic changes in lung cancer

Alterations	Small-cell carcinoma (%)	Adenocarcinoma (%)	Squamous cell carcinoma (%)
Mutation			
BRAF	0	<5	0
EGFR			
Whites	<1	10–20	<1
Asian	<5	35–45	<5
ERBB2/HER2	0	<5	0
KRAS			
Whites	<1	15–35	<5
Asian	<1	5–10	<5
PIK3CA	<5	<5	5–15
RB	>90	5–15	5–15
TP53	>90	30–40	50–80
Amplification			
EGFR	<1	5–10	10
ERBB2/HER2	<1	<5	<1
MET	<1	<5	<5
MYC	20–30	5–10	5–10
FGFR1	<1	<5	15–25
Gene rearrangement			
ALK	0	5	<1
RET	0	1–2	0
ROS1	0	1–2	0
NTRK1	0	<1	0
NRG1	0	<1	0

Source: From Ref. (14). Travis WD, Brambilla E, Burke AP, et al. *WHO Classification of Tumours of the Lung, Pleura, Thymus, and Heart*. 4th ed. Lyon, France: IARC; 2015.

amplification of *FGFR1*. Small-cell carcinoma typically harbors mutations in *RB* and *P53*, with frequent amplification of *MYC*.

KRAS Mutation

KRAS mutations are the most common signal transduction pathway driver mutations in lung adenocarcinomas in Whites. RAS proteins mediate cellular proliferation in many growth factor signaling pathways, including the EGFR pathway. Oncogenic missense mutations in *KRAS* result in the loss of intrinsic GTPase activity that is required to return the KRAS protein to its inactive form, resulting in a loss of intrinsic negative-feedback of RAS activity and constitutive activation of KRAS (15). *KRAS* mutations localize to codons 12, 13, and 61, and are detectable in approximately 30% of lung adenocarcinomas. *KRAS*-mutant adenocarcinomas typically occur in smokers and in the central region of the lung. In smokers, tobacco carcinogens might specifically induce *KRAS* mutations with subsequent activation of proliferative signaling pathways, while in never smokers as yet unidentified carcinogens might selectively induce *EGFR* mutations, thus activating the EGFR signaling pathway (15).

KRAS codon 12 mutations have been associated with inferior disease-free survival and increased lung cancer mortality (16). Furthermore, *KRAS* mutations are associated with a lack of response to EGFR-targeted agents in both lung and colorectal cancer. Thus far, no targeted treatments have demonstrated consistent clinical efficacy against *KRAS*-mutant NSCLC.

EGFR Mutation

Unlike *KRAS*, other genetic alterations are actionable in that they predict response to molecularly targeted drugs (8). Advances in this field have provided proof-of-principle for the concept of oncogene addiction, that despite the diverse array of genetic lesions typical of cancer, some tumors rely on a single dominant oncogene for growth and survival such that inhibition of this specific oncogene is sufficient to kill the tumor (17). In lung cancer, the first successful example of this approach was the use of anti-EGFR tyrosine kinase inhibitors (TKIs) in patients whose tumors harbored mutations in the *EGFR* gene. *EGFR* mutations typically occur in the receptor tyrosine kinase domain, leading to constitutive activation of downstream signaling and hypersensitivity to EGFR-TKIs, such as gefitinib or erlotinib. The two most common *EGFR* sensitizing mutations are the L858R point mutation in exon 21 and in-frame deletions in exon 19, which account for greater than 90% of *EGFR* mutations found in lung cancer. These *EGFR* mutations are highly specific for lung adenocarcinoma and are mutually exclusive with other major lung cancer driver mutations, including *KRAS, ALK, ROS1, RET, BRAF*, and *ERBB2/HER2*. For reasons that have not been determined, the prevalence of *EGFR* mutations in lung cancer show significant ethnic variations, ranging from 10% to 15% in whites to 30% to 50% in East Asians. In patients with advanced *EGFR*-mutated NSCLC, response rates to EGFR-TKIs are 60% to 70%, significantly higher than the 30% response rate achieved with conventional chemotherapy. EGFR-TKIs also yield a significant improvement in progression-free survival in patients with *EGFR*-mutated tumors, and EGFR-TKIs are now the standard treatment for this molecularly defined patient subgroup.

ALK Rearrangement

The discovery of chromosomal rearrangements of the *ALK* gene locus in adenocarcinoma of the lung has led to similar advances in therapy. Although *ALK* aberrations are common in anaplastic large cell lymphoma, the specific *EML4-ALK* rearrangement is almost exclusively found in lung adenocarcinoma with an acinar or solid growth pattern. *ALK* rearrangements are found in approximately 4% of NSCLCs, without any ethnic variations in prevalence. *ALK*-rearranged NSCLCs are highly sensitive to treatment with *ALK* inhibitors, such as crizotinib. In randomized clinical trials, crizotinib has demonstrated significant improvements in response rate and progression-free survival in patients with *ALK*-rearranged NSCLC when compared to standard chemotherapy. Similarly, high response rates have been seen with crizotinib in patients with *ROS1*-rearranged NSCLC.

Resistance to Targeted Therapy

The widespread implementation of molecularly targeted therapy has resulted in significant clinical benefits for selected subgroups of patients with advanced adenocarcinoma of the lung. However, there are limitations to targeted therapy. Acquired resistance inevitably develops to first-line TKIs directed against EGFR and ALK. For *EGFR*-mutated tumors, the most common form of acquired resistance is the development of a secondary, *EGFR* T790M point mutation in 50% of patients who have disease progression on an EGFR-TKI. Other mechanisms contributing to resistance to EGFR-TKIs include overexpression of other oncogene products (e.g., *MET*), bypass signaling pathways mediated by heat shock protein or TGFβ signaling, and induction of cellular differentiation pathways leading to histologic transformation to small-cell carcinoma.

Second- and third-generation EGFR-TKIs have been developed in response to the need for agents to override acquired resistance. For example, osimertinib is a mutation-selective EGFR-TKI that specifically targets T790M-positive tumors. Similarly, ceritinib and alectinib have been developed to target secondary *ALK* mutations in patients whose cancer has progressed on crizotinib (Table 2.2) (18).

Rebiopsy of driver mutation-positive tumors upon disease progression can guide the use of second- and third-line therapy by identifying specific mechanisms of resistance. Secondary mutations can be identified from biopsies of actual tumor deposits

Table 2.2 Recent U.S. FDA approvals of nonchemotherapy drugs for the treatment of lung cancer

Class	Drug	Year approved	Biomarker	Tumor indication	Sequence indication
Antiangiogenic agents	Bevacizumab (Avastin)	2006	None	Advanced non-squamous NSCLC	First-line; in combination with carboplatin/ paclitaxel
	Ramucirumab (Cyramza)	2014	None	Advanced NSCLC	Following failure of platinum-based chemotherapy; in combination with docetaxel
EGFR inhibitors	Erlotinib (Tarceva)	2013	Cobas EGFR mutation test	Advanced NSCLC with EGFR exon 19 deletion or L858R mutation	First-line
	Afatinib (Gilotrif)	2013	Therascreen EGFR RGQ PCR Kit	Advanced NSCLC with EGFR exon 19 deletion or L858R mutation	First-line
	Gefitinib (Iressa)	2015	Therascreen EGFR RGQ PCR Kit	Advanced NSCLC with EGFR exon 19 deletion or L858R mutation	First-line
	Osimertinib (Tagrisso)	2015	Cobas EGFR mutation test v2	Advanced NSCLC with EGFR T790M mutation	

(continued)

Table 2.2 Recent U.S. FDA approvals of nonchemotherapy drugs for the treatment of lung cancer (*continued*)

Class	Drug	Year approved	Biomarker	Tumor indication	Sequence indication
	Necitumumab (Portrazza)	2015	None	Advanced squamous cell lung cancer	First-line; in combination with cisplatin/ gemcitabine
ALK inhibitors	Crizotinib (Xalkori)	2011	ALK FISH+ (Vysis ALK FISH)	Advanced NSCLC with ALK rearrangement	
	Ceritinib (Zykadia)	2014	ALK+	Advanced NSCLC with ALK rearrangement	Crizotinib-refractory or intolerant
	Alectinib (Alecensa)	2015	ALK+	Advanced NSCLC with ALK rearrangement	Crizotinib-refractory or intolerant
ROS1 inhibitors	Crizotinib (Xalkori)	2016	ROS1+	Advanced NSCLC with ROS1 rearrangement	
Immune checkpoint inhibitors	Pembrolizumab (Keytruda)	2015	PD-L1 IHC+ (22C3 pharmDx)	Metastatic NSCLC	Following failure of platinum-based chemotherapy
	Nivolumab (Opdivo)	2015	None (PD-L1 IHC 28-8 pharmDx coapproved)	Metastatic NSCLC	Following failure of platinum-based chemotherapy

EGFR, epidermal growth factor receptor; FDA, Food and Drug Administration; NSCLC, non–small-cell lung cancer.
Source: Ref. (18). Spira A, Halmos B, Powell CA. Update in lung cancer 2015. *Am J Respir Crit Care Med*. 2016;194:661-671. Reprinted with permission of the American Thoracic Society.

(primary or metastatic) or from a "liquid biopsy" that evaluates circulating tumor DNA in the blood. Ongoing research is being directed toward the development of treatment approaches targeting other driver mutations found in lung cancer and the identification of strategies to overcome other mechanisms of acquired resistance.

EPIGENETICS

Epigenetic changes within the human genome, including chromatin remodeling, histone modification, and DNA methylation, can alter the expression of critical oncogenes and tumor suppressor genes and can have a profound impact on malignant transformation (19). Both global and gene-specific epigenetic changes are being evaluated as biomarkers for the early detection and prognosis of lung cancer.

Methylation

Hyper- and hypo-methylation of CpG islands within gene promoters is an epigenetic modification of DNA that can culminate in loss of gene transcription (20). Aberrant methylation of the promoter region of tumor suppressor genes, with resultant gene silencing, plays an important role in the pathogenesis of most types of human cancer, with individual tumor types having their own acquired pattern of methylation (21). In lung cancer, hypermethylation of CpG islands has been found in 15% to 80% of tumors, affecting many genes, including *APC*, *p16*, and *RASSF1A*. Techniques such as methylation-specific PCR and restriction landmark genomic scanning can be used to visualize different patterns of methylation that can distinguish tumor from normal tissue, and categorize clinically relevant subgroups. In sputum samples, the methylation pattern for a specific panel of genes has been reported to be predictive for the development of lung cancer among high-risk smokers (22,23).

Micro-RNA

miRNAs are small, noncoding RNA strands containing about 22 nucleotides that function in the transcriptional and posttranscriptional regulation of gene expression. It is estimated that miRNAs may regulate up to two-thirds of the human genome (19). More than 50% of miRNAs are located at cancer-related chromosomal regions, supporting the concept that miRNAs may act as oncogenes or tumor suppressor genes. The genome-wide expression profile of miRNAs is significantly different in primary lung cancers than in corresponding noncancerous lung tissues, and human lung cancers have extensive alterations of miRNA expression that may deregulate cancer-related genes. Thus, patterns of miRNA expression may be linked to relevant clinical parameters, such as prognosis and therapeutic response (24). For example, one study determined that expression of miRNA-21 consistently correlated with poor outcome in patients with early stage lung cancer (25), while another study suggested that patterns of plasma miRNA may be used for risk stratification in lung cancer screening programs (26). Overall, large-scale prospective trials will be required to establish the potential role of miRNA biomarkers in the clinical setting.

TUMOR MICROENVIRONMENT

The importance of cooperation between tumor cells and their surrounding microenvironment has been thoroughly reviewed by Hanahan and Weinberg (27,28). Tumor cells cooperate with surrounding cells to promote inflammation and to activate pathways involved in invasion, metastasis, and angiogenesis. Many of these processes represent potential targets for therapeutic interventions directed against tumor cells and/or the microenvironment. The tumor microenvironment is a complex system composed of stromal fibroblasts, macrophages, lymphocytes, other bone marrow-derived cells, and extracellular matrix that, in a reciprocal fashion, can contribute to tumor regression or progression.

TGFβ Signaling

The TGFβ signaling pathway mediates many of the interactions required for tumor cell progression (29). TGFβ, the ligand for the TGFβ-type II receptor (TGFβ-RII), is a family of pleiotropic cytokines (TGFβ 1, 2, 3) that regulate tissue homeostasis and prevent tumor initiation by inhibiting cellular proliferation, differentiation, and survival. TGFβ is secreted as a latent molecule and is activated by protease cleavage. TGFβ signaling primarily occurs through SMAD protein-dependent pathways in which binding to TGFβ-RII induces phosphorylation and activation of TGFβ-RI. TGFβ signaling may also proceed via less well defined SMAD-independent pathways. Depending upon context, TGFβ signaling may alternatively suppress tumor growth in early stage cancers or promote tumor cell invasion and metastasis in late-stage cancers. Both in vitro and in vivo models have demonstrated the importance of TGFβ signaling in the progression of lung adenocarcinoma from preinvasive lesions to invasive, metastatic tumors by mediating changes in both tumor cells and the stromal compartment.

Epithelial–Mesenchymal Transition

In order for epithelial tumor cells to metastasize, they must acquire mesenchymal cell properties, such as the loss of cell–cell adhesion, invasiveness, vascular intravasation and extravasation, and angiogenesis (30). This process of EMT involves numerous signaling pathways relevant to cancer, including those mediated by TGFβ, AKT, MEK-ERK, ZEB, SNAIL, FAS, and EZH2 (31). Studies in in vitro and in vivo model systems have demonstrated that both EMT within primary tumors and mesenchymal-to-epithelial transition (MET) within metastatic foci are required for lung cancer progression and metastasis.

Immune Checkpoints

The clinical significance of the immune cell component of the tumor microenvironment has been revealed by recent studies showing that the immune checkpoint mediator PD-L1, expressed by tumor cells, can bind to the PD-1 receptor on tumor infiltrating T-lymphocytes, resulting in T-cell inactivation (32). Through this mechanism, tumors can successfully evade immune surveillance. In 2015, two anti-PD-1 monoclonal antibodies, nivolumab, and pembrolizumab, were approved by the U.S. Food and Drug Administration (FDA) as second-line treatment for NSCLC after progression on standard chemotherapy (Table 2.2) (18). The response rate to these immune checkpoint inhibitors is approximately 20%, but many responses are durable and both agents have demonstrated an improvement in overall survival over standard second-line chemotherapy. Current research is focused on the identification of biomarkers to predict which patients will benefit the most from PD-1/PD-L1 targeted therapy. Thus far, PD-L1 expression by immunohistochemistry has yielded conflicting data, but the response to immune checkpoint inhibitors does appear to be directly correlated with the mutational load of the tumor, likely as a surrogate for increased neoantigen expression.

KEY POINTS

- Individual variation in the activity of endogenous enzymes that activate and eliminate specific tobacco carcinogens determines susceptibility to lung cancer in smokers.
- Genetic alterations within normal-appearing bronchial epithelial cells exposed to tobacco carcinogens can define lung cancer risk.

(continued)

(continued)

- Molecular profiles can be used to define subsets of lung cancer with variable sensitivity to specific treatments.
- Driver mutations in lung adenocarcinomas that can be targeted by effective treatment include sensitizing EGFR mutations, and ALK and ROS1 rearrangements.
- Epithelial-to-mesenchymal cellular transitions play an important role in the progression of lung cancer and the development of metastases.
- Interactions between tumor cells and the immune component of the tumor microenvironment are essential in immune checkpoint mediation and can be targeted for therapeutic benefit.

REFERENCES

1. Hecht SS. Lung carcinogenesis by tobacco smoke. *Int J Cancer*. 2012;131(12):2724-2732.
2. Gomperts BN, Walser TC, Spira A, Dubinett SM. Enriching the molecular definition of the airway "field of cancerization": establishing new paradigms for the patient at risk for lung cancer. *Cancer Prev Res (Phila)*. 2013;6(1):4-7.
3. Silvestri GA, Vachani A, Whitney D, et al. A bronchial genomic classifier for the diagnostic evaluation of lung cancer. *N Engl J Med*. 2015;373(3):243-251.
4. Spira A, Halmos B, Powell CA. Update in Lung Cancer 2014. *Am J Respir Crit Care Med*. 2015;192(3):283-294.
5. Borczuk AC, Gorenstein L, Walter KL, et al. Non-small-cell lung cancer molecular signatures recapitulate lung developmental pathways. *Am J Pathol*. 2003;163(5):1949-1960.
6. Borczuk AC, Powell CA. Expression profiling and lung cancer development. *Proc Am Thorac Soc*. 2007;4(1):127-132.
7. Cardarella S, Johnson BE. The impact of genomic changes on treatment of lung cancer. *Am J Respir Crit Care Med*. 2013;188(7):770-775.
8. Travis WD, Brambilla E, Nicholson AG, et al. The 2015 World Health Organization classification of lung tumors: impact of genetic, clinical and radiologic advances since the 2004 classification. *J Thorac Oncol*. 2015;10(9):1243-1260.
9. Travis WD, Brambilla E, Noguchi M, et al. International Association for the Study of Lung Cancer/American Thoracic Society/European Respiratory Society: international multidisciplinary classification of lung adenocarcinoma: executive summary. *Proc Am Thorac Soc*. 2011;8(5):381-385.

10. Clinical Lung Cancer Genome Project (CLCGP), Network Genomic Medicine (NGM). A genomics-based classification of human lung tumors. *Sci Transl Med*. 2013;5(209):209ra153.
11. Travis WD, Brambilla E, Noguchi M, et al. International Association for the Study of Lung Cancer/American Thoracic Society/European Respiratory Society international multidisciplinary classification of lung adenocarcinoma. *J Thorac Oncol*. 2011;6(2):244-285.
12. Travis WD, Asamura H, Bankier AA, et al. The IASLC Lung Cancer Staging Project: Proposals for Coding T Categories for Subsolid Nodules and Assessment of Tumor Size in Part-Solid Tumors in the Forthcoming Eighth Edition of the TNM Classification of Lung Cancer. *J Thorac Oncol*. 2016;11(8):1204-1223.
13. The Cancer Genome Atlas Research Network, Weinstein JN, Collisson EA, et al. The Cancer Genome Atlas Pan-Cancer analysis project. *Nat Genet*. 2013;45(10):1113-1120.
14. Travis WD, Brambilla E, Burke AP, et al. *WHO Classification of Tumours of the Lung, Pleura, Thymus, and Heart*. 4th ed. Lyon, France: IARC; 2015.
15. Sun S, Schiller JH, Gazdar AF. Lung cancer in never smokers—a different disease. *Nat Rev Cancer*. 2007;7(10):778-790.
16. Mascaux C, Iannino N, Martin B, et al. The role of RAS oncogene in survival of patients with lung cancer: a systematic review of the literature with meta-analysis. *Br J Cancer*. 2005;92(1):131-139.
17. Weinstein IB. Cancer. Addiction to oncogenes—the Achilles heal of cancer. *Science*. 2002;297(5578):63-64.
18. Spira A, Halmos B, Powell CA. Update in Lung Cancer 2015. *Am J Respir Crit Care Med*. 2016;194:661-671.
19. Nana-Sinkam SP, Powell CA. Molecular biology of lung cancer: diagnosis and management of lung cancer. 3rd ed. American College of Chest Physicians evidence-based clinical practice guidelines. *Chest*. 2013;143(5 suppl):e30S-39S.
20. Tessema M, Belinsky SA. Mining the epigenome for methylated genes in lung cancer. *Proc Am Thorac Soc*. 2008;5(8):806-810.
21. Toyooka S, Toyooka KO, Maruyama R, et al. DNA methylation profiles of lung tumors. *Mol Cancer Ther*. 2001;1(1):61-67.
22. Belinsky SA, Liechty KC, Gentry FD, et al. Promoter hypermethylation of multiple genes in sputum precedes lung cancer incidence in a high-risk cohort. *Cancer Res*. 2006;66(6):3338-3344.
23. Belinsky SA, Grimes MJ, Casas E, et al. Predicting gene promoter methylation in non-small-cell lung cancer by evaluating sputum and serum. *Br J Cancer*. 2007;96(8):1278-1283.
24. Yanaihara N, Caplen N, Bowman E, et al. Unique microRNA molecular profiles in lung cancer diagnosis and prognosis. *Cancer Cell*. 2006;9(3):189-198.
25. Saito M, Schetter AJ, Mollerup S, et al. The association of microRNA expression with prognosis and progression in early-stage, non-small cell lung adenocarcinoma: a retrospective analysis of three cohorts. *Clin Cancer Res*. 2011;17(7):1875-1882.

26. Boeri M, Verri C, Conte D, et al. MicroRNA signatures in tissues and plasma predict development and prognosis of computed tomography detected lung cancer. *Proc Natl Acad Sci USA*. 2011;108(9):3713-3718.
27. Hanahan D, Weinberg RA. Hallmarks of cancer: the next generation. *Cell*. 2011;144(5):646-674.
28. Hanahan D, Weinberg RA. The hallmarks of cancer. *Cell*. 2000; 100(1):57-70.
29. Borczuk AC, Sole M, Lu P, et al. Progression of human bronchioloalveolar carcinoma to invasive adenocarcinoma is modeled in a transgenic mouse model of K-ras-induced lung cancer by loss of the TGF-beta type II receptor. *Cancer Res*. 2011;71(21):6665-6675.
30. Powell CA, Halmos B, Nana-Sinkam SP. Update in lung cancer and mesothelioma 2012. *Am J Respir Crit Care Med*. 2013;188(2):157-166.
31. Gao D, Vahdat LT, Wong S, et al. Microenvironmental regulation of epithelial-mesenchymal transitions in cancer. *Cancer Res*. 2012; 72(19):4883-4889.
32. Couzin-Frankel J. Cancer immunotherapy. *Science*. 2013;342(6165): 1432-1433.
33. Borczuk AC, Kim HK, Yegen HA, et al. Lung adenocarcinoma global profiling identifies type II transforming growth factor-beta receptor as a repressor of invasiveness. *Am J Respir Crit Care Med*. 2005;172(6):729-737.
34. Beer DG, Kardia SL, Huang CC, et al. Gene-expression profiles predict survival of patients with lung adenocarcinoma. *Nat Med*. 2002;8(8):816-824.
35. Motoi N, Szoke J, Riely GJ, et al. Lung adenocarcinoma: modification of the 2004 WHO mixed subtype to include the major histologic subtype suggests correlations between papillary and micropapillary adenocarcinoma subtypes, EGFR mutations and gene expression analysis. *Am J Surg Pathol*. 2008;32(6):810-827.

Cellular and Molecular Pathology of Lung Cancer 3

Edwin R. Parra and Ignacio I. Wistuba

INTRODUCTION

Traditionally, clinical treatment options for lung cancer were based on the distinction between small cell lung carcinoma (SCLC, 13% of cases) and non–small-cell lung carcinoma (NSCLC, 83% of cases) (1), the two major types of lung cancer. Although this distinction is still relevant, this basic categorization of tumor types is no longer considered sufficient. Pathologists are under greater pressure to precisely subclassify lung cancers, even when presented with very small tumors or cytologic samples, because histologic subtyping is increasingly important for making molecular testing decisions and for the selection of appropriate therapy (1). Unfortunately, most patients with lung cancer present with advanced-stage disease and the overall prognosis is poor, with an overall 5-year survival rate of only 15% (2). Major advances in understanding the molecular pathogenesis of lung cancer have led to new strategies for early detection, diagnosis, staging, and therapy. The personalized or precision medicine approach has increasingly become a day-to-day reality in the treatment of lung cancer, and having a clear understanding of the molecular alterations within tumors will be crucial to improving patient outcomes (3–5). Pathologists play a crucial role in facilitating clear and timely communication between the clinical oncology care team and the molecular diagnostic laboratory. This chapter provides a broad overview of several of the driver oncogenes that are important in the pathogenesis of NSCLC and have emerged as targets for therapeutic approaches.

HISTOLOGIC SUBTYPING OF LUNG CANCER

Clinical treatment options were traditionally based on the distinction between SCLC and NSCLC, without major therapeutic interest in further subclassification. However, the advent of molecular profiling and targeted therapy renewed interest in the distinguishing between the major subtypes of NSCLC: adenocarcinoma (ADC, 39%) (2), squamous cell carcinoma (SqCC; 20%), and large cell lung carcinoma (LCLC, 3%) (4,6,7) (Figure 3.1).

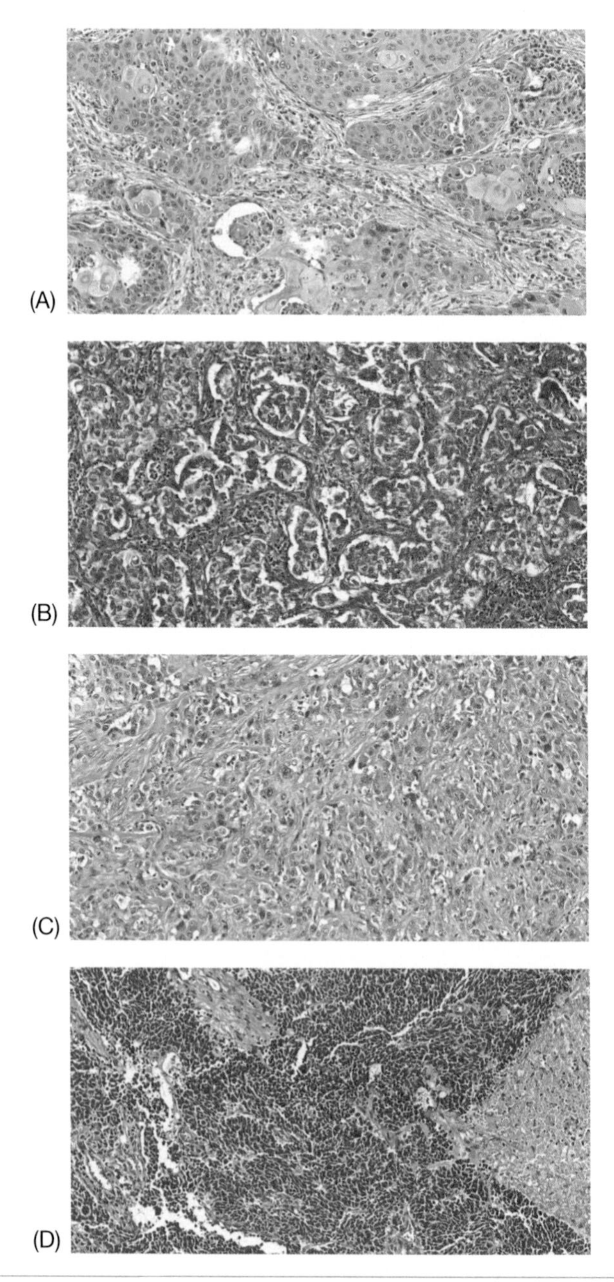

Figure 3.1 Microphotographs of H&E Stained Sections of the Four Major Subtypes of Lung Cancer: (A) Squamous Cell Carcinoma, (B) Adenocarcinoma, (C) Large Cell Carcinoma, and (D) Small Cell Carcinoma, H&E, x200

LCLC occurs throughout the lung and usually grows and spreads at a rapid rate. Other subtypes, including sarcomatoid carcinoma and neuroendocrine large cell carcinoma, represent a very small proportion of all NSCLC cases.

Squamous Cell Carcinoma

SqCC generally occurs in the central portion of the lung and is highly associated with tobacco smoking. Classical SqCC is generally recognized under light microscopy by its distinctive areas of keratinization and an associated inflammatory component, especially in tumors that have undergone cavitation (Figure 3.1). Less differentiated forms of SqCC, with smaller cells and without keratinization, may resemble basal cell layers of squamous epithelium (7). In these cases, immunohistochemistry (IHC) may be required to detect the presence of specific types of cytokeratin and the absence of neuroendocrine markers (Table 3.1).

Table 3.1 Immunohistochemical characterization of lung cancer

	Non–small cell carcinoma		
Marker	Adenocarcinoma	Squamous cell carcinoma	Small cell carcinoma
CK5/6	Negative	Positive	Negative
P40*	Negative	Positive	–
P63	Negative	Positive	Negative
TTF1*	Positive (77%)	Negative (11%)	Positive (87%)
CK7	Positive (97%)	–	Negative
CK20	Negative (9%)†	–	Negative
CK8	Positive (72%)	Negative	Positive (75%)
CEACAM6	Positive (33%)	–	Negative
Napsin A	Positive (90%)	–	Negative
TIMP2	Negative	–	Positive (82%)
CD56	Negative	–	Positive
Chromogranin	Negative	–	Positive
NSE	Negative	–	Positive
Synaptophysin	Negative	–	Positive

AIS, Adenocarcinoma in situ; CEACAM6, carcinoembryonic antigen-related cell adhesion molecule 6; CK, cytokeratin; NSE, neuron-specific enolase; TIMP2, tissue inhibitor of metalloproteinases 2; TTF1, thyroid transcription factor.

*Basic panel to distinguish between adenocarcinoma and squamous cell carcinoma.

†CK20 is frequently positive (67%) in AIS.

Adenocarcinoma

ADC is a relatively slow-growing lung cancer usually discovered in the periphery of the lung. It occurs most often in smokers, but it is the most common form of lung cancer found in nonsmokers (7). ADC includes a morphologically heterogeneous group of tumors characterized by gland formation (acinar pattern), papillary or micropapillary structures, or solid growth with mucin production (Figure 3.2) (7). Adenocarcinoma in situ (AIS), previously termed as bronchioloalveolar carcinoma, is defined as a small (≤3 cm) solitary tumor with a pure alveolar epithelial appearance, lepidic growth, and lack of invasion of the interstitium. AIS is further divided into mucinous and nonmucinous subtypes (Figure 3.2) (6). In clinical practice, however, the most common subtype is invasive ADC showing a combined pattern of growth, with conventional acinar or papillary ADC mixed with areas of AIS. Such tumors are classified as a mixed subtype ADC (6,7).

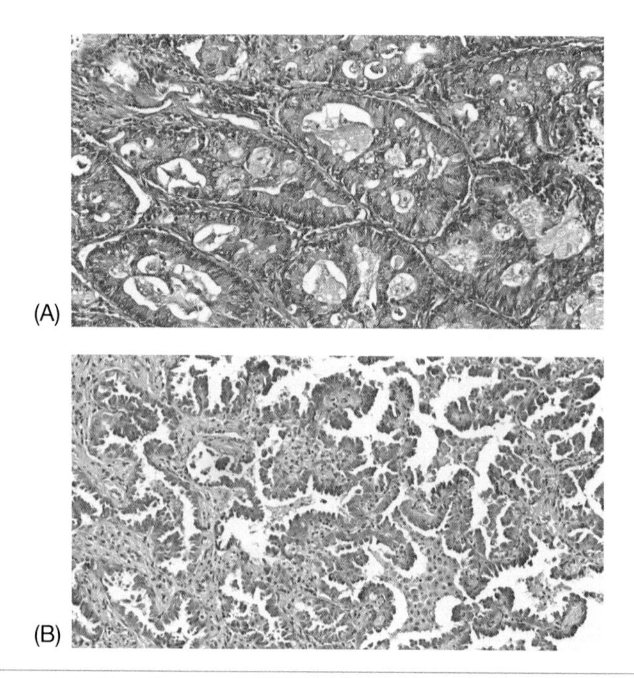

Figure 3.2 Microphotographs of H&E Stained Sections of the Common Subtypes of Lung Adenocarcinoma: (A) Acinar, (B) Papillary, (C) Micropapillary, (D) Solid, (E) Lepidic, Nonmucinous, and (F) Lepidic, Mucinous, H&E, x200

(continued)

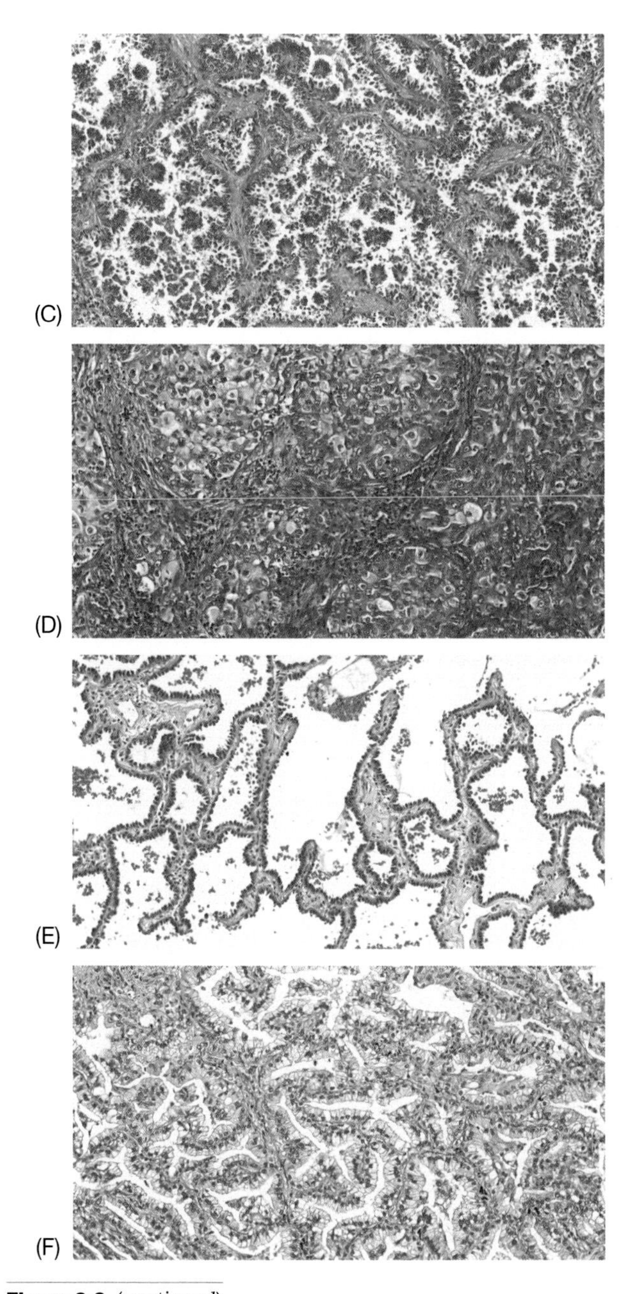

Figure 3.2 (*continued*)

Small Cell Lung Cancer

SCLC usually arises in the bronchi in the central portion of the lung. It is an aggressive cancer that spreads to lymph nodes and distant sites early in its course and tends to grow much faster than NSCLC (8). The major histologic feature that distinguishes SCLC from NSCLC is cell size. Typically, the cells in SCLC are roughly twice the size of lymphocytes when subjectively assessed under light microscopy. Additional features that distinguish SCLC from NSCLC include hyperchromatic appearance, small amounts of cytoplasm (i.e., high nucleus-to-cytoplasm ratio), cohesive sheets of small "blue" cells, crush artifact, necrosis, cellular fragility, and a high mitotic rate with an average of 80 mitoses/2 mm^2. When the classic features of SCLC are present, morphologic criteria alone are often diagnostic and support high interobserver reliability (8). Although IHC is useful in the diagnosis of SCLC, the most important stain is a good-quality hematoxylin and eosin (H&E) stain.

Immunohistochemistry

The most recent histologic classification of lung cancer published by the World Health Organization in 2015 incorporates the relevant genetic and IHC features of the different tumor subtypes (7). Major advances in lung cancer biology, diagnosis, and treatment have occurred in the past 10 years, and there is an even greater need for an integrated multidisciplinary approach to the diagnosis and management of NSCLC. Lung cancers are increasingly diagnosed and staged via transthoracic core needle biopsy or fine needle aspiration, endobronchial ultrasound (EBUS)-guided transbronchial needle aspiration, or endoscopic ultrasound (EUS)-guided fine needle aspiration (9). These techniques frequently result in small histologic or cytologic samples, which may be a limiting factor in distinguishing NSCLC subtypes and in obtaining an accurate histologic and molecular diagnosis.

Poorly differentiated ADC and SqCC can be indistinguishable by routine microscopy, particularly in small histologic and cytologic specimens. When presented with small samples, particularly when the tumor is poorly differentiated, we need to integrate morphology with IHC analysis to provide a precise diagnosis. In such situations, a useful IHC panel includes thyroid transcription factor (TTF1), the novel aspartic proteinases of the pepsin family (napsin A and B) and surfactants A and B, which are expressed in ADC, and p40, p63, and cytokeratin 5/6, which are expressed in SqCC (Figure 3.3 and Table 3.1) (7). In addition, staining for mucin is useful for the diagnosis of ADC.

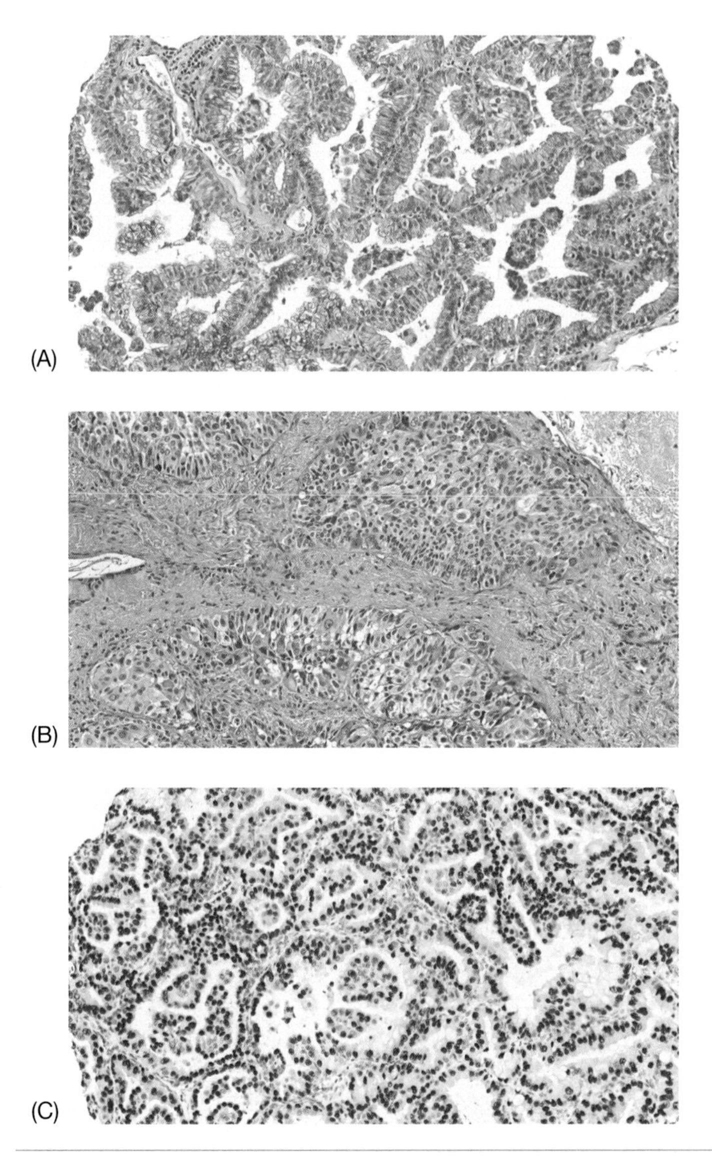

Figure 3.3 Microphotographs of Immunohistochemical Analysis to Distinguish Lung Adenocarcinoma (ADC) From Squamous Cell Carcinoma (SqCC): (A) H&E of ADC, (B) H&E of SqCC, (C) Thyroid Transcription Factor (TTF1) Positive in ADC, (D) TTF1 Negative in SqCC, (E) p40 Negative in ADC, and (F) p40 Positive in SqCC. H&E, Hematoxylin, and Eosin, x200 and IHC, Immunohistochemistry, x200

(*continued*)

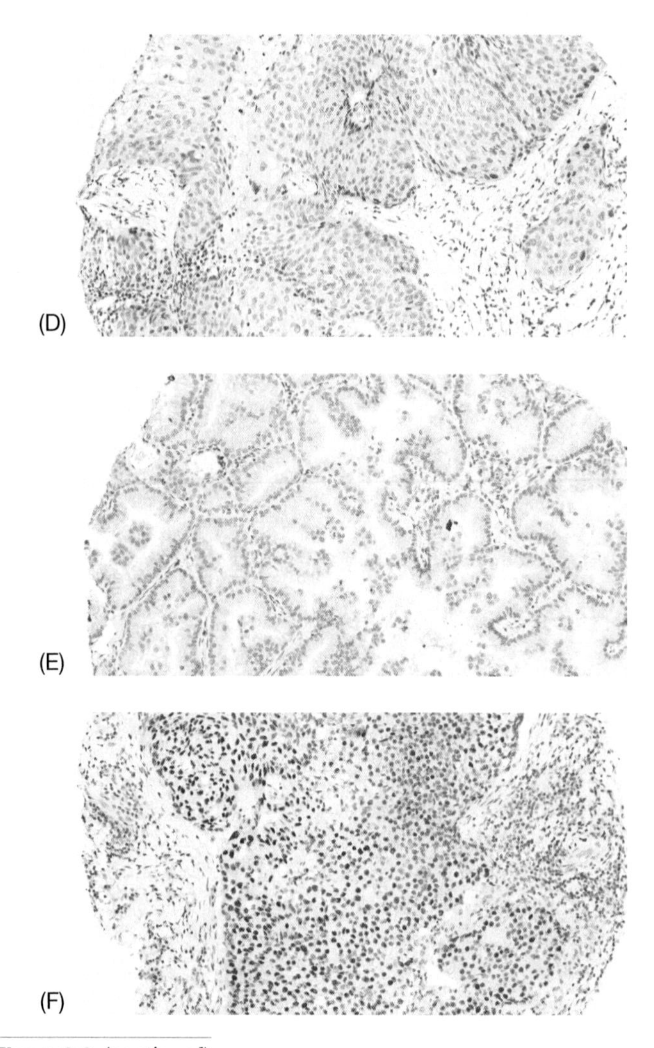

Figure 3.3 *(continued)*

Poorly differentiated metastases from distant sites may also need to be distinguished from primary NSCLC. Stains that are classically negative in NSCLC such as cytokeratin 20 (typically positive in colon cancer) and estrogen and progesterone receptors (typically positive in breast cancer) can help to distinguish the tissue of origin for an ADC found in the lung. SCLC can be positive for TTF1, but otherwise the staining pattern of SCLC should be distinct from that of NSCLC. As a neuroendocrine tumor, SCLC is typically positive for synaptophysin, CD56 neural cell adhesion molecule (NCAM), chromogranin, or neuron-specific enolase, whereas NSCLC is negative for these stains (Table 3.1) (7). While obtaining an accurate histologic diagnosis is important, it is also imperative to perform only essential IHC stains in order to ensure adequate tissue to maximize the yield for molecular testing.

MOLECULAR DIVERSITY IN NSCLC

At present, epidermal growth factor receptor (*EGFR*) mutation and anaplastic lymphoma kinase (*ALK*) rearrangement are the two best-characterized molecular alterations associated with targeted therapy in NSCLC, particularly ADC. However, the frequency of these two derangements combined is less than 20% in most patient populations. Thus, extensive efforts are ongoing to identify additional recurrent aberrations and to understand aspects of the biology of lung cancer that can be exploited for targeted therapy (Figure 3.4). On the basis of these efforts, other genomic alterations may become part of the routine analysis of NSCLC in the near future (5). Although the list of emerging genomic alterations is extensive, we present here those that may have clinical relevance as molecular targets in NSCLC (Table 3.2).

Epidermal Growth Factor Receptor

The *EGFR* gene is located on the short arm of chromosome 7 at position 12 (10). The protein encoded by this gene is a transmembrane glycoprotein that is a member of the protein kinase superfamily (10). EGFR is overexpressed in 40% to 80% of NSCLCs and many other epithelial cancers. Approximately 10% of patients with NSCLC in the United States and 35% in East Asia have tumor-associated *EGFR* mutations (11). The most common *EGFR* mutations, generally termed classic or sensitizing mutations, are in-frame deletions in exon 19 (around amino acid residues 747–750; 45% of *EGFR* mutations) and the L858R point mutation in exon 21 (40% of *EGFR* mutations) (12). The third most common type of *EGFR* mutation is in-frame insertions in exon 20 (5%–10%) (13). Other recurrent mutations include exon 18 point mutations at G719 (3%), exon 21 L861Q mutations (2%), and in-frame insertions in exon 19 (<1%) (12). *EGFR* mutations are more often found in tumors with ADC histology from female never-smokers (11,14). However, *EGFR* mutations can rarely be found in other lung cancer histologic subtypes in never-smokers. The paucity of classic *EGFR* mutations in SqCC of the lung has led to the widespread recommendation to obtain genotyping (usually complete or allele-specific sequencing of key regions of exons 18–21) only in non-squamous NSCLCs, except in cases with mixed histology or high clinical suspicion (e.g., never-smokers).

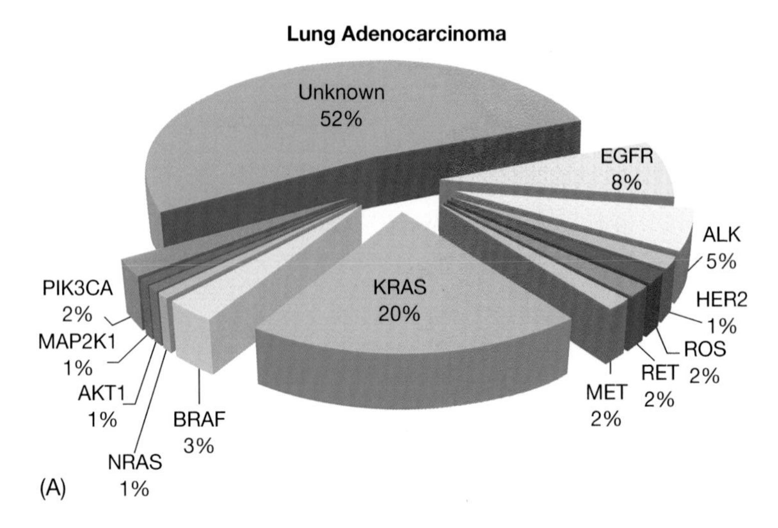

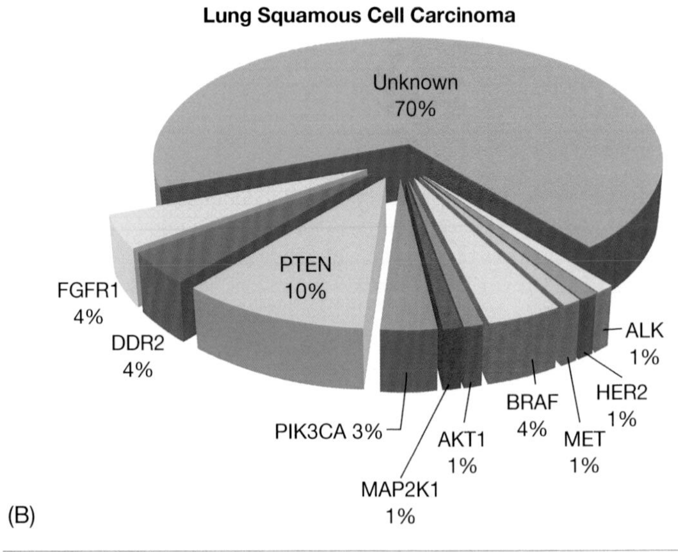

Figure 3.4 Relative Frequencies of Molecular Targets in Lung Adenocarcinoma (A) and Squamous Cell Carcinoma (B). The Number of Novel Molecular Targets Will Increase as Further Research Continues to Discover and Validate Them

The College of American Pathologists, the International Association for the Study of Lung Cancer, and the Association for Molecular Pathology recommend rapid testing for *EGFR* mutation and *ALK* rearrangement in all patients with advanced-stage ADC (15). The

Table 3.2 Characterization of molecular alterations in lung cancer

Alteration	Description	Prevalence	Pathologic characteristics	Drug	References
***EGFR* mutation**	Deletion exon 19; insertion/deletion exon 20; Mutation: L858R, T790M	10% United States; 35% Asia	Women, never-smokers, ADC	Gefitinib, erlotinib, afatinib, osimertinib	11, 12
***ALK* rearrangement**	Fusion: *EML4-ALK; KIF5B-ALK; TFG-ALK*	3%–7% United States/Asia	Never-smokers, ADC	Crizotinib, alectinib, ceritinib	19, 24
***ROS1* rearrangement**	Fusion: *SLC34A2-ROS1; CD74-ROS1; EZR-ROS1; TPM3-ROS1; SDC4-ROS1*	1%–2%	Younger, never-smokers, ADC	Crizotinib	27
***RET* rearrangement**	Fusion: *CCDC6-RET; NCOA4-RET; TRIM33-RET*	1%–2%	Younger, smokers, ADC	Cabozantinib, vandetinib	28, 31
***MET* mutation**	Mutation: juxtamembrane and semaphorin domains; exon 14 splice-site	2%–4%	NSCLC, SCLC	Crizotinib	40
***HER2* mutation**	Mutation: exon 20 (YVMA)	~5% Asia	Women, never-smokers, ADC, SqCC	Trastuzumab	42
***BRAF* mutation**	Mutation: exons 11, 15, 20	1%–4%	Smokers, ADC	Vemurafenib, dabrafenib, trametinib	48, 50
***KRAS* mutation**	Mutation: exons 1, 61, 63, 117, 119, 146	15%–20% United States/Europe/Asia	Smokers, ADC	Selumetinib, abemaciclib	54

ADC, adenocarcinoma; NSCLC, non–small-cell lung cancer; SCLC, small cell lung cancer; SqCC, squamous cell carcinoma.

etiology of the initial genomic insult that either leads to or selects for *EGFR* mutations in lung tissue remains elusive. Interestingly, rare inherited germline *EGFR* mutations, such as T790M and V843I, are associated with increased familial clustering of *EGFR*-mutated NSCLC in which tumors develop when a somatic classic *EGFR* mutation associates with the inherited allele.

Tumors with *EGFR* mutations are susceptible to treatment with EGFR tyrosine kinase inhibitors (EGFR-TKIs) such as gefitinib and erlotinib (16). However, relapse eventually occurs and resistance to 1st generation EGFR-TKIs is usually associated with a second mutation in exon 20 (T790M or D7961Y), *MET* amplification, or *PI3KCA* mutation (5). Interestingly, "transformation" to SCLC has also been described in a subset of ADC exhibiting resistance to EGFR-TKIs (5). Gene sequencing is the most comprehensive method of *EGFR* mutation testing. IHC for EGFR is not currently recommended because the expression of EGFR by IHC does not necessarily correlate with the presence or absence of an *EGFR* mutation or responsiveness to EGFR-directed therapy (15).

Anaplastic Lymphoma Kinase

ALK was originally discovered in chromosomal translocations leading to the production of fusion proteins consisting of the C-terminal kinase domain of ALK and the N-terminal portions of a variety of other genes (17). The *ALK* gene is located on the short arm of chromosome 2 at position 23 (17). Translocation of *ALK* has been identified in approximately 3% to 7% of NSCLCs in both white and Asian populations (18,19). Nucleophosmin (*NPM1*) is the most common fusion partner of ALK, primarily in hematologic malignancies, accounting for 80% of *ALK* translocations, but at least six other fusion partners have been identified (20).

In NSCLC, the most common *ALK* fusion partner is the echinoderm microtubule-associated protein-like 4 (*EML4*) gene. *EML4-ALK* is an aberrant fusion gene that encodes for a chimeric protein with constitutive kinase activity (21). *EML4-ALK* fusions are more commonly found in younger patients who have never smoked or have a history of light smoking (<10 pack years) (19,20), and in patients with ADC with acinar or signet ring cell histology (18,22). In lung SqCC, the estimated prevalence of *ALK* rearrangement is approximately 1%. Other fusion partners for *ALK*, such as *KIF5B* and *TFG*, have also been described in NSCLC (23). In the majority of cases, *ALK* rearrangements are mutually exclusive with other oncogenic mutations, such as those in *EGFR* and *KRAS* (18,19).

Clinical trials demonstrate that patients with *ALK*-rearranged NSCLC can be successfully treated with crizotinib, an ALK inhibitor, and that crizotinib is superior to chemotherapy in both the first- and second-line settings (24). In addition, next-generation ALK inhibitors, such as alectinib and ceritinib, have shown excellent efficacy for patients with *ALK*-rearranged NSCLC. However, ultimately acquired resistance develops to ALK inhibitors. Potential mechanisms of resistance to ALK inhibitors include secondary mutations or copy number gain of the *ALK* gene and activation of bypass pathways, including EGFR, KRAS, KIT, MET, and IGF-1R. Therapeutic strategies to overcome these resistance mechanisms have been proposed, including next-generation ALK inhibitors, agents that inhibit bypass pathways, and heat shock protein 90 inhibitors (25).

In clinical practice, fluorescence in situ hybridization (FISH) is the primary method used to identify gene copy number changes and structural variations due to *ALK* rearrangements. For NSCLC, FISH using the Vysis ALK Break Apart Probe Kit (Abbott Molecular) was approved as a companion diagnostic test along with crizotinib on the basis of the clinical responses seen in patients with *ALK*-rearranged tumors (26). The use of IHC for ALK protein detection is based on the premise that ALK protein is normally absent in the lung and therefore, the overexpression of ALK protein infers an underlying rearrangement of the *ALK* gene, leading to constitutive activation and subsequent overexpression of the protein (26). Although IHC is used as a prescreening method to detect ALK protein, confirmation by FISH is required because IHC is subject to technical issues such as tissue fixation, antibody clone used, endogenous peroxidase activity, necrosis/crush artifact, and interobserver variability.

ROS1

The *ROS1* proto-oncogene is located on the long arm of chromosome 6 at position 22. It is a member of the insulin receptor gene family and is a type I integral membrane protein with tyrosine kinase activity, which may function as a growth or differentiation factor receptor. *ROS1* rearrangements lead to constitutively active fusion proteins and are detected in approximately 1% to 2% of NSCLCs (27). *ROS1* rearrangements are associated with ADC, are most commonly found in light or never-smokers and young patients (<50 years of age) (27), and are mutually exclusive with *EGFR* mutations, *KRAS* mutations, and *ALK* rearrangements (28). Several types of *ROS1* rearrangements, such as *SLC34A2-ROS1*, *CD74-ROS1*, *EZR-ROS1*, *TPM3-ROS1*, and *SDC4-ROS1*, have been described in NSCLC (23,28).

In recent studies, patients with advanced NSCLC harboring an *ROS1* rearrangement derived great benefit from treatment with crizotinib, which targets ROS1 in addition to ALK (27). For this reason, the U.S. Food and Drug Administration (FDA) recently expanded the use of crizotinib to patients with metastatic NSCLC whose tumors harbor an *ROS1* rearrangement. Crizotinib is the first and only FDA-approved treatment for patients with *ROS1*-rearranged NSCLC.

RET

The *RET* gene is located on the long arm of chromosome 10 at position 11.2. It encodes for a tyrosine kinase that is involved in cellular proliferation, migration, and differentiation (29). Although *RET* point mutations and fusions have long been recognized in medullary and papillary thyroid carcinoma, respectively, *RET* rearrangements involving kinesin family member 5B (*KIF5B*) were only recently discovered in NSCLC (28,30). Alternative *RET* fusion partners, such as *CCDC6-RET*, *NCOA4-RET*, and *TRIM33-RET*, have since been described (31). In early studies, *RET* rearrangements were identified in approximately 1% to 2% of NSCLCs (28,32). *RET* fusions are associated with specific clinicopathologic features, such as smoking status, young age (≤60 years), and ADC histology, especially poorly differentiated tumors (31). *RET* rearrangements are largely mutually exclusive with genetic alterations in other oncogenic drivers, such as *EGFR*, *KRAS*, *ALK*, and *ROS1* (28,31,32), suggesting that *RET*-rearrangement defines a new, distinct, molecular subset of NSCLC.

RET fusions are oncogenic, and in vitro studies show that small-molecule inhibitors, such as vandetanib, sorafenib, and sunitinib, can inhibit *RET* fusion products (32). A recent study reported that cabozantinib, an RET inhibitor, may represent a promising targeted therapy for *RET* fusion-positive lung ADC (33). Cabozantinib, which is FDA-approved for the treatment of metastatic thyroid cancer, may also prove to be an effective treatment for metastatic NSCLC.

FISH is generally used to detect *RET* and *ROS1* rearrangements using *RET* and *ROS1* Dual Color Break Apart Probes (ZytoVision, Bremerhaven, Germany) (34). IHC has also been used to detect *RET* and *ROS1* rearrangements in NSCLC, with results that are comparable to FISH and reverse transcription polymerase chain reaction (RT-PCR) (34). Although the IHC interpretive criteria for predicting underlying rearrangements is not yet clearly defined, IHC can be used as a screening tool for further confirmatory testing.

MET

The *MET* gene encodes a receptor with tyrosine kinase activity (35). MET is activated by binding its ligand, hepatocyte growth factor, and regulates many physiologic processes including cellular proliferation, motility, invasion, and survival (35). The *MET* gene is located on the long arm of chromosome 7 at position 31, and in lung cancer, *MET* mutations are found in extracellular and juxtamembrane domains (36). The extracellular domain, encoded by exon 2, is required for receptor dimerization and activation (37). The presence of these mutations has been clearly defined in lung cancer; however, because of certain histologic and ethnic variations, their biologic relevance remains unclear.

In NSCLC, overexpression of MET and hepatocyte growth factor in tumor tissue is associated with higher pathologic tumor stage and worse prognosis (38), and multiple studies have reported primary *MET* amplification ranging from 2% to 20% in NSCLC, particularly in EGFR-TKI-naive patients (39). A recent study elucidated a mechanism of activation of *MET* via diverse exon 14 splicing alterations (*METex14*), which occurs in multiple tumor types, including NSCLC (40). The same study showed that *METex14* mutations are detected more frequently in lung ADC (3%) than in SqCC (1%) (40). Importantly, in vitro studies showed sensitivity to MET inhibitors in cells harboring *METex14* alterations, and patients whose tumors harbored these alterations have derived meaningful clinical benefit from MET inhibitors (40). In addition to targeting ALK and ROS1, crizotinib is also a potent MET inhibitor. Initial studies of crizotinib in patients with intermediate or high *MET* gene amplification demonstrated tumor responses and stable disease, which were unusually prolonged in patients with high *MET* amplification. Because *MET* amplification can also contribute to acquired resistance to EGFR-TKI therapy, combinations of MET inhibitors are being investigated in this patient population. The FDA has not yet approved any clinical tests for MET overexpression, but mutations in *MET* can be detected by several standard laboratory methods including FISH and PCR.

Human Epidermal Growth Factor Receptor 2

The proto-oncogene human epidermal growth factor receptor 2 (*HER2*), also known as *ERBB2*, *NEU*, and *EGFR2*, encodes for a member of the EGFR family of receptor tyrosine kinases, which plays important roles in cellular growth, differentiation, and survival. *HER2* is located on chromosome 17 at position 12 (41). The HER2 protein has no ligand-binding domain and, therefore, cannot bind growth factors. However, HER2 does bind tightly to other ligand-bound EGFR family members to form a heterodimer, stabilizing ligand binding and enhancing kinase-mediated activation of downstream signaling pathways, such as those involving mitogen-activated protein kinase (MAPK) and phosphatidylinositol-3 kinase (PI3K). Activating mutations in the tyrosine kinase domain of *HER2* have recently been reported in less than 5% of NSCLCs (2% of ADCs and 1% of SqCCs) (42,43). *HER2* mutations in lung cancer are associated with Asian ethnicity, female sex, never-smokers, and ADC histology, particularly a lepidic histologic pattern (42,43). However, *HER2* mutations can also be found in other subsets of NSCLC, including in former and current smokers (42,43). The vast majority of *HER2* mutations are represented by a 12-base pair duplication/insertion of the amino acid sequence YVMA in exon 20 at codon 776 (44). The exon 20 insertion induces increased HER2 kinase activity and enhanced signaling through downstream pathways, resulting in increased tumor cell survival, invasiveness, and tumorigenicity (45).

There is no obvious association between *HER2* amplification and *HER2* mutation, and previous trials demonstrated no benefit of trastuzumab in *HER2*-amplified NSCLC. However, newer studies suggest that patients with tumors harboring *HER2* insertions often respond to trastuzumab plus chemotherapy or to afatinib. A recent preclinical study demonstrated antitumor activity with the irreversible pan-HER inhibitor neratinib and the mammalian target of rapamycin (mTOR) inhibitor temsirolimus (45). Larger clinical trials are ongoing to further define efficacy of these agents in this lung cancer subtype.

Currently, HER2 testing can be carried out by several methods including IHC, FISH, chromogenic in situ hybridization (CISH), and silver-enhanced in situ hybridization (SISH). These tests are performed on tumor samples that are fixed in buffered formalin-fixed, paraffin-embedded (FFPE). A new test to measure total HER2 as well as HER2 homodimers and heterodimers is also available as a predictor of efficacy for anti-HER2 therapies (46). IHC detects HER2 protein overexpression using monoclonal or polyclonal antibodies that bind to the protein. Currently in the United States, there are two FDA-approved methods for HER2 assessment: HerceptTest™ (Dako) and HER2/neu (4B5) rabbit monoclonal primary antibody (Ventana).

BRAF

The *BRAF* oncogene is located on the long arm of chromosome 7 at position 34. It encodes a serine/threonine kinase that is part of the RAS/MAPK signaling pathway, a key molecular cascade that regulates important cellular functions such as proliferation, differentiation, migration, and apoptosis (47). Mutations in *BRAF* are more commonly seen in melanoma (50%–70%) than in lung cancer (1%–4%) (48,49). In contrast to melanoma, in which the majority of *BRAF* mutations occur at V600 in exon 15 of the kinase domain, *BRAF* mutations in lung cancer occur at other positions in exons 11 and 15 of the kinase domain, such as G469A and D594G, and they are mutually exclusive with *EGFR* and *KRAS* mutations (49). *BRAF* mutations in NSCLC are most frequently found in ADC and are more common in former and current smokers (49).

Clinically, BRAF inhibitors, such as vemurafenib and dabrafenib, have potent and selective activity against V600-mutant BRAF (50,51). Dabrafenib is being studied, in combination with the MAPK inhibitor trametinib, in patients with previously treated advanced NSCLC whose tumors contain the V600E mutation (50,51). Various approaches have been validated for *BRAF* V600 mutation detection, including Sanger sequencing, mismatch ligation assay, denaturing high-performance liquid chromatography, mutation-specific RT-PCR, IHC, next-generation sequencing (NGS), and mass spectrometry. Each method has its own sensitivity, specificity, cost, and response delay. Sanger sequencing is considered the reference test, but some data indicate that this method fails to efficiently detect *BRAF* mutations in many melanomas (52).

KRAS

KRAS is an oncogene located on the short arm of chromosome 12 at position 12.1. It encodes for the KRAS protein, which is involved primarily in regulating cell division as part of the RAS/MAPK pathway (53). Activating *KRAS* point mutations have been detected in 15% to 25% of patients with lung ADC. *KRAS* mutations are extremely uncommon in lung SqCC and SCLC (54). Mutations in *KRAS* have important cell-type-specific effects on carcinogenesis (55). The mutations found most frequently in *KRAS* are located at positions 12 and 13 in exon 1, and less frequently in codons 61, 63, 117, 119, and 146 (56). *KRAS* mutations are strongly associated with tumors in former and current smokers (57). However, they are rare in never-smokers and less common in East Asian than American and European patients (58). *KRAS* mutation is one of the most important predictors of resistance to EGFR-TKIs in patients with NSCLC (54). Molecular analysis has revealed that patients with activating *KRAS* mutations in codons 12, 13, or 61 do not derive benefit from EGFR-TKI therapy and had a 96% chance of disease progression (59,60). The current assays for *KRAS* genotyping include nucleic acid sequencing, allele-specific PCR methods, single-strand conformational polymorphism analysis, and probe hybridization (61).

BIOMARKERS FOR IMMUNOTHERAPY

Advances in cancer immunotherapy have generated excitement across all fields of oncology, including lung cancer. The challenges to discovering predictive biomarkers for cancer immunotherapy are significant and include the wide variety of cell types involved, multiple mechanisms of T-cell regulation, and genetic heterogeneity of tumors. Recent studies of novel agents, particularly immune checkpoint inhibitors, have shown promising results in achieving meaningful and durable treatment responses with manageable toxicity (62). New IHC markers for immune checkpoint proteins, such as programmed death-ligand 1 (PD-L1), PD-L2, OX-40, indoleamine 2,3-dioxygenase (IDO1), VISTA, and B7-H3, are being added to the pathologic analysis of NSCLC (63).

Immune checkpoints modulate the immune response to effectively balance self-tolerance and tissue destruction. Many tumors express immune checkpoints or their ligands to inhibit antitumor immune responses. One of the most important immune checkpoints is PD-L1, which is expressed in at least one-quarter of patients with NSCLC (64). Several monoclonal antibodies have been developed to block either PD-1 or PD-L1. Two PD-1 inhibitors, nivolumab and pembrolizumab, are now FDA-approved for the second-line treatment of NSCLC (65). With respect to PD-L1 inhibitors, BMS-936559, MPDL3280A, and Durvalumab are currently being evaluated in clinical trials in patients with NSCLC (63). Although several studies have demonstrated a correlation between PD-L1 expression in NSCLC cells and clinical responses to anti-PD-1 and anti-PD-L1 antibodies (65,66), some patients with tumors negative for PD-L1 expression have had a good response to immune checkpoint therapy. Recently, investigators showed that across several cancer types, including NSCLC, patients with tumors expressing PD-L1 at high levels in both malignant cells and tumor-associated immune cells (TAICs) had responses to anti-PD-L1 therapy (66). Taken together, these findings suggest that factors other than PD-L1 in the tumor microenvironment, including tumor-infiltrating lymphocytes (TILs) and tumor-associated macrophages (TAMs) (67,68), may drive responses to anti-PD-1 and anti-PD-L1 therapies.

The presence or absence of TILs and PD-L1 has promoted a new tumor stratification system based on the tumor microenvironment (68). This stratification classifies tumors into four categories: type I or adaptive immune resistance (TIL+/PD-L1+), type II or immunologic ignorance (TIL–/PD-L1–), type III or immunologic tolerance (TIL+/PD-L1–), and type IV or intrinsic induction (TIL–/PD-L1+) (68). The clinical validation of such a tumor stratification scheme for immunotherapy will encourage pathologists to incorporate new tools, such as multispectral immunofluorescence analysis of immunologic markers, into clinical practice.

MOLECULAR DIAGNOSTIC ASSAYS

The earliest approaches to molecular diagnostics in lung cancer were characterized by the use of a combination of assays, such as IHC, Sanger sequencing, RT-PCR, and FISH, that each interrogated genomic changes in a specific gene. These assays have led to a better understanding of disease pathogenesis and the development of personalized medicine in lung cancer. Newer methods, including multiplex hot spot mutational testing and NGS, have the capability of providing broader molecular profiling to define the full genomic context of an individual tumor.

Immunohistochemistry

Numerous studies have examined the use of specific antibodies for IHC detection of known driver oncogenes. IHC provides a rapid assessment of ALK or ROS1 protein expression as an initial screening method before FISH testing (Figure 3.5) (31). These antibodies are designed to detect wild-type ALK or ROS1 proteins based on the concept that the majority of tumors harboring recurrent rearrangements involving *ALK* or *ROS1* will have elevated levels of expression of the corresponding protein. Several ALK and ROS1 IHC antibodies have demonstrated good sensitivity and specificity when compared to FISH (69,70). In contrast, screening for *RET* fusions with IHC has not been successful.

Sanger Sequencing

Direct DNA sequencing after PCR-based amplification was one of the first methods used to detect mutations in lung cancer, such as those involving *KRAS* and *EGFR*. The procedure involves a single-stranded DNA template and DNA extension, via DNA polymerase, from a bound primer using standard deoxynucleotides. DNA fragments are then exposed to capillary electrophoresis and fluorochromes are used for automated sequence analysis (71). This method was previously used extensively in clinical pathology, but has now been replaced by multiplex or high-throughput assays such as reverse transcription polymerase change reaction, fluorescence in situ hybridization, multiplex hot spot mutational testing, and next-generation sequencing.

Reverse Transcription Polymerase Chain Reaction

The RT-PCR method is used for the detection of gene fusions in RNA extracted from a patient's tumor (31). Gene expression is detected via the creation of complementary DNA (cDNA) transcripts from mRNA and the amplification of cDNA is measured quantitatively with the use of fluorescent probes (72). Quantitative RT-PCR is considered the gold standard for measuring the number of copies of specific cDNA targets. The extensive use of this technique has resulted in the development of various protocols that enable the generation of quantitative data using fresh, frozen, or archived paraffin samples from whole-tissue biopsies, microdissected samples, single cells, or tissue-cultured cells (73). The advantages of this

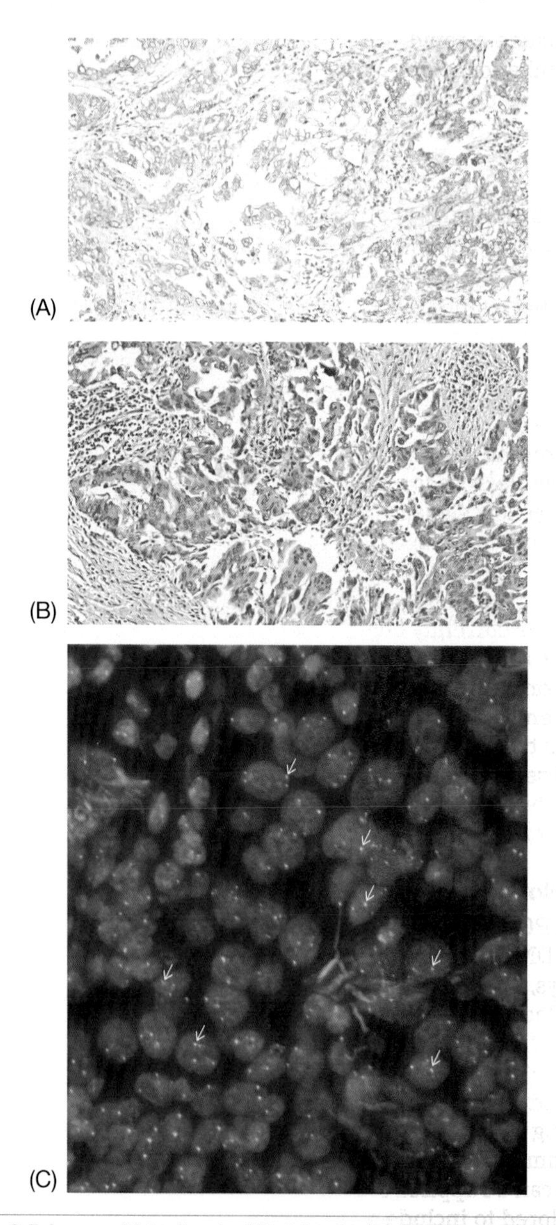

Figure 3.5 **Immunohistochemical Staining for ROS1 (A) and ALK (B) Protein Expression in Lung Adenocarcinoma. FISH Analysis of *ALK* Rearrangement in Lung Adenocarcinoma—Positive FISH Break Apart Test Is Shown With Split Red and Green Signals (Arrows) Denoting the Presence of an *ALK* Rearrangement. IHC, Immunohistochemistry x200, FISH x400**

method include a rapid processing time and the requirement for a small number of cells. However, RT-PCR is specific for particular fusion gene pairings and will not detect alternate partners. Other limitations include the high level of technical skill required to perform the assay and the need for high-quality RNA (74).

Fluorescence In Situ Hybridization

FISH is the most commonly used assay in the clinic for the detection of gene fusions in lung cancer. As mentioned earlier, FISH is the traditional method for the detection of *ALK* fusions (18), leading to the accelerated approval of crizotinib by the FDA with a companion FISH diagnostic assay. The FISH assay for *ALK* involves the use of break-apart probes, labeling the fusion breakpoint with an orange fluorochrome on the 3′ (telomeric) end and a green fluorochrome on the 5′ (centromeric) end. In the nonrearranged state, these probes lie close to each other on the chromosome and appear as a fused yellow signal. In contrast, the presence of a gene rearrangement, chromosomal inversion, or translocation results in split orange and green signals (Figure 3.5) (75). FISH detection of *ROS1* and *RET* fusions is similar to that of *ALK*, and assay validation for these genes is currently ongoing (27, 76).

For *MET* amplification, probes are designed against *MET* (red), which lies on chromosome 7, and the centromere of chromosome 7 (*CEP7*; green) (77). Normal tissues will have an average of two *MET* signals and two control-probe or *CEP7* signals, while MET amplification will result in multiple *MET* signals. FISH assays require significant technical skill for both the performance and interpretation of the assay, as well as expertise in preparing and storing tissues.

Multiplex Hot Spot Mutational Testing

Multiplex PCR is the simultaneous amplification of two or more DNA or cDNA targets in a single reaction container. Multiplex PCR assays, such as the FDA-approved Cobas® *EGFR* Mutation Test v2 (Roche), are capable of identifying 42 mutations across exons 18, 19, 20, and 21 of the *EGFR* gene. The SNaPshot™ assay (Applied Biosystems) can detect at least 50 mutation sites in up to 14 individual cancer genes, and the Sequenom assay is capable of detecting 238 or more somatic mutations across 19 different genes commonly associated with cancer (78). All of these testing platforms can be applied to DNA extracted from FFPE tissues and can be tailored to include a panel specific for each cancer type.

Next-Generation Sequencing

NGS is arguably one of the most significant technologic advances in the biologic sciences in the last 30 years. It refers to an assessment of the genome at different levels of alteration, including targeted-exome, whole-exome (WES), and whole-genome (WGS) sequencing, as well as whole-transcriptome (RNA sequencing) and whole-epigenome analyses (79). NGS methods have already been proven to be valuable in the clinic, helping physicians make difficult diagnoses by providing a comprehensive view of their patients' genetic profiles. WGS and WES provide a broader scope by sequencing either the complete genome of a sample or all of the protein-coding genes (exome), respectively (80). Different NGS platforms use various technologies to sequence millions of small fragments of DNA in parallel. Bioinformatic analyses are then used to piece together these fragments by mapping the individual reads to the human reference genome. Each of the

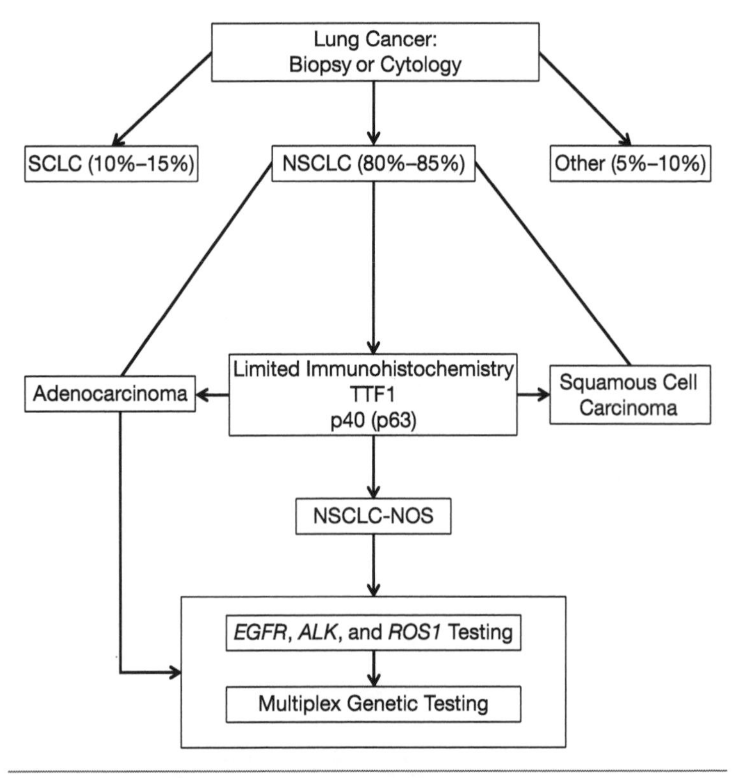

Figure 3.6 Algorithm for Histologic Subtyping and Molecular Testing of Lung Cancer. Adenocarcinoma (TTF1 Positive) and NSCLC-NOS (IHC Negative) Should Be Tested for *EGFR* Mutation, and *ALK* and *ROS1* Rearrangements. If These Tests Are Negative, Tumor Could Be Tested With a Larger Panel of Genetic Abnormalities

NSCLC-NOS, non–small-cell lung carcinoma—not otherwise specified; SCLC, small cell lung carcinoma; TTF1, thyroid transcription factor.

3 billion bases in the human genome is sequenced multiple times, providing high-quality, accurate data and insight into unexpected DNA findings (80). For multiplex platforms and NGS, the genomic alterations that are evaluated can often be customized based on histology and clinical needs.

Histologic and Molecular Diagnostic Workflow for NSCLC

As we have described, several types of molecular testing for NSCLC are currently available. The histologic and cytologic samples available for molecular testing in patients with advanced, metastatic NSCLC are frequently small specimens, including core needle biopsies and fine needle aspirates, which may limit molecular and genomic analysis. The role of the pathologist in this process is becoming increasingly important. The pathologist must adequately integrate routine histopathologic assessment and molecular testing into the clinical pathology lab to allow for accurate tumor diagnosis and subsequent selection of the most appropriate therapy. Use of a workflow algorithm for specimen management can help to incorporate accurate and timely results into clinical management (Figure 3.6).

KEY POINTS

- The participation of the pathologist in assessing tumor architecture, cytology, and specimen quality is important for the selection of appropriate molecular diagnostic testing.
- The pathologist needs to be involved in the interpretation and analysis of molecular diagnostic tests.
- *EGFR* mutation, *ALK* rearrangement, and *ROS1* rearrangement are the best-characterized molecular alterations in NSCLC and serve as targets for FDA-approved therapy. All patients with lung ADC or tumors with an ADC component need to be tested for these genomic alterations.
- Small tumor samples, such as those obtained via core needle biopsy or fine needle aspiration should be considered for testing.
- An important consideration with respect to the future of molecular testing in lung cancer is the growing number of therapeutic targets, such as *RET* rearrangements, *MET* amplification or mutation, and immune checkpoints.
- Testing algorithms are important to enhance the efficiency of molecular diagnostic testing and to optimize results from small samples.

REFERENCES

1. Langer CJ, Besse B, Gualberto A, et al. The evolving role of histology in the management of advanced non-small-cell lung cancer. *J Clin Oncol*. 2010;28:5311-5320.
2. Dela Cruz CS, Tanoue LT, Matthay RA. Lung cancer: epidemiology, etiology, and prevention. *Clinics Chest Med*. 2011;32:605-644.
3. Travis WD, Brambilla E, Noguchi M, et al. Diagnosis of lung adenocarcinoma in resected specimens: implications of the 2011 International Association for the Study of Lung Cancer/American Thoracic Society/European Respiratory Society classification. *Arch Pathol Lab Med*. 2013;137:685-705.
4. Travis WD, Brambilla E, Riely GJ. New pathologic classification of lung cancer: relevance for clinical practice and clinical trials. *J Clin Oncol*. 2013;31:992-1001.
5. Fujimoto J, Wistuba II. Current concepts on the molecular pathology of non-small cell lung carcinoma. *Semin Diagn Pathol*. 2014;31:306-313.
6. Travis WD, Brambilla E, Noguchi M, et al. International Association for the Study of Lung Cancer/American Thoracic Society/European Respiratory Society international multidisciplinary classification of lung adenocarcinoma. *J Thorac Oncol*. 2011;6:244-285.
7. Travis WD, Bambrilla E, Burke AP, et al., eds. *WHO Classification of Tumours of the Lung, Pleura, Thymus and Heart* (IARC WHO Classification of Tumours). 4th ed. Geneva, Switzerland: World Health Organization; 2015.
8. Travis WD. Update on small cell carcinoma and its differentiation from squamous cell carcinoma and other non-small cell carcinomas. *Mod Pathol*. 2012;25(suppl 1):S18-S30.
9. Shah PL, Singh S, Bower M, et al. The role of transbronchial fine needle aspiration in an integrated care pathway for the assessment of patients with suspected lung cancer. *J Thorac Oncol*. 2006;1:324-327.
10. Voldborg BR, Damstrup L, Spang-Thomsen M, et al. Epidermal growth factor receptor (EGFR) and EGFR mutations, function and possible role in clinical trials. *Ann Oncol*. 1997;8:1197-1206.
11. Pao W, Miller V, Zakowski M, et al. EGF receptor gene mutations are common in lung cancers from "never smokers" and are associated with sensitivity of tumors to gefitinib and erlotinib. *Proc Natl Acad Sci USA*. 2004;101:13306-13311.
12. Shigematsu H, Lin L, Takahashi T, et al. Clinical and biological features associated with epidermal growth factor receptor gene mutations in lung cancers. *J Natl Cancer Inst*. 2005;97:339-346.
13. Yasuda H, Park E, Yun CH, et al. Structural, biochemical, and clinical characterization of epidermal growth factor receptor (EGFR) exon 20 insertion mutations in lung cancer. *Science Translat Med*. 2013;5:216ra177.
14. Paez JG, Jänne PA, Lee JC, et al. EGFR mutations in lung cancer: correlation with clinical response to gefitinib therapy. *Science*. 2004;304:1497-1500.

15. Lindeman NI, Cagle PT, Beasley MB, et al. Molecular testing guideline for selection of lung cancer patients for EGFR and ALK tyrosine kinase inhibitors: guideline from the College of American Pathologists, International Association for the Study of Lung Cancer, and Association for Molecular Pathology. *Arch Pathol Lab Med.* 2013;137:828-860.
16. Lynch TJ, Bell DW, Sordella R, et al. Activating mutations in the epidermal growth factor receptor underlying responsiveness of non-small-cell lung cancer to gefitinib. *N Engl J Med.* 2004;350:2129-2139.
17. Roskoski R Jr. Anaplastic lymphoma kinase (ALK): structure, oncogenic activation, and pharmacological inhibition. *Pharmacol Res.* 2013;68:68-94.
18. Kwak EL, Bang YJ, Camidge DR, et al. Anaplastic lymphoma kinase inhibition in non-small-cell lung cancer. *N Engl J Med.* 2010;363:1693-1703.
19. Wong DW, Leung EL, So KK, et al; University of Hong Kong Lung Cancer Study Group. The EML4-ALK fusion gene is involved in various histologic types of lung cancers from non-smokers with wild-type EGFR and KRAS. *Cancer.* 2009;115: 1723-1733.
20. Soda M, Choi YL, Enomoto M, et al. Identification of the transforming EML4-ALK fusion gene in non-small-cell lung cancer. *Nature.* 2007;448:561-566.
21. Shaw AT, Yeap BY, Mino-Kenudson M, et al. Clinical features and outcome of patients with non-small-cell lung cancer who harbor EML4-ALK. *J Clin Oncol.* 2009;27:4247-4253.
22. Mano H. Non-solid oncogenes in solid tumors: EML4-ALK fusion genes in lung cancer. *Cancer Sci.* 2008;99:2349-2355.
23. Rikova K, Guo A, Zeng Q, et al. Global survey of phosphotyrosine signaling identifies oncogenic kinases in lung cancer. *Cell.* 2007;131:1190-1203.
24. Solomon BJ, Mok T, Kim DW, et al. PROFILE 1014 Investigators. First-line crizotinib versus chemotherapy in ALK-positive lung cancer. *N Engl J Med.* 2014;371:2167-2177.
25. Kogita A, Togashi Y, Hayashi H, et al. Activated MET acts as a salvage signal after treatment with alectinib, a selective ALK inhibitor, in ALK-positive non-small cell lung cancer. *Int J Oncol.* 2015;46:1025-1030.
26. Thunnissen E, Bubendorf L, Dietel M, et al. EML4-ALK testing in non-small cell carcinomas of the lung: a review with recommendations. *Virchows Arch.* 2012;461:245-257.
27. Bergethon K, Shaw AT, Ou SH, et al. ROS1 rearrangements define a unique molecular class of lung cancers. *J Clin Oncol.* 2012;30:863-870.
28. Takeuchi K, Soda M, Togashi Y, et al. RET, ROS1 and ALK fusions in lung cancer. *Nat Med.* 2012;18:378-381.
29. Knowles PP, Murray-Rust J, Kjaer S, et al. Structure and chemical inhibition of the RET tyrosine kinase domain. *J Biol Chem.* 2006;281:33577-33587.

30. Ju YS, Lee WC, Shin JY, et al. A transforming KIF5B and RET gene fusion in lung adenocarcinoma revealed from whole-genome and transcriptome sequencing. *Genome Res*. 2012;22:436-445.
31. Wang R, Hu H, Pan Y, et al. RET fusions define a unique molecular and clinicopathologic subtype of non-small-cell lung cancer. *J Clin Oncol*. 2012;30:4352-4359.
32. Kohno T, Ichikawa H, Totoki Y, et al. KIF5B-RET fusions in lung adenocarcinoma. *Nat Med*. 2012;18:375-377.
33. Drilon A, Wang L, Hasanovic A, et al. Response to Cabozantinib in patients with RET fusion-positive lung adenocarcinomas. *Cancer Discov*. 2013;3:630-635.
34. Lee SE, Lee B, Hong M, et al. Comprehensive analysis of RET and ROS1 rearrangement in lung adenocarcinoma. *Mod Pathol*. 2015;28:468-479.
35. Trusolino L, Bertotti A, Comoglio PM. MET signalling: principles and functions in development, organ regeneration and cancer. *Nat Rev Mol Cell Biol*. 2010;11:834-848.
36. Kong-Beltran M, Seshagiri S, Zha J, et al. Somatic mutations lead to an oncogenic deletion of met in lung cancer. *Cancer Res*. 2006;66:283-289.
37. Kong-Beltran M, Stamos J, Wickramasinghe D. The Sema domain of Met is necessary for receptor dimerization and activation. *Cancer Cell*. 2004;6:75-84.
38. Benedettini E, Sholl LM, Peyton M, et al. Met activation in non-small cell lung cancer is associated with de novo resistance to EGFR inhibitors and the development of brain metastasis. *Am J Pathol*. 2010;177:415-423.
39. Beau-Faller M, Ruppert AM, Voegeli AC, et al. MET gene copy number in non-small cell lung cancer: molecular analysis in a targeted tyrosine kinase inhibitor naïve cohort. *J Thorac Oncol*. 2008;3:331-339.
40. Frampton GM, Ali SM, Rosenzweig M, et al. Activation of MET via diverse exon 14 splicing alterations occurs in multiple tumor types and confers clinical sensitivity to MET inhibitors. *Cancer Discov*. 2015;5:850-859.
41. Popescu NC, King CR, Kraus MH. Localization of the human erbB-2 gene on normal and rearranged chromosomes 17 to bands q12-21.32. *Genomics*. 1989;4:362-366.
42. Buttitta F, Barassi F, Fresu G, et al. Mutational analysis of the HER2 gene in lung tumors from Caucasian patients: mutations are mainly present in adenocarcinomas with bronchioloalveolar features. *Int J Cancer*. 2006;119:2586-2591.
43. Shigematsu H, Takahashi T, Nomura M, et al. Somatic mutations of the HER2 kinase domain in lung adenocarcinomas. *Cancer Res*. 2005;65:1642-1646.
44. Li C, Hao L, Li Y, et al. Prognostic value analysis of mutational and clinicopathological factors in non-small cell lung cancer. *PLOS ONE*. 2014;9:e107276.
45. Wang SE, Narasanna A, Perez-Torres M, et al. HER2 kinase domain mutation results in constitutive phosphorylation and activation of

HER2 and EGFR and resistance to EGFR tyrosine kinase inhibitors. *Cancer Cell*. 2006;10:25-38.

46. Shi Y, Huang W, Tan Y, et al. A novel proximity assay for the detection of proteins and protein complexes: quantitation of HER1 and HER2 total protein expression and homodimerization in formalin-fixed, paraffin-embedded cell lines and breast cancer tissue. *Diagn Mol Pathol*. 2009;18:11-21.
47. Wan PT, Garnett MJ, Roe SM, et al; Cancer Genome Project. Mechanism of activation of the RAF-ERK signaling pathway by oncogenic mutations of B-RAF. *Cell*. 2004;116:855-867.
48. Cardarella S, Ogino A, Nishino M, et al. Clinical, pathologic, and biologic features associated with BRAF mutations in non-small cell lung cancer. *Clin Cancer Res*. 2013;19:4532-4540.
49. Paik PK, Arcila ME, Fara M, et al. Clinical characteristics of patients with lung adenocarcinomas harboring BRAF mutations. *J Clin Oncol*. 2011;29:2046-2051.
50. Gautschi O, Pauli C, Strobel K, et al. A patient with BRAF V600E lung adenocarcinoma responding to vemurafenib. *J Thorac Oncol*. 2012;7:e23-e24.
51. Falchook GS, Long GV, Kurzrock R, et al. Dabrafenib in patients with melanoma, untreated brain metastases, and other solid tumours: a phase 1 dose-escalation trial. *Lancet*. 2012;379:1893-1901.
52. Halait H, Demartin K, Shah S, et al. Analytical performance of a real-time PCR-based assay for V600 mutations in the BRAF gene, used as the companion diagnostic test for the novel BRAF inhibitor vemurafenib in metastatic melanoma. *Diagn Mol Pathol*. 2012;21:1-8.
53. McBride OW, Swan DC, Tronick SR, et al. Regional chromosomal localization of N-ras, K-ras-1, K-ras-2 and myb oncogenes in human cells. *Nucleic Acids Res*. 1983;11:8221-8236.
54. Tam IY, Chung LP, Suen WS, et al. Distinct epidermal growth factor receptor and KRAS mutation patterns in non-small cell lung cancer patients with different tobacco exposure and clinicopathologic features. *Clin Cancer Res*. 2006;12:1647-1653.
55. Guerra C, Mijimolle N, Dhawahir A, et al. Tumor induction by an endogenous K-ras oncogene is highly dependent on cellular context. *Cancer Cell*. 2003;4:111-120.
56. Popescu NC, Amsbaugh SC, DiPaolo JA, et al. Chromosomal localization of three human ras genes by in situ molecular hybridization. *Somat Cell Mol Genet*. 1985;11:149-155.
57. Soung YH, Lee JW, Kim SY, et al. Mutational analysis of EGFR and K-RAS genes in lung adenocarcinomas. *Virchows Arch*. 2005;446:483-488.
58. Sun Y, Ren Y, Fang Z, et al. Lung adenocarcinoma from East Asian never-smokers is a disease largely defined by targetable oncogenic mutant kinases. *J Clin Oncol*. 2010;28:4616-4620.
59. Massarelli E, Varella-Garcia M, Tang X, et al. KRAS mutation is an important predictor of resistance to therapy with epidermal growth

factor receptor tyrosine kinase inhibitors in non-small-cell lung cancer. *Clin Cancer Res*. 2007;13:2890-2896.

60. Riely GJ, Ladanyi M. KRAS mutations: an old oncogene becomes a new predictive biomarker. *J Mol Diagn*. 2008;10:493-495.
61. Bolton L, Reiman A, Lucas K, et al. KRAS mutation analysis by PCR: a comparison of two methods. *PLOS ONE*. 2015;10:e0115672.
62. Anagnostou VK, Brahmer JR. Cancer immunotherapy: a future paradigm shift in the treatment of non-small cell lung cancer. *Clin Cancer Res*. 2015;21:976-984.
63. Creelan BC. Update on immune checkpoint inhibitors in lung cancer. *Cancer Control*. 2014;21:80-89.
64. Taube JM, Klein A, Brahmer JR, et al. Association of PD-1, PD-1 ligands, and other features of the tumor immune microenvironment with response to anti-PD-1 therapy. *Clin Cancer Res*. 2014;20:5064-5074.
65. Patnaik A, Kang SP, Rasco D, et al. Phase I study of pembrolizumab (MK-3475; anti-PD-1 monoclonal antibody) in patients with advanced solid tumors. *Clin Cancer Res*. 2015;21:4286-4293.
66. Herbst RS, Soria JC, Kowanetz M, et al. Predictive correlates of response to the anti-PD-L1 antibody MPDL3280A in cancer patients. *Nature*. 2014;515:563-567.
67. Berghoff AS, Ricken G, Widhalm G, et al. PD1 (CD279) and PD-L1 (CD274, B7H1) expression in primary central nervous system lymphomas (PCNSL). *Clin Neuropathol*. 2014;33:42-49.
68. Teng MW, Ngiow SF, Ribas A, et al. Classifying cancers based on T-cell infiltration and PD-L1. *Cancer Res*. 2015;75:2139-2145.
69. Sholl LM, Sun H, Butaney M, et al. ROS1 immunohistochemistry for detection of ROS1-rearranged lung adenocarcinomas. *Am J Surg Pathol*. 2013;37:1441-1449.
70. Wang J, Cai Y, Dong Y, et al. Clinical characteristics and outcomes of patients with primary lung adenocarcinoma harboring ALK rearrangements detected by FISH, IHC, and RT-PCR. *PLOS ONE*. 2014;9:e101551.
71. Sanger F, Coulson AR. A rapid method for determining sequences in DNA by primed synthesis with DNA polymerase. *J Mol Biol*. 1975;94:441-448.
72. Bustin SA. Absolute quantification of mRNA using real-time reverse transcription polymerase chain reaction assays. *J Mol Endocrinol*. 2000;25:169-193.
73. Jozefczuk J, Adjaye J. Quantitative real-time PCR-based analysis of gene expression. *Methods Enzymol*. 2011;500:99-109.
74. Murakami Y, Mitsudomi T, Yatabe Y. A screening method for the ALK fusion gene in NSCLC. *Front Oncol*. 2012;2:24.
75. Camidge DR, Kono SA, Flacco A, et al. Optimizing the detection of lung cancer patients harboring anaplastic lymphoma kinase (ALK) gene rearrangements potentially suitable for ALK inhibitor treatment. *Clin Cancer Res*. 2010;16:5581-5590.

76. Go H, Jung YJ, Kang HW, et al. Diagnostic method for the detection of KIF5B-RET transformation in lung adenocarcinoma. *Lung Cancer*. 2013;82:44-50.
77. Go H, Jeon YK, Park HJ, et al. High MET gene copy number leads to shorter survival in patients with non-small cell lung cancer. *J Thorac Oncol*. 2010;5:305-313.
78. Sequist LV, Heist RS, Shaw AT, et al. Implementing multiplexed genotyping of non-small-cell lung cancers into routine clinical practice. *Ann Oncol*. 2011;22:2616-2624.
79. Cardarella S, Johnson BE. The impact of genomic changes on treatment of lung cancer. *Am J Respir Crit Care Med*. 2013;188:770-775.
80. Buermans HP, den Dunnen JT. Next generation sequencing technology: advances and applications. *Biochim Biophys Acta*. 2014; 1842:1932-1941.

4 Lung Cancer Screening

Steven E. Lommatzsch and James Jett

INTRODUCTION

Lung cancer is the leading cause of cancer-related death in the United States (1). The association between tobacco use and lung cancer has been reported since the 1950s, and smoking cessation is the key intervention for preventing lung cancer (2). However, tobacco cessation is difficult to achieve, with only 20% to 30% of smokers who attempt to quit remaining tobacco free for at least 2 years (3). The wide use of tobacco is the main reason that lung cancer continues to burden society. At the time of diagnosis, the majority of patients with lung cancer have stage III or IV disease, and over half have distant metastases (4). Since most early stage lung tumors are asymptomatic, only 15% of lung cancers are localized at the time of detection (1). Due to the high frequency of late stage at diagnosis, the 5-year survival rate for lung cancer is only 16%, with little recent improvement (5). The high prevalence and mortality of lung cancer highlights the great impact that successful screening could have on this disease.

Cancer Screening Bias

Lead-time bias and overdiagnosis present potential problems for lung cancer screening. Lead-time bias occurs when screening detects a cancer earlier, but does not alter time of death. In other words, screening improves survival time from diagnosis to death, but does not change the mortality (the number of people dying of the disease). Overdiagnosis refers to the diagnosis of a slow-growing cancer that would be unlikely to progress in a clinically relevant way and would not have impacted on the patient's longevity. Thus, these cancers would not have presented as disease if it were not for the screening test. Overdiagnosis is a particular concern when a screening test leads to invasive diagnostic testing or therapy, since potential complications from these procedures may cause more harm than good.

Conflict of interest: Dr. Jett has a research grant paid to National Jewish Health from Oncimmune, Inc. (Biomarker).

CHEST RADIOGRAPHY FOR LUNG CANCER SCREENING

Early Studies

In the early 1980s, several clinical trials evaluating chest radiography (chest x-ray) and sputum cytology for lung cancer screening reported no reduction in lung cancer mortality (6). The Mayo Lung Project was one of the largest early trials to study lung cancer screening. From 1971 to 1983, this study enrolled 9,211 men 45 years of age or older who were smoking more than a pack of cigarettes per day. Participants were randomized into two groups: (a) those undergoing chest radiography and sputum cytology every 4 months for 6 years, or (b) those getting standard of care, which included annual chest radiography. Despite a higher rate of detection of lung cancer, lower stage at diagnosis, and greater candidacy for surgical resection in the intervention group, there was no difference in all-cause or lung cancer-specific mortality between the two groups (7). The detection of lower stage cancers and an improvement in survival time from diagnosis to death without impacting mortality demonstrated lead-time bias in this study. Long-term follow-up reported that the higher prevalence of lung cancer in the intervention group (585 vs. 500 lung cancers) persisted long after completion of the screening period, suggesting overdiagnosis (8).

The Prostate, Lung, Colorectal, and Ovarian Trial

The prostate, lung, colorectal, and ovarian (PLCO) trial, published in 2011, gave further support to prior studies demonstrating a lack of utility of chest radiography as a lung cancer screening tool (9). The PLCO study enrolled 154,901 subjects between the ages of 55 and 74 years with the goal of determining the impact of screening for prostate, lung, colorectal, and ovarian cancer on mortality. The selection criteria did not include a history of smoking. Subjects in the control arm underwent imaging only if the treating physician felt it was indicated, while those in the intervention arm underwent screening with a chest radiograph annually for 4 years. All subjects remained in follow-up for 13 years. At the end of the study period, there were no differences between the arms in lung cancer detection rate, clinical stage at time of diagnosis, or mortality. The lack of mortality benefit was also noted in high-risk subjects with a smoking history of at least 30 pack-years, either current smokers or those who had quit within the past 15 years. Thus, this study confirms that chest radiography is not an effective method for lung cancer screening in the general population.

COMPUTED TOMOGRAPHY (CT) FOR LUNG CANCER SCREENING

Early Studies

The negative results of studies of chest radiography led to the evaluation of CT for lung cancer screening. Helical, multidetector row CT scanners have much greater sensitivity than standard chest radiographs for lung abnormalities, but repeated imaging results in exposure to larger amounts of radiation. The advent of low-dose CT (LDCT) lessened this concern due to the use of much lower doses of radiation than standard chest CT scans (<2 mSv vs. 7 mSv).

In 2005, the Mayo Clinic published a 5-year prospective study using annual LDCT as a screening tool in high-risk patients (10). Each of the 1,520 participants had at least a 20 pack-year smoking history and had been smoking within the past 10 years. Data from the earlier Mayo Lung Project with chest radiography was used as the control arm for comparison to LDCT. Sixty-eight lung cancers were diagnosed, 31 on the initial LDCT screen, 34 on subsequent screens, and three in the screening interval. Compared to historical controls using chest radiography, more of the lung cancers found on incidence LDCT were stage IA (47% vs. 21%) and fewer were stage III/IV (33% vs. 45%). In addition, among the lung cancers detected on subsequent screens, 61% were stage I tumors (10). Overall, the rate of early-stage cancer detected by LDCT screening was significantly higher than the 15% early-stage detection rate noted in current practice (1), suggesting a favorable stage shift with LDCT screening.

The Early Lung Cancer Action Program (ELCAP) was a larger analysis of 31,567 subjects who underwent annual LDCT screening (11). Once again, screen-detected lung cancers were mostly stage I (85%), but the lack of a control arm undermined the ability to detect any improvement in mortality (11). One early effort at randomization was the Detection and Screening of Early Lung Cancer by Novel Imaging Technology and Molecular Assays (DANTE) trial. The DANTE study enrolled 2,450 men from 60 to 74 years old with at least a 20 pack-year smoking history who were randomized to either annual CT screening or no screening. Long-term follow-up data from this study showed that lung cancer-specific mortality was similar in both arms (LDCT, 543 per 100,000 person-years vs. control, 544 per 100,000 person-years) (12). Although the DANTE study was limited by its small sample size and unisex enrollment, LDCT did not appear to improve lung cancer-specific or all-cause mortality.

The National Lung Screening Trial (NLST)

The randomized National Lung Screening Trial (NLST) enrolled 53,454 men and women between 55 and 75 years of age with at least a 30 pack-year smoking history and use of tobacco within the last 15 years at 33 centers in the United States. Participants were randomized to undergo either LDCT or standard chest radiography annually for 3 years. A positive finding was defined as any noncalcified nodule ≥4 mm in longest dimension on axial CT images or any noncalcified density on chest radiography. More subjects had positive findings by LDCT than chest radiography (24.2% vs. 6.9%), but the majority of nodules in both groups were benign: 96.4% with LDCT vs. 94.5% with chest radiography (13). Despite the large number of benign nodules, the malignancy detection rate was higher with LDCT than with chest radiography. During the 3-year screening period, LDCT detected 649 lung cancers as compared to 279 with chest radiography. This trend continued through the follow-up period (median follow-up of 6.5 years) with 1,060 lung cancers diagnosed in the LDCT arm and 941 in the chest radiography arm, suggesting potential overdiagnosis during the LDCT screening period. There was also a notable stage shift between the two arms. In the LDCT arm, 40% of the cancers detected were stage IA and 22% were stage IV as compared to 21% stage IA and 36% stage IV in the chest radiography arm (13).

For the first time, the NLST revealed a significantly lower lung cancer-specific mortality rate with LDCT screening with a relative risk reduction of 20.3% compared to chest radiography (247 deaths per 100,000 person-years vs. 309 deaths per 100,000 person-years) (13). In other words, 320 individuals need to be screened to prevent one death from lung cancer. All-cause mortality was also significantly lower in the LDCT arm (6.7% risk reduction; 95% CI, 1.2 to 13.6; $P = .02$) (13). It should be noted that the NLST did not dictate a standardized diagnostic algorithm for subjects with positive screening results. Recommendations on further diagnostic evaluation or timing of follow-up scans were provided to subjects and their referring health care providers based on the specific findings of screening studies. Despite this lack of uniformity in the subsequent evaluation of abnormal findings, both the use of invasive procedures in patients with ultimately benign lesions and the complication rate from such interventions were very low.

Despite the clear mortality benefit demonstrated in the NLST, the use of LDCT as a screening tool continues to be debated due to the high false-positive rate and unclear cost-effectiveness. There is also concern about the potential for overdiagnosis with LDCT screening. Adenocarcinoma was the most commonly detected histologic subtype of lung cancer diagnosed, with bronchioloalveolar carcinoma (BAC; adenocarcinoma in situ, [AIS]) being found much more commonly with LDCT than with chest radiography (14.7% vs. 4.7%) (13). Since BAC/AIS is a slow growing, noninvasive tumor, there is concern that its diagnosis would not impact on mortality, but could lead to potential harm due to unnecessary interventions (14).

On-Going Studies

The Dutch-Belgian Randomized Lung Cancer Screening Trial (NELSON) is a randomized, controlled trial comparing LDCT screening to no screening in high-risk participants between 50 and 75 years of age (15). It differs from the NLST trial in two major ways: (a) high-risk tobacco exposure is defined as a smoking history of at least 15 cigarettes per day for 25 years or at least 10 cigarettes per day for 30 years, and former smokers must have quit less than 10 years ago; and (b) radiologic criteria for a positive scan include volumetric nodule changes over time with the goal being to reduce subsequent imaging and invasive diagnostic testing. The NELSON trial is powered to detect a 25% decrease in lung cancer-specific mortality after 10 years. Since 2003, 15,822 subjects have been randomized. Preliminary results from 7,155 subjects screened with LDCT found 196 screen-detected cancers in 187 subjects, for a sensitivity of 84.6%, and specificity of 98.6% (15). Of lung cancers detected with LDCT, 64% were stage I, a finding that is similar to that reported in the NLST (16). Several other randomized trials of LDCT screening for lung cancer are on-going, including the United Kingdom Lung Cancer Screening Trial (UKLS), the Multicentric Italian Lung Detection Trial (MILD), the Italian Lung Cancer CT Screening Trial (ITALUNG), and the German Lung Cancer Screening Intervention Study (LUSI).

CT Screening Recommendations

The U.S. Preventive Services Task Force (USPSTF) published a statement on the utility of LDCT lung cancer screening in 2013 that was based on the results of the NLST and on mathematical modeling. The USPSTF recommended "annual screening for lung cancer with low-dose CT in adults aged 55 to 80 years who have a 30 pack-year smoking history and currently smoke or have quit within the past 15 years" (17). The overall strength of this recommendation was "Grade B," meaning that the data created a high certainty of at least a moderate net benefit or a moderate degree of certainty of a moderate to substantial net benefit.

In 2015, the U.S. Centers for Medicare and Medicaid Services (CMS) determined that Medicare would cover the cost of lung cancer screening with annual LDCT in adults from 55 to 77 years of age who have a 30 pack-year smoking history and currently smoke or have quit within the past 15 years. Medicare coverage also includes a visit with a physician or qualified nonphysician practitioner for counseling and shared decision making on the benefits and risks of lung cancer screening. Importantly, the CMS statement requires counseling on smoking cessation as part of the screening process.

CT SCREENING INTERPRATATION GUIDELINES

Since the invention of CT in 1972, advances in technology have resulted in the development of helical and multidetector row CT scanners that decrease scan time and low-dose scanners that still provide high-resolution images. Both of these developments were essential for the progress of lung cancer screening since they allow faster, more convenient imaging with high resolution and less radiation exposure (18). Another key advance in CT-based lung cancer screening is the development of a standardized system of cancer risk assessment that could guide recommendations for follow-up imaging.

The international, multidisciplinary Fleischner Society has published guidelines to evaluate CT-detected lung nodules in both high- and low-risk patients (19). The Fleischner guidelines offer a detailed, systematic approach for the evaluation of incidentally discovered, not screen-detected, pulmonary nodules. These recommendations center on several factors affecting the risk of malignancy, including size, density of attenuation, border characteristics, calcification, and growth over time (20). It should be noted, that this system was intended for data obtained from standard-dose CT, not LDCT, in a population that is not undergoing screening. For subjects undergoing annual screening with LDCT more selective guidelines are needed to avoid excessive follow-up imaging of lower-risk findings.

Lung Imaging Reporting and Data System (Lung-RADS™)

The American College of Radiology developed the Lung Imaging Reporting and Data System (Lung-RADS) to standardize pulmonary nodule reporting and management within the context of LDCT screening (www.acr.org/Quality-Safety/Resources/LungRADS). The Lung-RADS differs from Fleischner guidelines in that it assumes future screening LDCT scans will be completed on a yearly basis (Table 4.1). In the Lung-RADS system, a positive nodule is defined as ≥6 mm, as compared to ≥4 mm in the Fleischner guidelines. McKee et al. evaluated the performance of Lung-RADS in 2,180 patients by comparing institutional standard LDCT interpretation to a retrospective reevaluation of the scans

Table 4.1 American College of Radiology Lung Imaging Reporting Data System (Lung-RADS)

Category	Category descriptor	Category code	Radiologic finding	Management
Incomplete		0	Prior CT required for comparison or lungs cannot be fully examined	Additional lung cancer screening CT and/or comparison CT is needed
Negative	No nodules or definitely benign nodules	1	No lung nodule or nodule with specific benign calcifications or fat-containing nodule	Continue annual LDCT screening in 12 months
Benign appearance or behavior	Nodules with very low likelihood of becoming active cancer due to size or lack of growth	2	Solid nodule: <6 mm or new <4 mm Part solid nodule: <6 mm on baseline screening Nonsolid nodule: <20 mm or ≥20 mm and unchanged or slow growing Category 3 or 4 nodule unchanged for ≥3 months	Continue annual LDCT screening in 12 months

(*continued*)

Table 4.1 American College of Radiology Lung Imaging Reporting Data System (Lung-RADS) (*continued*)

Category	Category descriptor	Category code	Radiologic finding	Management
Probably benign	Probably benign finding—short-term follow-up recommended; includes nodules with low likelihood of becoming active cancer	3	Solid nodule: ≥6 to <8 mm at baseline or new 4 mm to <6 mm Part solid nodule: ≥6 mm with solid component <6 mm or new <6 mm Nonsolid nodule: ≥20 mm at baseline or new nodule on repeat screening	Follow-up LDCT in 6 months
Suspicious	Finding suggestive of malignancy, for which additional diagnostic testing and/or tissue sampling is recommended	4A	Solid nodule: ≥8 to <15 mm at baseline or growing <8 mm or new 6 to <8 mm Part solid nodule: ≥6 mm with solid component ≥6 to <8 mm or new/growing <4 mm solid component Endobronchial nodule	Follow-up LDCT in 3 months; consider PET/CT if ≥8 mm solid component

(*continued*)

Table 4.1 American College of Radiology Lung Imaging Reporting Data System (Lung-RADS) (*continued*)

Category	Category descriptor	Category code	Radiologic finding	Management
		4B	Solid nodule: ≥15 mm or new/growing and ≥8 mm Part solid nodule: solid component >8 mm or new/growing >4 mm solid component	Chest CT with or without contrast, PET/CT, and/or tissue sampling depending on probability of malignancy and comorbidities
		4X	Category 3 or 4 nodule with additional features that increase likelihood of malignancy	
Other	Clinically significant or potentially significant finding (nonlung cancer)	S	Modifier—add to category 0–4	As appropriate for the specific finding
Prior lung cancer	Patient with a prior lung cancer diagnosis who returns to screening	C	Modifier—add to category 0–4	

Source: Adapted from American College of Radiology: http://www.acr.org/~/media/ACR/Documents/PDF/QualitySafety/Resources/LungRADS/AssessmentCategories.pdf

using Lung-RADS (21). Overall, the positive predictive value (PPV) for malignancy was 17.3% with Lung-RADS vs. 6.9% with standard NLST guidelines. This improvement in PPV was largely due to the higher cutoff of 6 mm for defining a positive finding in the Lung-RADS leading to a decrease in false-positive scans. Pinsky et al. retrospectively applied Lung-RADS criteria to the NLST's baseline scan and found not only a reduction in the false-positive rate (12.8% for Lung-RADS vs. 26.6% for NLST interpretations), but also a decrease in sensitivity (84.9% for Lung-RADS vs. 93.5% for NLST) (22). In addition, this study reported a marked reduction in the number of subsequent CT scans required when Lung-RADS was applied, with the avoidance of an estimated 5,707 follow-up scans. Currently, Lung-RADS is recommended for use in lung cancer screening programs, but prospective studies of the performance of Lung-RADS in real-world situations are still needed.

PRESCREENING LUNG CANCER RISK ASSESSMENT

It is extremely important to select the appropriate population to consider for LDCT lung cancer screening, since the vast majority of CT-detected pulmonary nodules will be benign even in a high-risk cohort (10–13). The Pan-Canadian Early Detection of Lung Cancer Study validated this point by reporting that only 144 out of 12,029 pulmonary nodules detected on CT screening scans were malignant (23). The goal of this study was to develop an accurate model that could predict the probability that a nodule detected on LDCT screening would be malignant. The authors concluded that the ideal screening subject should have a higher probability of developing a malignant pulmonary nodule than the general population. Using such a risk prediction model to identify candidates for screening would increase the PPV of the screening test.

A good risk prediction model should have appropriate discrimination, calibration, and accuracy. With regard to lung cancer, discrimination is the ability of the model to distinguish those who died from lung cancer from those who did not. Calibration is the probability that an individual will die from cancer in a defined period of time (e.g., a 30% chance of death over the next 10 years). The closer this risk assessment is to the observed death rate, the more reliable the model. Accuracy refers to how well the risk prediction model functions, as measured by internal and external validation. Internal validation is determined in the patient cohort from which the model was derived, while external validation comes from applying the model to other cohorts.

Validated lung cancer risk assessment tools include the Tammemagi Model, the Bach Model, the Spitz Model, and the Liverpool Lung Project Model. Tammemagi et al. used the prospective data from the PLCO trial to compare a cohort of 70,962 nonsmokers to a cohort of 38,254 subjects who had a smoking history (24). The parameters included in the model were age, socioeconomic status, education, body mass index, recent chest radiography, smoking status, pack-years, and years of being tobacco free. In the validation cohort, the model demonstrated high reliability (area under the curve, 0.784) (www.brocku.ca/lung-cancer-risk-calculator).

All models evaluating lung cancer risk include length, quantity, and quit time of tobacco use. The large sample size of the NLST afforded the development of an absolute-risk prediction model for lung cancer mortality by retrospectively applying these characteristics (25). The prediction model for the LDCT arm stratifies the 5-year risk of death from lung cancer into five groups spanning low to high risk. When this risk stratification model was applied to the screened cohort, the number of false-positive results declined from 1,648 in the lowest risk group to 65 in the group having the highest risk of lung cancer-related death. Since screening of the lowest risk group prevented only 1% of lung cancer deaths, this risk-assessment model suggests that lung cancer screening may be indicated only in higher risk subjects.

Tobacco use is the strongest risk predictor for the development of lung cancer. Tanner et al. demonstrated an association between smoking and increased mortality in a subgroup analysis of the NLST cohort (26). This study found that current smokers had a higher risk of lung cancer-related death than former smokers (HR 2.14–2.29). Based on these risk-assessment models, multiple organizations have released statements on the minimum tobacco exposure required to be an optimal candidate for LDCT lung cancer screening (Table 4.2).

Table 4.2 Organizational recommendations on lung cancer screening

Organization	Recommendation	Publication date
American Cancer Society (27)	Annual LDCT screening in adults aged 55–74, who have at least a 30 pack-year smoking history and currently smoke or have quit within the past 15 years. Thorough informed consent and shared decision making should be offered prior to screening, along with smoking cessation counseling.	March 2013

(continued)

Table 4.2 Organizational recommendations on lung cancer screening (*continued*)

Organization	Recommendation	Publication date
American College of Chest Physicians/ American Society for Clinical Oncology (28)	Annual LDCT screening in adults aged 55–74, who have at least a 30 pack-year smoking history and currently smoke or have quit within the past 15 years. Screening should only be performed in settings capable of offering comprehensive care similar to that provided in the NLST trial.	May 2013
U.S. Preventative Services Task Force (29)	Annual LDCT screening in adults aged 55–80, who have at least a 30 pack-year smoking history and currently smoke or have quit within the past 15 years. Screening should be discontinued once a patient has not smoked for more than 15 years, develops a life expectancy-limiting illness, or refuses curative thoracic surgery, if indicated.	December 2013
European Respiratory Society/ European Society of Radiology (30)	Annual LDCT screening in adults aged 55–80, who have at least a 30 pack-year smoking history and currently smoke or have quit within the past 15 years. Multidisciplinary medical resources, shared decision making, and smoking cessation interventions should be offered.	April 2015

RISKS OF LUNG CANCER SCREENING

Lung cancer screening with LDCT carries multiple risks, including cumulative radiation exposure, complications from diagnostic procedures, financial cost, and anxiety from incidental findings.

Radiation Exposure

Although one LDCT scan results in only ≤2 mSv of radiation exposure as compared to 7 mSv with standard chest CT (31), there remains concern regarding the cumulative effect of serial scans. The risk of radiation-related malignancy versus the risk of death from lung cancer was evaluated in a systematic review, which concluded that the benefit of screening in higher-risk subjects outweighs the risk of cumulative radiation exposure (32).

Unnecessary Interventions

About 27% of the NLST-screened population underwent additional imaging or invasive procedures, including thoracotomy, thoracoscopy, mediastinoscopy, bronchoscopy, and needle biopsy. Within the LDCT arm, 16 participants (0.06%) died within 60 days of their procedure, and 10 of these may have died from lung cancer rather than from complications of the procedure (13). Although the rate of serious complications was already low in the NLST, defining a higher cutoff point for a positive nodule, as is being done with Lung-RADS, should lead to even fewer interventions and thus, fewer complications.

Cost

The cost of LDCT screening is a major concern given the number of additional tests that will result from its implementation. A cost-effectiveness analysis of the NLST found that LDCT screening costs an additional $1,631 per person as compared to no screening (33). The estimated life years per person gained through LDCT screening was calculated to be 0.0316, which led to a predicted value of $52,000 per life year gained. This cost is similar to that incurred by screening for breast or colorectal cancer. Another study using simulation modeling showed that the cost in a commercially insured population for LDCT lung cancer screening was actually lower than that of screening for other cancers (34). This study reported that the cost of LDCT screening was $0.76 per member per month (PMPM) as compared to $0.95, $1.10, and $2.50 for colorectal, cervical, and breast cancer screening, respectively (34).

If the screening program incorporates smoking cessation counseling, cost-effectiveness improves by 20% to 45% (34). The improved cost-effectiveness stems from an increase in the number of quality-adjusted life years (QALY) saved. The NLST data for current smokers ($n = 15{,}489$) was analyzed using longitudinal regression models to predict annual smoking cessation rates in relation to abnormalities detected on LDCT scans. There was a statistically significant association between smoking cessation and the type of abnormality detected. Specifically, a subject with a LDCT revealing a new or growing nodule concerning for cancer was at lower risk of remaining a continuing smoker (OR 0.66, 95% CI 0.61–0.72; $P < .001$) (35). Several other studies, including the NELSON trial, evaluated the effect of LDCT screening on smoking cessation. To date, there has been no consistently detected difference in cessation rates between those undergoing screening versus those in the control arm of a prospective study (36). Smoking cessation counseling is a requirement for CMS reimbursement, but clearly, more effective measures are needed to achieve higher smoking cessation rates.

Incidental Findings

Another area of concern regarding LDCT screening is the identification of abnormalities unrelated to lung cancer. The goal of the NLST was to decrease lung cancer mortality by detecting cancer at an early, curable stage. However, LDCT also identified other abnormalities, such as coronary calcifications, thoracic aortic aneurysms, and thyroid masses, with greater frequency than chest radiography (7.5% vs. 2.1%) (13). These data suggest that LDCT screening would result in more testing and referrals to address these incidental findings, increasing the total cost of care and the potential for harmful complications from added interventions.

LUNG CANCER BIOMARKERS

A biomarker is any biological substance indicating the risk, presence, or activity of a particular disease. Sources of biomarkers include breath, sputum, urine, and blood (37). A classic example of a biomarker is cholesterol for the risk assessment of coronary artery disease. The identification and validation of a biomarker for the risk assessment of lung cancer would be invaluable. Additionally, with the growing implementation of lung cancer screening, there is great interest in defining biomarkers that could distinguish lung cancer from benign pulmonary nodules.

Pepe et al. described the five phases of biomarker development (38). Very few biomarkers for the detection of lung cancer have progressed to prospective screening (phase 4), and none have demonstrated a reduction of the burden of disease (phase 5). While the list of putative lung cancer biomarkers is extensive, the most promising blood biomarkers evaluated for clinical use include micro-RNA, proteins, and autoantibodies.

Micro-RNA

Micro-RNA (miRNAs) are short noncoding RNAs that are released by tumor cells or the tumor microenvironment into the circulation and are highly stable and quantifiable in plasma or serum (39). Sozzi et al. developed a plasma-based miRNA signature classifier (MSC) consisting of 24 miRNAs, which they tested in a validation set of 69 patients with screen-detected lung cancer and 870 control subjects enrolled in the Multicenter Italian Lung Detection Trial (40). The MSC had a sensitivity and specificity for lung cancer detection of 87% and 81%, respectively, with a PPV of 27% and negative predictive value (NPV) of 99%. The LDCT arm in this study had a false-positive rate of 19.4% with LDCT alone, while the combination of LDCT and MSC reduced the false-positive rate to 3.7% (40). Prospective screening trials using a variety of miRNA assays are currently underway.

Protein Signatures

Blood protein classifiers measure the presence of proteins associated with various lung carcinomas. A panel of 11 proteins was tested in a retrospective validation study evaluating indeterminate pulmonary nodules 8 to 30 mm in diameter. Using a cancer prevalence estimate of 23%, this multicenter, case-control study of 141 patients with pulmonary nodules, including 78 cancers, identified likely benign nodules with a 90% NPV, and 26% PPV (41). This protein-based classifier is now being evaluated in a prospective trial in over 700 patients with noncalcified nodules. Another panel of seven proteins was developed in a cohort of 94 patients with non-small cell lung cancer and 269 long-term smokers with benign pulmonary nodules (42). The test performed better for squamous cell cancer and the utility of this test to improve the PPV of LDCT screening is currently being explored.

Autoantibodies

Autoantibodies are identifiable in patients with a wide variety of cancers and may be present months to years before clinical diagnosis. Classic examples of autoantibodies in lung cancer are the anticalcium channel antibodies in Lambert–Eaton myasthenic syndrome and the antineuronal nuclear antibody (anti-Hu) in neurologic paraneoplastic syndromes associated with small cell lung cancer. Thus, detection of autoantibodies could be a potential avenue for earlier malignancy detection. A panel of autoantibodies to lung cancer-associated antigens (Early CDT Lung) was validated in case-control studies that demonstrated a sensitivity of 36% to 39% and specificity of 89% to 91% (43). A clinical audit of the Early CDT Lung panel was performed in 1,613 patients at high risk for lung cancer, some of whom had indeterminate pulmonary nodules (44). Six-month follow-up was performed for all participants. Sixty-one (4%) were diagnosed with lung cancer and 25 of these were blood test-positive (true positive), resulting in a sensitivity of 41%. Thirty-six lung cancers had a negative biomarker test (false negative), resulting in a specificity of 87%. A positive Early CDT Lung test was associated with a five-fold increase in the chance of having lung cancer. Among lung cancers with a positive test, 57% were Stage I or II (43). Currently, two large prospective trials evaluating the clinical utility of the Early CDT Lung biomarker assay are underway (45,46).

Biomarker Summary

While LDCT screening results in a 20% reduction in lung cancer-specific mortality, it is estimated that only 25% to 30% of patients with lung cancer in the United States would meet the current criteria for LDCT screening (47). Thus, a validated biomarker assay could have a substantial impact by identifying other lung cancers when they are asymptomatic or in an early stage. Biomarkers could also be used to identify high-risk individuals who should undergo LDCT screening outside of the current guidelines. At this time, there are no standard biomarkers that have been fully validated for use in clinical practice for determining the risk of lung cancer or for delineating benign from malignant pulmonary nodules.

CONCLUSION

Lung cancer screening has developed beyond a topic of research interest to one with practical utility. Nevertheless, it is important to continue to refine the screening system in order to yield more precise data. The implementation of LDCT screening must include good communication with patients regarding the risks and benefits of this intervention. A screening program should also be committed to smoking cessation counseling, as this will have the greatest impact on the incidence of lung cancer in any population and will improve the cost-effectiveness of the screening program. A multidisciplinary team is required to guide the choice of diagnostic interventions for screen-detected pulmonary nodules. This team should include radiologists, radiation oncologists, thoracic surgeons, medical oncologists, pathologists, and pulmonologists. Hopefully, improvements in lung cancer risk assessment with modeling, derived not only from patient demographics and characteristics but also from validated biomarker assays, will afford more precise determinations of who will benefit from screening.

In summary, the positive results of the NLST have led to a cascade of approvals from a variety of national and international organizations (Table 4.2) and an agreement for financial compensation through the CMS in the United States. The current recommendation is to offer annual screening for lung cancer with LDCT in adults age 55 to 77 years who have at least a 30 pack-year smoking history and currently smoke or have quit within the past 15 years. Of course, the potential risks of screening need to be balanced against the potential benefits, such as harm that may result from procedures done on those who ultimately do not have cancer. However, as demonstrated in the NLST, such complications are relatively rare. Overdiagnosis is also a concern since LDCT will discover clinically insignificant malignancies that create anxiety and potential morbidity for the patient, and added costs for the health system.

Counseling patients before screening on the potential outcomes will help with coping and allow rational decision making; thus, counseling in a formalized visit with a provider is mandated by CMS. Financial cost to the health system can be decreased through smoking cessation counseling and by limiting screening to those at the highest risk for lung cancer. In addition, annual LDCT screening should stop once a patient has not smoked for 15 years or develops a health issue that substantially limits his or her life expectancy or reaches the upper age limit of 77 years. The CMS guidelines for lung cancer screening are presented in Table 4.3. Adherence to these mandates is required by any program in the United States that wishes to be reimbursed for lung cancer screening.

Table 4.3 CMS lung cancer screening guidelines

Patient criteria	Provider criteria	Facility criteria
• Age 55–77 years • No signs or symptoms of lung cancer • Tobacco smoking history of at least 30 pack-years • Current smoker or one who has quit smoking within the last 15 years • Willingness to undergo diagnostic or curative procedures/surgery, if indicated • Willingness to adhere to annual LDCT screening as long as indicated	• Written order supplied for LDCT scan • Lung cancer screening counseling and shared decision-making visit that is furnished by a physician or qualified nonphysician practitioner • Counseling that includes benefits and harms of screening, follow-up diagnostic testing, overdiagnosis, false-positive rate, total radiation exposure, and impact of comorbidities on ability to undergo diagnostic and treatment procedures • Counseling on importance of adherence to annual lung cancer LDCT screening • Counseling on the importance of maintaining cigarette smoking abstinence if former smoker; or the importance of smoking cessation if current smoker; furnishing of information about tobacco cessation interventions	• Performs LDCT with volumetric CT dose index of ≤3.0 mGy for standard size patients with appropriate reductions for smaller patients and appropriate increases for larger patients • Utilizes a standardized lung nodule identification, classification, and reporting system • Collects and submits data to a CMS-approved registry for each LDCT lung cancer screening performed • All CMS-approved registries must have the capacity and capability to collect data from any Medicare-eligible imaging facility that furnishes lung cancer screening with LDCT

Source: Adapted from www.cms.gov/Medicare/Medicare-General-Information/MedicareApprovedFacilitie/Lung-Cancer-Screening-Registries.html.

KEY POINTS

- The NLST showed that lung cancer screening with annual low-dose CT (LDCT) provides a relative risk reduction of 20% in lung cancer-specific mortality when compared to chest radiography.
- The U.S. CMS covers annual screening for lung cancer with LDCT in adults from 55 to 77 years old who have at least a 30 pack-year smoking history and currently smoke or have quit within the past 15 years.
- Appropriate patient selection and counseling are required to provide effective lung cancer screening. CMS has mandated patient counseling on smoking cessation and the risks of LDCT screening.
- The American College of Radiology has developed Lung-RADS™, a pulmonary nodule management plan that standardizes recommendations for findings on screening LDCT.
- LDCT uses much less radiation (<2mSv) than prior CT scan techniques.
- Chest radiography and sputum cytology are not effective lung cancer screening methods.
- Biomarkers for the early detection of lung cancer are being developed, but none have been validated for clinical application.

REFERENCES

1. Siegel R, Miller K, Jemal A. Cancer statistics 2015. *CA Cancer J Clin*. 2015;65:5-29.
2. Study Group on Smoking and Health. Joint report of smoking and health. *Science*. 1957;125:1129-1133.
3. Centers for Disease Control and Prevention. Quitting smoking amount adults—United States, 2001–2010. *MMWR Morb Mortal Wkly Rep*. 2011;60:1513-1519.
4. Mulshine J, Sullivan D. Lung cancer screening. *N Engl J Med*. 2005;352:2714-2720.
5. Siegel R, Ward E, Brawley O, Jemal A. Cancer statistics, 2011: the impact of eliminating socioeconomic and racial disparities on premature cancer deaths. *CA Cancer J Clin*. 2011;61:212-236.
6. Smith JJ, Berg CD. Lung cancer screening: promise and pitfalls. *Semin Oncol Nurs*. 2008;24:9-15.

7. Fontana R, Sanderson D, Woolner L, et al. Lung cancer screening: the Mayo program. *J Occup Med*. 1986;28:746-750.
8. Marcus P, Bergstralh E, Zweig M, et al. Extended lung cancer incidence follow-up in the Mayo Lung Project and overdiagnosis. *J Natl Cancer Inst*. 2006;98:748-756.
9. Oken M, Hocking W, Kvale P, et al. Screening by chest radiograph and lung cancer mortality: the Prostate, Lung, Colorectal, and Ovarian (PLCO) randomized trial. *JAMA*. 2011;306:1865-1873.
10. Swensen S, Jett J, Hartman T, et al. CT screening for lung cancer: fiver-year prospective experience. *Radiology*. 2005;235:259-265.
11. The International Early Lung Cancer Action Program Investigators. Survival of patients with stage I lung cancer detected on CT screening. *N Engl J Med*. 2006;355:1763-1771.
12. Infante M, Cavuto S, Lutman F, et al. Long-term follow-up results of the DANTE trial, a randomized study of lung cancer screening with spiral computed tomography. *Am J Respir Crit Care Med*. 2015;191:1166-1175.
13. National Lung Screening Trial Research Team, Aberle D, Adams A, et al. Reduced lung-cancer mortality with low-dose computed tomographic screening. *N Engl J Med*. 2011;365:395-409.
14. Russell P, Wainer Z, Wright G, et al. Does lung adenocarcinoma subtype predict patient survival? A clinicopathologic study based on the new International Association for the Study of Lung Cancer/American Thoracic Society/European Respiratory Society international multidisciplinary lung adenocarcinoma classification. *J Thorac Oncol*. 2011;6:1496-1504.
15. Horeweg N, Scholten E, de Jong P, et al. Detection of lung cancer through low-dose CT screening (NELSON): a prespecified analysis of screening test performance and interval cancers. *Lancet Oncol*. 2014;15:1342.
16. Klaveren R, Oudkerk M, Prokop M, et al. Management of lung nodules detected by volume CT scanning. *N Engl J Med*. 2009;361:2221-2229.
17. Moyer V, on behalf of U.S. Preventive Services Task Force. Screening for lung cancer: US Preventive Services Task Force recommendation statement. *Ann Intern Med*. 2014;160:330-338.
18. Itoh S, Ikeda M, Isomura T, et al. Screening helical CT for mass screening of lung cancer: application of low-dose and single-breath-hold scanning. *Radiat Med*. 1998;16:75-83.
19. MacMahon H, Austin J, Gamsu G. Guidelines for management of small pulmonary nodules detected on CT scans: a statement from the Fleischner Society. *Radiology*. 2005;237:395-400.
20. Swensen S, Silverstein M, Ilstrup D, Schleck C, Edell E. The probability of malignancy in solitary pulmonary nodules. Application to small radiologically indeterminate nodules. *Arch Intern Med*. 1997;157:849-855.

21. McKee B, Regis S, McKee A, Flacke S, Wald C. Performance of ACR Lung-RADS in a clinical CT lung screening program. *J Am Coll Radiol.* 2015;12:273-276.
22. Pinsky P, Gierada D, Black W, et al. Performance of Lung-RADS in the National Lung Screening Trial. *Ann Intern Med.* 2015;162:485-491.
23. McWilliams A, Tammemagi M, Mayo J, et al. Probability of cancer in pulmonary nodules detected on first screening CT. *N Engl J Med.* 2013;369:910-919.
24. Tammemagi M, Pinsky P, Caporaso N, et al. Lung cancer risk prediction: Prostate, Lung, Colorectal and Ovarian Cancer Screening Trial models and validation. *J Natl Cancer Inst.* 2011;103:1058-1068.
25. Kovalchik S, Tammemagi M, Berg C, et al. Targeting of low-dose CT screening according to the risk of lung-cancer death. *N Engl J Med.* 2013;369:245-254.
26. Tanner N, Kanodra N, Gebregziabher M, et al. The association between smoking abstinence and mortality in the National Lung Screening Trial. *Am J Respir Crit Care Med.* 2015. doi:10.1164/rccm.201507-1420OC
27. Wender R, Fontham ETH, Barrera E, et al. American Cancer Society lung cancer screening guidelines. *CA Cancer J Clin.* 2013;63:106-117.
28. Detterbeck FC, Mazzone PJ, Naidich DP, Bach PB. Screening for lung cancer: diagnosis and management of lung cancer, 3rd ed: American College of Chest Physicians evidence-based clinical practical guidelines. *Chest.* 2013;143(suppl 5):e78S-92S.
29. Final Update Summary: Lung Cancer Screening. U.S. Preventive Services Task Force. July 2015.
30. Kauczor H, Bonomo L, Gaga M, et al. ESR/ERS white paper on lung cancer screening. *Eur Respir J.* 2015;46:28-39. e-published April 30, 2015.
31. Mettler F Jr, Huda W, Yoshizumi T, Mahesh M. Effective doses in radiology and diagnostic nuclear medicine: a catalog. *Radiology.* 2008;248:254-263.
32. Bach P, Mirkin J, Oliver T, et al. Benefits and harms of CT screening for lung cancer: a systematic review. *JAMA.* 2012;307:2418-2429.
33. Black W, Gareen I, Soneji S, et al. Cost-effectiveness of CT screening in the National Lung Screening Trial. *N Engl J Med.* 2014;371:1793-1802.
34. Villanti A, Jiang Y, Abrams D, Pyenson B. A cost-utility analysis of lung cancer screening and the additional benefits of incorporating smoking cessation interventions. *PLOS ONE.* 2013;8:e71379.
35. Tammemagi M, Berg C, Riley T, Cunningham C, Taylor K. Impact of lung cancer screening results on smoking cessation. *J Natl Cancer Inst.* 2014;106:dju084.
36. Ashraf H, Tonnesen P, Holst P, Dirksen A, Thorsen H, Døssing M. Effect of CT screening on smoking habits at 1-year follow-up in the Danish Lung Cancer Screening Trial (DLCST). *Thorax.* 2009;64:388-392.

37. Hassanein M, Callison J, Callaway-Lane C, Aldrich M, Grogan E, Massion P. The state of molecular biomarkers for the early detection of lung cancer. *Cancer Prevent Res*. 2012;5:992-1006.
38. Pepe M, Etzioni R, Feng Z, et al. Phases of biomarker development for early detection of cancer. *J Natl Cancer Inst*. 2001;93:1054-1061.
39. Boeri M, Sestini S, Fortunato O, et al. Recent advances of microrna-based molecular diagnostics to reduce false-positive lung cancer imaging. *Expert Rev Molec Diagn*. 2015;15:801-813.
40. Sozzi G, Boeri M, Rossi M, et al. Clinical utility of a plasma-based mirna signature classifier within computed tomography lung cancer screening: a correlative mild trial study. *J Clin Oncol*. 2014;32:768-773.
41. Vachani A, Pass H, Rom W, et al. Validation of a multiprotein plasma classifier to identify benign lung nodules. *J Thorac Oncol*. 2015;10:629-637.
42. Mehan M, Williams S, Siegfried J, et al. Validation of a blood protein signature for non-small cell lung cancer. *Clin Proteomics*. 2014;11:32.
43. Boyle P, Chapman C, Holdenrieder S, et al. Clinical validation of an autoantibody test for lung cancer. *Ann Oncol*. 2011;22:383-389.
44. Jett J, Peek L, Fredericks L, Jewell W, Pingleton W, Robertson J. Audit of the autoantibody test, early CDT(r)-lung, in 1600 patients: an evaluation of its performance in routine clinical practice. *Lung Cancer*. 2014;83:51-55.
45. Sullivan F, Schembri S. Progress with an rct of the detection of autoantibodies to tumor antigens in lung cancer using the early CDT-lung test in Scotland. *J Thorac Oncol*. 2015;10:S306.
46. Jett J, Dyer D, Kern J. Screening for lung cancer with early CDT-lung and computed tomography. *J Thorac Oncol*. 2015;10:S306.
47. Pinsky P, Berg C. Applying the national lung screening trial eligibility criteria to the US population: what percent of the population and of incident lung cancers would be covered? *J Med Screening*. 2012;19:154-156.

5 Diagnosis and Staging of Lung Cancer

Shirish M. Gadgeel

INTRODUCTION

Lung cancer is a major cause of cancer-related mortality in the United States and worldwide and is expected to remain so in the near future (1). In the United States, the incidence of lung cancer in males is 83 per 100,000 and in females it is 55 per 100,000. The median age at presentation is around 71 years and about 10% of cases occur in patients below the age of 50 (2). In the United States, lung cancer is the most common cause of cancer-related death in both men and women. The primary reason for the high mortality rate associated with lung cancer is the advanced stage of disease in the majority of patients at the time of diagnosis.

CLINICAL FEATURES OF LUNG CANCER

The clinical presentation of lung cancer is highly variable. Patients with early stage disease usually don't have any symptoms related to the cancer. This lack of symptoms in early stage patients is related to the sparse pain fiber innervation of the lungs and the significant respiratory reserve provided by two lungs. Approximately 10% to 20% of lung cancer patients are asymptomatic at presentation (3–5). Such cancers are often detected during evaluation with chest radiography or CT scan obtained for an unrelated medical problem, such as preoperative assessment.

Evaluation of a Solitary Pulmonary Nodule

One common presentation of lung cancer in asymptomatic patients is the detection of a lung nodule, either solitary or multiple, on a chest imaging study. As lung cancer screening becomes more prevalent, asymptomatic lung nodules will be detected more frequently (6). The definition of a solitary pulmonary nodule is a pulmonary opacity surrounded completely by lung parenchyma that measures no more than 3 cm. A lesion larger than 3 cm is called a lung mass. The primary issue for consideration in the evaluation of a lung nodule is whether or not it is malignant. The work-up of a lung nodule is based on the patient factors, such as age, smoking history, occupational history, presence or absence of chronic obstructive pulmonary disease (COPD) and availability of prior imaging studies, and nodule factors, such as size, calcification, density, and border characteristics (7).

Further work-up of a lung nodule is guided by the probability that the nodule is malignant. The risk of malignancy is categorized as low-risk or high-risk either based on published risk models or the physician's judgement (8,9). Studies have shown that a physician's clinical judgement is not significantly inferior to guideline-based risk categorization (10). Following risk categorization, further assessment of an incidentally identified pulmonary nodule is based on guidelines, such as those published by the Fleischner Society (11,12). In general, lung nodules less than 8 mm in diameter are followed with repeat scans in 6 to 12 months (shorter intervals for higher risk patients), with further evaluation, such as a PET scan or a biopsy, performed only if the nodule increases in size over time. For nodules greater than 8 mm, further work-up, such as PET scan, biopsy, or even surgical resection, is considered if other risk factors suggest that the risk of malignancy is high. If the overall risk of malignancy is low, then repeat imaging at 3- to 6-month intervals is appropriate.

Common Symptoms

The most common symptoms caused by lung cancer are cough, dyspnea, weight loss, and chest pain (Table 5.1) (3–5). Unfortunately, most patients have metastases to regional lymph nodes or distant sites by the time symptoms develop. In addition, delays in reporting new symptoms or changes in existing symptoms frequently hamper the diagnosis of early stage lung cancer. In a series from Britain, the median time between the onset of symptoms and a patient seeking medical attention was 12 months (5). Various reasons account for delays in diagnosis, including the

Table 5.1 Common presenting symptoms of non–small-cell lung cancer

Symptom	Frequency (%)
Cough	45–75
Dyspnea	40–60
Weight loss	20–70
Chest pain	30–45
Hemoptysis	25–35
Bone pain	6–25
Fatigue	0–20

nonspecific nature of the symptoms and the attribution of symptoms to more commonly occurring ailments such as COPD. Symptoms of lung cancer can be related to the primary tumor, metastases, overall tumor burden (constitutional symptoms), or paraneoplastic syndromes.

Symptoms Related to the Primary Tumor

The most common symptom related to the primary tumor is cough, which eventually develops in most patients. Cough may be associated with hemoptysis. Cough can result from a variety of etiologies, including a central lung mass involving the airway, post-obstructive pneumonia, pleural effusion, or comorbid illnesses. Many patients with lung cancer have underlying COPD, which can cause a chronic cough. In these patients, gradual worsening of the cough may not be appreciated, resulting in a delay in the diagnosis.

Chest pain or discomfort is a common symptom that may occur even in early stage lung cancer without frank evidence of invasion of the pleura, chest wall, or mediastinum. Such pain does not localize to a specific area, and the origin of this discomfort is unclear since the lung parenchyma is not supplied with pain-sensing nerves. Patients may develop retrosternal pain from hilar or mediastinal lymphadenopathy or, less commonly, from pericardial involvement. Pain from chest wall involvement is usually more localized and severe, and is related to rib erosion or intercostal nerve compression.

Dyspnea or worsening dyspnea is another common symptom of lung cancer. Dyspnea may be related to either the lung cancer directly or to concomitant illnesses, such as COPD, pneumonia, or heart disease. Bronchial obstruction and pleural effusion are among the most common causes of dyspnea that result directly from lung cancer. Other causes include lymphangitic spread of the cancer and pulmonary embolus.

Symptoms Related to Local-Regional Invasion or Spread

Patients may develop specific constellations of symptoms related to the invasion of local structures by the primary tumor or regional lymph nodes. The two most well defined are superior vena cava (SVC) syndrome and Pancoast tumor. SVC syndrome results in signs and symptoms directly related to compression or invasion of the SVC by the primary lung tumor or paratracheal lymph nodes, resulting in edema in the face, neck, arms, and upper chest (13). SVC syndrome is more common with central, bulky tumors, such as squamous cell carcinoma and small cell lung cancer (SCLC). The most common symptoms of SVC syndrome are cough, hoarseness, and dyspnea from laryngeal and upper airway edema. The most serious consequence of SVC syndrome is cerebral edema resulting in headache, confusion, and even coma. Prompt diagnosis and initiation of therapy to shrink the responsible tumor are of paramount importance. However, initiating therapy before diagnosis is discouraged unless laryngeal or cerebral edemas are deemed to be life-threatening. In select situations, stenting the SVC to relieve the obstruction should be considered.

Pancoast tumors comprise less than 5% of all lung cancers (14). These tumors are located in the apex of the lung and the symptom complex results from invasion of the structures in the thoracic inlet, including the first and second ribs, upper thoracic spine, brachial plexus, sympathetic chain, and subclavian vessels. Therefore, patients have ipsilateral shoulder pain, arm weakness, hand muscle atrophy, Horner's syndrome, and upper extremity edema. An important aspect of Pancoast syndrome that may delay diagnosis is that the symptoms frequently direct the attention of medical providers to the neck and shoulder rather than to the lung. In addition, routine chest radiography may not adequately visualize an apical lung mass, further delaying diagnosis.

Symptoms Related to Metastases

Symptoms from metastases are highly variable since lung cancer can metastasize to almost any organ in the body. The most common sites of metastases are lungs, pleura, brain, adrenal glands, bones, and liver. Thus, some of the symptoms attributed to metastases are bone pain, abdominal pain, shortness of breath, and neurologic symptoms.

Constitutional symptoms, such as depression, fatigue, anorexia, weight loss, anxiety, and insomnia, are among the most frequent and troubling problems for patients with lung cancer. These symptoms are generally observed in patients with advanced stage disease, but can also be seen in patients with earlier stage tumors.

Paraneoplastic Syndromes

Clearly defined paraneoplastic syndromes occur in about 10% of lung cancer patients, and are more commonly associated with SCLC than non–small-cell lung cancer (NSCLC) (Table 5.2) (15). These syndromes are an indirect effect of the cancer, primarily caused by either hormones or cytokines secreted ectopically by the tumor or by antibodies directed against tumor antigens that cross react with normal tissues. The symptoms caused by paraneoplastic syndromes usually precede the diagnosis of lung cancer, and the presence of a paraneoplastic syndrome does not correlate with the size or extent of the cancer. Most paraneoplastic

Table 5.2 Paraneoplastic syndromes in lung cancer
Endocrine syndromes
Hypercalcemia
Syndrome of inappropriate antidiuretic hormone production
Cushing's syndrome
Neurological syndromes
Encephalomyelitis
Limbic encephalitis
Subacute cerebellar degeneration
Opsoclonus–myoclonus
Cancer-associated retinopathy
Sensory neuropathy
Sensori-motor neuropathy
Myasthenia gravis
Lambert–Eaton syndrome
Other syndromes
Anorexia–cachexia
Acanthosis nigrans
Dermatomyositis
Hypertrophic osteoarthropathy
Digital clubbing
Trousseau's syndrome

syndromes improve with effective treatment of the cancer, with the exception of most of the neurological syndromes in which the neuronal damage cannot be reversed.

Anorexia-cachexia: The most common paraneoplastic syndrome is cancer-related anorexia-cachexia, which is thought to be primarily related to the release of cytokines and other hormones. However, cachexia can occur for a variety of other reasons in patients with lung cancer. Approximately 60% of lung cancer patients have significant weight loss (>5% of baseline body weight) at the time of diagnosis (16).

Endocrine syndromes: Endocrine syndromes, such as hypercalcemia due to the secretion of parathyroid hormone-related peptide (PTHrP) or the syndrome of inappropriate antidiuretic hormone secretion (SIADH) can cause presenting symptoms. Hypercalcemia is present in 2% to 6% of lung cancer patients at diagnosis and develops in more than 10% during the course of the illness (15). The mechanisms of hypercalcemia include bone metastases and the secretion of PTHrP. Squamous cell lung cancer is the most common histology associated with hypercalcemia. Unlike other paraneoplastic syndromes, PTHrP secretion is less commonly seen in SCLC than in NSCLC. Clinically relevant hyponatremia due to SIADH occurs in up to 16%

of patients with SCLC, but is not common in NSCLC. SIADH does not correlate with stage and is associated with a worse prognosis (17). In addition, patients whose sodium levels don't improve with anticancer treatment have a worse outcome.

Neurologic syndromes: Another important category of paraneoplastic syndromes are neurologic syndromes. Neurologic paraneoplastic disorders such as Eaton-Lambert syndrome or limbic encephalopathy, usually present prior to the diagnosis of the cancer. Paraneoplastic neurologic syndromes are rare, but do occur in 3% to 5% of patients with SCLC. Almost all neurologic syndromes result from onconeural antibodies generated against antigens present on the cancer cells that cross react with specific neural tissues. However, the inability to detect these antibodies in the serum does not exclude the possibility of symptoms caused by a paraneoplastic syndrome.

DIAGNOSIS AND STAGING

In a patient suspected of having lung cancer, the goals of the initial work-up are to obtain an accurate diagnosis, define the histologic subtype, define the stage of disease, and obtain adequate tissue for the assessment of molecular alterations that may guide treatment (Table 5.3). Staging evaluation includes imaging of the common sites of metastases, such as liver, adrenals, bones, and brain, and assessment of the patient's performance status.

A detailed history and physical examination is of paramount importance since it not only guides subsequent diagnostic and

Table 5.3 Assessment of patients with newly diagnosed lung cancer

Assessment of lung cancer patients*
History and physical examination
Complete blood count
Liver function tests (AST, ALT, bilirubin, alkaline phosphatase)
Renal function tests (BUN, creatinine)
Electrolytes, including calcium
CT of the chest, including liver and adrenal glands, with IV contrast
FDG-PET
MRI or CT of brain with and without IV contrast
Diagnostic biopsy
Molecular diagnostic studies, as dictated by histology and stage
Performance status

AST, aspartate aminotransferase; ALT, alanine aminotransferase; BUN, blood urea nitrogen; FDG, fluorodeoxyglucose; IV, intravenous.
*Specific tests in an individual patient will vary based on stage of the disease and comorbid illnesses.

staging studies, but also provides information on the patient's general health, which is crucial for the development of a rational management plan. Laboratory tests are important for the assessment of bone marrow, liver, and kidney function, as well as the evaluation for the presence of metabolic abnormalities such as hyponatremia or hypercalcemia.

Imaging Studies

The primary purpose of imaging studies in patients with known or suspected lung cancer is to define the stage of the disease. Imaging studies are also done to assess symptoms that cannot be explained by clinical examination. It is extremely important to recognize that specific imaging studies should be guided by the clinical status of the individual patient. For example, further staging studies, such as a PET scan, are usually not necessary in patients already known to have metastatic disease, particularly those with a poor performance status. Staging studies could be initiated in patients who are suspected of having lung cancer even before a pathological diagnosis of lung cancer has been made since the imaging studies may help guide diagnostic procedures. Frequently, the results of imaging studies are not conclusive, since imaging studies can only identify abnormalities that may be malignant, but cannot definitively diagnose cancer. In most cases, it is important to obtain a tissue diagnosis to confirm regional or distant metastases, especially in situations where curative therapy could be offered if suspicious lesions are found to be nonmalignant.

CT: Usually, the first imaging test obtained is CT of the chest, which should include the liver and adrenal glands, and should be done with intravenous contrast. In addition to assessment for distant metastases, another important objective of CT is to assess mediastinal involvement by the tumor, either through direct invasion or metastases to mediastinal lymph nodes. Most studies of the utility of CT have used ≥1 cm in short axis as the criterion for defining a "positive" lymph node. In an analysis of over 7,000 patients conducted by the American College of Chest Physicians (ACCP), the sensitivity and specificity for detecting mediastinal lymph node metastasis were 55% and 81%, respectively (18). This suggests that CT is an imperfect tool for identifying lymph node metastases and should not be relied upon as the sole criterion for lymph node involvement.

PET: Fluorodeoyglucose (FDG)-PET is performed in nearly all patients with suspected stage I to III disease since PET can detect metastases in both regional lymph nodes and extrathoracic sites that are not detectable by conventional staging methods (19).

Based on randomized clinical trials, PET can identify potential regional and distant metastases in about 20% more patients than conventional staging (20). Several studies have suggested that FDG-PET can reduce the number of unnecessary lung cancer surgeries due to its greater sensitivity for regional and distant metastases (21). In addition, PET can eliminate the need for other staging procedures. For example, in randomized studies PET performed better than radionuclide bone scans for the detection of bone metastases, so a bone scan can be omitted from the staging work-up if a PET is obtained (22). However, FDG-PET also has a false positive rate of about 10%, and therefore, it is important to obtain pathologic confirmation that a suspicious area is malignant prior to making therapeutic decisions. This is particularly relevant in patients with a solitary or uncommon site of suspected metastasis. In one study in which all patients with a solitary, extrapulmonary, FDG-avid site and otherwise resectable NSCLC underwent biopsy of the suspected metastasis, almost 50% of patients were found to have an unrelated malignancy or a benign lesion (23). In patients with a central tumor or evidence of hilar lymph node involvement pathological assessment of mediastinal lymph nodes is recommended even if CT and PET are negative, since the risk of mediastinal lymph node involvement in such patients is about 25% (24). The sensitivity, specificity, positive predictive value, and negative predictive value of PET for mediastinal lymph node staging is about 80%, 88%, 75%, and 91%, respectively (18). PET is not recommended for patients with a small (≤2 cm), peripheral lung cancer with no other abnormality detected by conventional staging methods (cT1aN0M0). The likelihood of regional or distant metastases in this situation is only about 4%. In addition, PET scans are not recommended for patients who are already known to have documented metastatic disease.

Brain imaging: Brain metastases are an important cause of morbidity and mortality in patients with lung cancer. Due to the very high risk of brain metastases in SCLC, brain imaging is recommended irrespective of the stage of disease. In contrast, brain metastases are detected in ≤10% of patients with newly diagnosed NSCLC and a negative clinical evaluation (25). There is a higher risk of brain metastases in patients with adenocarcinoma and those with mediastinal lymph node involvement. CT or MRI scans are generally obtained in patients with stage III or IV NSCLC and in any earlier stage patient in whom adjuvant therapy is being considered. Another important reason to obtain brain imaging in the current era of targeted therapy is that the brain is a common site of progression and many, but not all, of the available targeted agents have limited therapeutic activity in the brain. MRI is more sensitive than CT in detecting brain metastases, particularly smaller lesions and those in the posterior fossa (26).

Staging Classification

The Tumor-Node-Metastasis (TNM) staging system defined by the American Joint Committee on Cancer (AJCC), seventh edition, has been validated for use in both NSCLC and SCLC (27,28). However, for SCLC the Veterans Affairs Lung Study Group (VALSG) staging system has been in use for many years, so nearly all clinical management data has been derived from trials using this classification scheme (29). In the VALSG system, patients are categorized as having limited-stage or extensive-stage disease. The AJCC staging system has been less commonly used since it relies on surgical confirmation and patients with SCLC are rarely considered for surgery since they almost always have metastatic or locally advanced disease at diagnosis.

TNM Staging

The current TNM staging system is presented in Appendix A. Basically, a primary tumor less than 7 cm in size that is confined to the lung (T1-2) and has not spread to lymph nodes (N0) or distant sites (M0) is classified as stage I. A primary tumor less than 7 cm that is confined to the lung (T1-2), but does have hilar or peribronchial lymph node involvement (N1) or a primary tumor ≥7 cm or with chest wall involvement or within 2 cm of carina (T3) without lymph node involvement (N0) is classified as stage II. A primary tumor of any size (T1-4) with mediastinal or supraclavicular lymph node involvement (N2-3) or a primary tumor that invades the mediastinum (T4) is classified as stage III. Further classification into stage IIIA or IIIB is based on the presence of supraclavicular or contralateral mediastinal lymph node metastases (N3—IIIB) or primary tumor invasion of the mediastinum with mediastinal or supraclavicular lymph node metastases (T4 N2-3—IIIB). The presence of any systemic metastases (M1) is classified as stage IV. The level of metastases is further grouped as M1a, if the only metastatic sites are the lung and/or the pleura, or M1b, for extrathoracic sites of disease. Patients with M1a disease have a better prognosis than those with M1b disease.

Practical Staging

The TNM stage classifications are based primarily on prognosis, not on therapy. A more practical approach to staging patients with NSCLC is to consider the disease either local, regional, or distant, since the status of the cancer at these sites guides therapy (Table 5.4). In general, for patients with local disease

Table 5.4 Staging and management of lung cancer

Stage (TNM stage*)	Therapy
NSCLC	
Local (stages I and II)	Surgery ± adjuvant chemotherapy
Regional (stages IIIA and IIIB)	Chemotherapy + RT
Distant (stage IV)	Systemic therapy (chemotherapy, targeted therapy, immunotherapy)
SCLC	
Limited† (stages I, II, III)	Chemotherapy + RT
Extensive† (stage IV)	Chemotherapy

*According to *AJCC*, 7th ed. Silvestri GA, Gonzalez AV, Jantz MA, et al. Methods for staging non-small cell lung cancer: diagnosis and management of lung cancer, 3rd ed.: American College of Chest Physicians evidence based clinical practice guidelines. *Chest*. 2013;143(5 suppl):e211S-e250S (18).
†According to the VALSG. Fischer B, Lassen U, Mortensen J, et al. Preoperative staging of lung cancer with combined PET-CT. *N Engl J Med*. 2009;361:32-39 (20).

(TNM stages I and II), surgical resection with or without adjuvant chemotherapy is considered the standard-of-care. In patients with regional disease (TNM stages IIIA and IIIB), concurrent chemotherapy and radiation therapy (RT) with curative intent is usually the treatment of choice. Finally, in patients with distant disease (TNM stage IV), systemic, palliative therapy is the primary treatment. The initial goal of the staging evaluation is to identify distant metastases. In the absence of distant metastases, the next step is to assess for mediastinal involvement either by direct invasion of the primary tumor or by metastasis to mediastinal lymph nodes.

Treatment Delays

If there has been an excessive delay between staging evaluation and the initiation of therapy, then staging scans should be repeated before initiating therapy. Mohammed et al. studied 40 patients who underwent more than one scan (CT and/or PET) before treatment and found that 31% had evidence of disease progression on scans done at least 8 weeks apart (30). Therefore, baseline scans should be repeated prior to the start of therapy if there has been a gap of more than 6 to 8 weeks since initial staging studies.

Diagnostic Biopsy

Selecting the most appropriate site to biopsy is crucial. The biopsy not only yields a diagnosis, but also provides information on the stage of disease and tumor material for the analysis of molecular markers used in the selection of therapy. Treatment of NSCLC is significantly influenced by the specific histologic subtype (squamous vs. non-squamous) and the presence of driver genetic alterations, such as EGFR mutation or ALK gene rearrangement (31). Therefore, it is imperative to obtain sufficient tissue to perform these analyses. Generally, biopsy of a metastatic site is preferred over the primary tumor since it also provides conclusive evidence of metastatic spread. In addition, a core biopsy is preferred over a fine needle aspirate since core samples are more likely to yield enough tissue not only for the diagnosis of lung cancer, but also for histologic subtyping and for the analysis of driver genetic alterations. The two most commonly performed diagnostic procedures for suspected lung cancer are image-guided (CT or ultrasound) biopsy of the primary tumor or an accessible metastatic site or bronchoscopic biopsy of the primary with or without biopsy of mediastinal lymph nodes. Thoracentesis with cytologic evaluation of pleural fluid is very helpful in patients with a pleural effusion.

Mediastinal Staging

Assessment of the mediastinum is an important aspect of staging patients with potentially resectable lung cancer. Metastatic spread to the mediastinal lymph nodes is generally considered a contraindication to primary surgical resection. Initial noninvasive mediastinal assessment is done with both CT and PET. However, since both the false-positive and false-negative rates with PET are about 10%, pathologic confirmation of mediastinal lymph node involvement is crucial in patients with otherwise resectable lung cancer. In the past, the only procedure available to define mediastinal lymph node metastases before surgery was mediastinoscopy. However, less invasive endobronchial ultrasound (EBUS)-guided or endoscopic ultrasound (EUS)-guided biopsies are now being used with increasing frequency both for initial diagnosis and staging of the mediastinum.

Mediastinoscopy

Mediastinoscopy is a surgical procedure conducted under general anesthesia to assess the contents of the mediastinum and biopsy mediastinal lymph nodes. The lymph nodes that can be accessed by mediastinoscopy include high (levels IIR and IIL) and low (levels IVR and IVL) paratracheal and anterior subcarinal (level VII) lymph nodes. The lymph nodes that are not accessible are above the suprasternal notch (level I), anterior to the SVC or posterior in paraesophageal area (level III), posterior subcarinal (level VII), aorto-pulmonary window (level V), para-aortic (level VI), and lower mediastinal (levels VIII and IX). An extended cervical mediastinoscopy can access levels V and VI. The ACCP conducted an analysis of over 9,000 patients form various series and found that the sensitivity of mediastinoscopy is 78% with a negative predictive value of 91% (18).

Endobronchial Ultrasound/Endoscopic Ultrasound

EBUS-guided mediastinal lymph node biopsies are now common. This procedure can assess the same lymph nodes as mediastinoscopy. In many centers, EBUS is combined with EUS, which permits access to level VIII and IX lymph nodes. In the ACCP analysis, the sensitivity and specificity for this combined procedure were 91% and 100%, respectively, with a negative predictive value of 96% (18).

In a recent randomized trial in patients who were being considered for lung cancer resection and had negative lymph nodes on imaging studies, EUS/EBUS followed by mediastinoscopy was superior to mediastinoscopy alone for the detection of mediastinal lymph node metastases and the avoidance of unnecessary surgery (32). Mediastinal lymph node involvement was identified in 35% of the 117 patients who underwent mediastinoscopy and 46% of the 123 patients who underwent endosonography. Of the patients who did not have mediastinal lymph nodes detected by EBUS, six were found to have involvement on subsequent mediastinoscopy. Thus, the combined approach detected mediastinal lymph node metastases in 50% of patients. The rate of unnecessary thoracotomies, defined as unexpected mediastinal lymph node involvement or tumor invasion of the mediastinum at surgery, was 18% in the mediastinoscopy alone group and 7% in the combined staging group.

Histologic Classification and Molecular Markers

Historically, the only histologic distinction required for therapeutic decision making in lung cancer was whether the patient had NSCLC or SCLC. However, clinical trials over the last 10 years have now clearly demonstrated that histology is a predictor of both efficacy and toxicity for specific agents (31). For example, patients with squamous cell carcinoma do not appear to benefit from treatment with pemetrexed and have excessive toxicity with bevacizumab. These findings have highlighted the need to obtain adequate tissue at the time of biopsy.

Another reason to obtain adequate biopsy tissue is to allow the performance of appropriate molecular analyses. Over the past 10 years, genetic alterations that drive the proliferation and survival of lung cancer cells have been identified and specific agents that target these alterations have been developed and demonstrated to yield significant therapeutic benefit. For patients with tumors harboring either EGFR sensitizing mutations or ALK rearrangements, clinical trials have reported that targeted agents improve clinical outcomes when compared to standard cytotoxic chemotherapy. In addition to EGFR and ALK, the National Comprehensive Cancer Network now recommends testing for several other genetic abnormalities in patients with lung adenocarcinoma, including ROS1 and RET rearrangements, BRAF mutation, and cMET amplification, or mutation (33).

FUNCTIONAL ASSESSMENT

Performance status remains one of the most important prognostic factors in patients with lung cancer (Tables 5.5 and 5.6). Performance status can be impaired by the cancer itself or by comorbid illnesses. Appropriate determination of performance status and the reasons for any impairment is very important for defining management strategies, including whether or not staging studies should be obtained and whether or not patients should receive any anticancer therapy. In those who are fit to receive therapy, the performance status helps guide the intensity of therapy. For example, although concurrent chemotherapy and definitive RT is considered the standard-of-care for patients with stage III NSCLC, an individual patient's severely impaired performance status may dictate the use of palliative RT alone to control symptoms related to local tumor extension. For patients with advanced lung cancer and impaired performance status, systemic anticancer therapy may be a stronger consideration if the patient's impairment is related to the cancer, which might improve with therapy, while palliative care might be most appropriate if it is due to irreversible comorbid disease.

Performance status is also important in patients with early stage lung cancer. Patients being considered for thoracic surgery require preoperative assessment of both pulmonary and cardiac function (34). In recent years, patients with early stage lung cancer who are not candidates for lobectomy can be treated with other options, such as limited surgical resection or stereotactic radiation therapy. Therefore, appropriate assessment and continual reassessment of functional status and organ function are crucial for all patients with lung cancer throughout the course of their disease.

Table 5.5 Karnofsky performance status scale

Able to carry on normal activity and to work; no special care needed	100	Normal no complaints; no evidence of disease.
	90	Able to carry on normal activity; minor signs or symptoms of disease.
	80	Normal activity with effort; some signs or symptoms of disease.
Unable to work; able to live at home and care for most personal needs. Varying amount of assistance needed	70	Cares for self; unable to carry on normal activity or to do active work.
	60	Requires occasional assistance, but is able to care for most personal needs.
	50	Requires considerable assistance and frequent medical care.
Unable to care for self; requires equivalent of institutional or hospital care; disease may be progressing rapidly	40	Disabled; requires special care and assistance.
	30	Severely disabled; hospital admission is indicated although death not imminent.
	20	Very sick; hospital admission necessary; active supportive treatment necessary.
	10	Moribund; fatal processes progressing rapidly.
	0	Dead.

Table 5.6 Zubrod performance status scale

Grade	Performance status
0	Fully active, able to carry on all predisease performance without restriction.
1	Restricted in physically strenuous activity but ambulatory and able to carry out work of a light or sedentary nature, e.g., light house work, office work.

(*continued*)

Table 5.6 Zubrod performance status scale (*continued*)

Grade	Performance status
2	Ambulatory and capable of all self-care but unable to carry out any work activities; up and about more than 50% of waking hours.
3	Capable of only limited self-care; confined to bed or chair more than 50% of waking hours.
4	Completely disabled; cannot carry on any self-care; totally confined to bed or chair.
5	Dead.

KEY POINTS

- Symptoms are not common in early stage lung cancer.
- Symptoms from lung cancer can be categorized as those related to the primary tumor, regional progression, distant metastases, overall tumor burden, or paraneoplastic syndromes.
- Initial evaluation of patients with lung cancer should include thorough history and physical examination, laboratory tests, and appropriate imaging studies, including CT of the chest, PET, and brain MRI.
- The goals of a biopsy are to diagnose the disease, define the histologic subtype, and obtain adequate tissue for molecular analysis. The general principle is to biopsy the site that would define the highest stage of disease as this allows for the establishment of both the diagnosis and stage of disease.
- Histologic diagnosis, stage, molecular profile, and performance status are the most important factors for determination of the therapeutic approach to patients with lung cancer.

REFERENCES

1. American Cancer Society. Cancer facts and figures 2016. Available at: http://www.cancer.org/research/cancerfactsstatistics/cancerfacts figures2016/index
2. Ramalingam S, Pawlish K, Gadgeel S, et al. Lung cancer in young patients: analysis of a Surveillance, Epidemiology, and End Results database. *J Clin Oncol*. 1998;16:651-657.

3. Chute CG, Greenberg ER, Baron J, et al. Presenting conditions of 1539 population-based lung cancer patients by cell type and stage in New Hampshire and Vermont. *Cancer*. 1985;56:2107-2111
4. Koyi H, Hillerdal G, Brandén E. A prospective study of a total material of lung cancer from a county in Sweden 1997–1999: gender, symptoms, type, stage, and smoking habits. *Lung Cancer*. 2002;36:9-14.
5. Buccheri G, Ferrigno D. Lung cancer: clinical presentation and specialist referral time. *Eur Respir J*. 2004;24:898.
6. The National Lung Screening Trial Research Team, Aberle DR, Adams AM, et al. Reduced lung-cancer mortality with low-dose computed tomographic screening. *N Engl J Med*. 2011;365:395-409.
7. Murrmann GB, van Vollenhoven FH, Moodley L. Approach to a solid solitary pulmonary nodule in two different settings-"Common is common, rare is rare." *J Thorac Dis*. 2014;6:237-248.
8. Gould MK, Donington J, Lynch WR, et al. Evaluation of individuals with pulmonary nodules: when is it lung cancer? Diagnosis and management of lung cancer, 3rd ed.: American College of Chest Physicians evidence-based clinical practice guidelines. *Chest*. 2013;143:e93s-e120s.
9. Gould MK, Ananth L, Barnett PG, Veterans Affairs SNAP Cooperative Study Group. A clinical model to estimate the pretest probability of lung cancer in patients with solitary pulmonary nodules. *Chest*. 2007;313:383-388.
10. Balekian AA, Silvestri GA, Simkovich SM, et al. Accuracy of clinicians and models for estimating the probability that a pulmonary nodule is malignant. *Ann Am Thorac Soc*. 2013;10:629-635.
11. MacMahon H, Austin JH, Gamsu G, et al. Guidelines for management of small pulmonary nodules detected on CT scans: a statement from the Fleischner Society. *Radiology*. 2005;237:395.
12. Naidich DP, Bankier AA, MacMahon H, et al. Recommendations for the management of subsolid pulmonary nodules detected at CT: a statement from the Fleischner society. *Radiology*. 2013;266:304-317.
13. Lepper PM, Ott SR, Hoppe H, et al. Superior vena cava syndromes in thoracic malignancies. *Respir Care*. 2011;56:653-666.
14. Glassman LR, Hyman K. Pancoast tumor: a modern perspective on an old problem. *Curr Opin Pulm Med*. 2013;19:340-343.
15. Kanaji N, Watanabe N, Kita N, et al. Paraneoplastic syndromes associated with lung cancer. *World J Clin Oncol*. 2014;5:197-223.
16. Tuca A, Jimenez-Fonseca P, Gascon P. Clinical evaluation and optimal management of cancer cachexia. *Crit Rev Oncol Hematol*. 2013;88:625-636.
17. Hansen O, Sorensen P, Hansen KH. The occurrence of hyponatremia in SCLC and the influence on prognosis: a retrospective study of 453 patients treated in a single institution in a 10-year period. *Lung Cancer*. 2010;68:111-114.

18. Silvestri GA, Gonzalez AV, Jantz MA, et al. Methods for staging non-small cell lung cancer: diagnosis and management of lung cancer, 3rd ed.: American College of Chest Physicians evidence based clinical practice guidelines. *Chest*. 2013;143(5 suppl):e211S-e250S.
19. Sahiner I, Vural GU. Positron emission tomography/computerized tomography in lung cancer. *Quant Imaging Med Surg*. 2014;4:195-206.
20. Fischer B, Lassen U, Mortensen J, et al. Preoperative staging of lung cancer with combined PET-CT. *N Engl J Med*. 2009;361:32-39.
21. van Tinteren H, Hoekstra OS, Smith EF, et al. Effectiveness of positron emission tomography in the preoperative assessment of patients with suspected non-small-cell lung cancer: the PLUS multicenter randomized trial. *Lancet*. 2002;359:1388-1393.
22. Hsia TC, Shen YY, Yen RF, et al. Comparing whole body ^{18}F-2-deoxyglucose positron emission tomography and technetium-99m methylene diphosphatebone scan to detect bone metastases in patients with non-small cell lung cancer. *Neoplasma*. 2002;49:267-271.
23. Lardinois D, Weder W, Roudas M, et al. Etiology of solitary extrapulmonary positron emission tomography and computed tomography findings in patients with lung cancer. *J Clin Oncol*. 2005;23:6846-6853.
24. Gdeedo A, Van Schil P, Corthouts B, et al. Comparison of imaging TNM [(i) TNM] and pathological TNM [pTNM] in staging of bronchogenic carcinoma. *Eur J Cardiothorac Surg*. 1997;12:224-227.
25. Colice GL, Birkmeyer JD, Black WC, et al. Cost effectiveness of head CT in patients with lung cancer without clinical evidence of metastases. *Chest*. 1995;108:1264-1271.
26. Davis PC, Hudgins PA, Peterman SB, Hoffman JC. Diagnosis of cerebral metastases: double dose delayed CT vs contrast-enhanced MRI imaging. *AJNR*. 1991;156:1039-1046.
27. Goldstraw P, Crowley J, Chansky K, et al. The IASLC Lung Cancer Staging Project: proposals for the revision of the TNM stage groupings in the forthcoming (seventh) edition of TNM classification of malignant tumors. *J Thorac Oncol*. 2007;2:706-714.
28. Shepherd FA, Crowley J, Van Houtte P, et al. The International Association for the Study of Lung Cancer lung cancer staging project: proposals regarding the clinical staging of small cell lung cancer in the forthcoming (seventh) edition of the tumor, node, metastasis classification of lung cancer. *J Thorac Oncol*. 2007;2:1066-1077.
29. Stahel R, Ginsberg R, Havemann K, et al. Staging and prognostic factors in small cell lung cancer: a consensus report. *Lung Cancer*. 1989;5:119-126.
30. Mohammed N, Kestin LL, Grills IS, et al. Rapid disease progression with delay in treatment of non-small cell lung cancer. *Int J Radiat Oncol Biol Phys*. 2011;79:466-472.
31. Johnson DH, Schiller JH, Bunn PA. Recent clinical advances in lung cancer management. *J Clin Oncol*. 2014;32:973-982.

32. Annema JT, van Meerbeeck JP, Rintoul RC, et al. Mediastinoscopy vs endosonography for mediastinal nodal staging of lung cancer: a randomized trial. *JAMA*. 2010;304:2245-2252.
33. Ettinger DS, Wood DE, Akerley W, et al. Non-small cell lung cancer NCCN evidence blocks. Available at: http://www.nccn.org/professionals/physician_gls/pdf/nscl_blocks.pdf
34. Salati M, Brunelli A. Preoperative assessment of patients for lung cancer surgery. *Curr Opin Pulm Med*. 2012;18:289-294.

6 Management of Early Stage Non–Small-Cell Lung Cancer

Jessica S. Donington and Jean Lee

INTRODUCTION

Treatment for early stage non–small-cell lung cancer (NSCLC) is no longer "one-size fits all" with stage being the only determinant of the most effective therapy. Tumor histology, size, and location, as well as numerous epidemiologic factors, each contribute significantly to prognosis and therapy. For the majority of patients with early stage NSCLC, anatomic resection by lobectomy or more extensive surgery, provides the greatest chance for cure and is the initial treatment of choice. This approach has been challenged in patients with medical comorbidities, advanced age, and/or small or indolent tumors. Adjuvant chemotherapy has been shown to improve survival in those with completely resected stage II/III, and large (≥4 cm) stage IB tumors. This chapter outlines treatment strategies for patients with stage I and II NSCLC, including surgical approaches, adjuvant chemotherapy, and ablative therapy (e.g., stereotactic body radiation therapy [SBRT], radiofrequency ablation [RFA], microwave ablation [MWA], and cryotherapy).

SURGERY

Early stage NSCLC, defined as stage I and stage II disease, is most commonly treated with surgery as the initial modality. The current tumor node metastasis (TNM) staging guidelines by the American Joint Committee on Cancer (AJCC), seventh edition, define these as tumors up to 7 cm in size with or without ipsilateral hilar lymph node involvement, but without mediastinal lymph node disease. Tumors greater than 7 cm are considered to be stage II in the absence of lymph node involvement (1). A preoperative diagnostic biopsy of a highly suspicious pulmonary nodule is not necessarily required prior to definitive resection. There are two key components to surgery for early stage NSCLC, complete resection of the primary tumor and evaluation of draining lymph node basins in the ipsilateral hilum and mediastinum. Surgical intervention for NSCLC is not without risk and complications occur in up to 30% of patients. Appropriate assessment and mediation of interventional risk have evolved dramatically in the past decade.

Preoperative Assessment

Patients with NSCLC have more tobacco-related comorbidities than patients with other solid tumors and, therefore, physiologic assessment is essential to determine appropriate treatment strategies. The goal of preoperative assessment is to identify patients at increased risk for operative complications and long-term disability. The evaluation focuses heavily on cardiac and pulmonary physiology. Risk assessment can be complex, with subtleties related to patient age, cognition and mobility, tumor size and location, and the mode of intervention. Therefore, high-risk patients are best approached in multidisciplinary fashion.

Coronary artery disease (CAD) is more common in patients with NSCLC than the general population. The underlying rate of CAD in patients with NSCLC is 11% to 17% and the risk for major cardiac complication following lung resection is 2% to 3% (2). The American Heart Association/American College of Cardiology recommend the revised cardiac risk index (RCRI) tool for assessing cardiac risk in most patients undergoing noncardiac surgery. This has been further refined in a thoracic surgery-specific population through the development of the thoracic RCRI (ThRCRI), which also takes into account the extent of resection (3). Any patient with a score greater than 1.5, a newly suspected cardiac condition, limited exercise tolerance, or requiring cardiac medications should undergo a formal evaluation by a cardiologist prior to surgical intervention.

Pulmonary function tests (PFTs), primarily the forced expired volume in 1 second (FEV_1), is the tool used most frequently for preoperative pulmonary assessment. Diffusion capacity for carbon monoxide (DLCO) is less commonly measured, but equally predictive of outcome. However, the two values do not always correlate with each other, so both FEV_1 and DLCO should be measured as a routine part of preoperative planning. Impaired FEV_1 and DLCO are both independent predictors of pulmonary morbidity, but their associated predicted postoperative (ppo) values appear to be more accurate guides. The $ppoFEV_1$ and ppoDLCO should be calculated in all patients with abnormal lung function (FEV_1 or DLCO <80% predicted). Calculations for $ppoFEV_1$ and ppoDCLO can be based on either lung perfusion scan or planned extent of anatomic resection.

- Perfusion: $ppoFEV_1$ or ppoDLCO = preoperative FEV_1 or DLCO × (1 − fraction of total perfusion of the resected lung)

- Anatomic: ppoFEV$_1$ or ppoDLCO = preoperative FEV$_1$ or DLCO × (1 − no. of functional segments resected/total no. of functional segments)

Postoperative predicted FEV$_1$ and DLCO greater than 40% portend a good prognosis for resection, but the inverse is not necessarily true; patients with ppoFEV$_1$ or ppoDLCO less than 40% may require additional evaluation in the form of cardiopulmonary exercise testing, and alternative treatment strategies may need to be considered. Commonly used low-technology exercise tests include stair climbing and a shuttle walk. Peak oxygen consumption ($V0_2$ max) is the most specific cardiopulmonary test and values less than 10 mL/kg/min are considered prohibitive for surgery, while values greater than 20 mL/kg/min indicate low risk for perioperative complications (2).

Lobectomy

Open Lobectomy

The majority of open lobectomies are performed using a posterior lateral thoracotomy, entering the pleural cavity through the 5th intercostal space. Median sternotomy and anterior thoracotomy can also be used, but exposure to the pulmonary hilum is suboptimal. Local control and overall survival following anatomic lobectomy for early stage NSCLC have improved over the past 50 years with substantial improvement in operative morbidity and mortality. In the American College of Surgeons Oncology Group (ACOSOG) Z0030 trial, 5-year disease-free survival was 68% for patients with resected early stage disease (4). Completeness of resection and lymph node involvement are the primary predictors of long-term survival. By definition, lobectomy involves individual identification and division of the lobar arteries, veins, and bronchus. In the modern era, most lobectomies are completed with endoscopic staplers. Resections by thoracotomy carry significant risk, with up to 37% of patients experiencing a postoperative complication (5). Most of these are minor, such as atrial arrhythmia or a prolonged air leak, but more serious complications, including respiratory failure, can occur and increase in frequency with decreasing baseline pulmonary function. The operative mortality following lobectomy is reported to be 1% to 3% (5,6), with pneumonia and respiratory failure as the most common causes of death.

Systematic Mediastinal Nodal Evaluation

Resection of the draining lymph nodes is vital for pathologic NSCLC staging, and is an integral part of surgical therapy. The demonstration of a survival improvement with adjuvant chemotherapy following resection of stage II and III NSCLC (7) places added importance to adequate intraoperative lymph node evaluation. Hilar and mediastinal lymph nodes are assigned stations as defined by the AJCC seventh edition TNM lung cancer staging system (1). The definitions of lymph node classifiers (N) remained essentially unchanged from the previous version and will remain unchanged in the next proposed system (see Appendix B). All interlobar and intralobar lymph nodes (stations 10–14, N1) encountered during dissection of the hilum and fissure are removed and sent for pathologic evaluation.

A thorough evaluation of mediastinal lymph nodes is essential and can be performed as a systematic sampling in which one or several lymph nodes are biopsied at each of the ipsilateral mediastinal stations (stations 2R, 4R, 7, and 9R on the right; levels 5, 6, 7, and 9L on the left), or a formal mediastinal lymphadenectomy in which all associated nodes and soft tissues between anatomic landmarks are removed. The collection and evaluation of at least 10 hilar and mediastinal lymph nodes are recognized as a quality measure for NSCLC resections by the American College of Surgeons Commission on Cancer, but controversy remains as to whether lymph node sampling or full dissection is superior, and if there is any survival benefit for the more aggressive approach. The ACOSOG randomized trial (ACOSOG Z0030) looked specifically at lymph node dissection versus sampling in greater than 1,000 patients with early stage NSCLC undergoing resection and failed to identify significant differences in morbidity or survival between the approaches (4). However, the authors cautioned that the trial focused on patients with clinical stage I disease and the results may not apply to those with higher stage tumors that would be more prone to metastasize.

Video-Assisted Thoracoscopic Surgery Lobectomy

Video-assisted thoracoscopic surgery (VATS), like thoracotomy, is a surgical approach and not a unique therapeutic intervention. The VATS approach to lobectomy typically involves two to three port sites and a 5 to 8 cm access incision. The distinction between VATS and mini-thoracotomy is the lack of rib spreading and the use of thoracoscopic visualization as opposed to visualization through the access incision (8). The rigid nature of the thoracic cavity makes it particularly well suited to scope-based approaches. The use of "pleuroscopy" has been reported since the early 20th century (9), but the practicality of thoracoscopic techniques increased dramatically in the 1980s with improvements in video technology and the introduction of double lumen endotracheal tubes to facilitate single-lung ventilation. Initial reports of VATS lobectomy appeared in the 1990s, documenting their safety and outlining techniques (10–13). Subsequently, numerous large series have reported recurrence and survival data equivalent to that achieved with open lobectomy (14–18). These studies have demonstrated that VATS lobectomy is a safe procedure with a rate of conversion to open lobectomy of 5% to 10%. Importantly, it has also been found that the conversion from VATS to open lobectomy is not associated with increased perioperative morbidity or mortality (19).

VATS lobectomy is the same oncologic operation as open lobectomy, including removal of the entire lobe that contains the tumor with individual ligation of vessels and the bronchus, and systematic evaluation of hilar and mediastinal lymph nodes. Most large VATS lobectomy series describe a similar pattern of perioperative complications as open lobectomy, but at reduced rates (14–16). The most widely recognized benefits of VATS are reduction in pain and length of hospital stay. The patients who appear to benefit the most from minimally invasive techniques are those at high risk due to marginal lung function. Multiple analyses from the Society of Thoracic Surgeons' General Thoracic Surgery database (STS-GTSDB) have demonstrated similar rates of cardiopulmonary complications and death after VATS and open lobectomy for standard-risk patients, but significant decreases in these poor outcomes in high risk patients who undergo VATS as opposed to open thoracotomy (20,21).

One downside of VATS when compared to open lobectomy may be a decrease in the thoroughness of hilar lymph node evaluation. Analysis of clinical stage I tumors from the STS-GTSDB found similar rates of N0 to N2 upstaging with VATS and open lobectomy (4.9% vs. 5.0%), but a lower rate of N0 to N1 upstaging with VATS (6.7% vs. 9.3%) (22). Forty percent of lobotomies reported in the STS-GTSDB are currently performed thoracoscopically (8), but this database is heavily weighted toward academic centers and large practices, so it is thought that the actual rate of VATS lobectomy use in the United States is likely lower. Dense pleural adhesion and the inability to tolerate single-lung ventilation are the only definitive contraindications to VATS resections. Dense mediastinal scarring, central tumors, and tumors larger than the access incision are relative contraindications. Emerging technologies include single-port lobectomy and spontaneous breathing, nonintubated techniques, but thus far there are few reports of lobectomy using these procedures.

Robotic-Assisted Lobectomy

The main advantage of robotic technology for anatomic lung resections mirrors that of the VATS approach, namely smaller, non–rib-spreading incisions resulting in less operative trauma, and decreased pain and length of hospital stay. The benefits of a robotic approach over VATS include binocular visualization, wristed instruments that allow for more precise dissection, and no requirement for an access incision. Additionally, given the totally portal nature of the procedure, carbon dioxide insufflation of the hemithorax can be used to further collapse the lung providing a larger working area.

Robotic lobectomy requires similar positioning as the open or VATS approach with the patient in the lateral decubitus position. There are three or four access ports for the robot and one assistant port for suctioning, stapling, and retraction. The dissection of the hilum and fissure is performed in a similar manner as with the VATS and open approaches with the bronchovascular structures being dissected and individually divided with staplers. Initial series reporting on robotic lobectomy for NSCLC have demonstrated the safety and feasibility of this approach, without increased morbidity or mortality (23–25). While large longitudinal studies addressing long-term oncologic outcomes are needed, initial reports show comparable stage-specific survival rates with VATS and robotic approaches (26,27). Cost comparisons between robotic and VATS techniques are difficult due to the larger upfront cost of a robotic system; however, both approaches appear to have an overall cost benefit compared to open thoracotomy due to the significant decrease in hospital length of stay (28).

Sublobar Resection

Sublobar resections have always been a compromise procedure for patients with early stage NSCLC who lack the pulmonary function to tolerate lobectomy. However, since the 1950s lobectomy has been the standard-of-care for treatment of resectable early stage NSCLC, even for patients with small tumors (<2 cm). In 1996, the Lung Cancer Study Group (LCSG) reported the only randomized trial that compared lobectomy to lesser resections for early stage NSCLC (29). This study found a threefold increase in local recurrence with sublobar resection compared to lobectomy. The main concerns regarding these results are that this trial completed accrual in 1988, prior to the introduction of FDG-PET, and that CT scans were obtained in less than 30% of patients. So while this trial has guided surgical care for 20 years, its findings are becoming less relevant due to improvements in the radiographic diagnosis and staging of lung cancer and advancements in our understanding of the biology of this disease.

Recently, there has been a resurgence of interest in the intentional use of sublobar resections for small and indolent clinical stage I NSCLC. The primary advantage of sublobar resection is the preservation of pulmonary parenchyma, which should translate into better postoperative pulmonary function, improved quality of life, and increased ability to tolerate a second curative procedure for a subsequent bronchogenic carcinoma.

Several recent, single institution, retrospective analyses that compared sublobar resection to lobectomy in patients with limited cardiopulmonary reserve contradict the earlier findings from the LCSG study, demonstrating that in well-selected patients with stage I NSCLC sublobar resection achieves similar survival rates as lobectomy. Most series highlight important requirements to assume an equivalent outcome between sublobar resections and lobectomy, including

- Tumor size less than 2 cm
- Indolent histologic subclassification
- Segmentectomy rather than wedge resection
- Surgical margins of at least 2 cm or as large as the tumor

Increased rates of detection of small peripheral tumors and ground-glass opacities (GGOs) associated with favorable histology have led to the increasing use of sublobar resections in many centers to include patients with adequate physiologic reserve (30). Both American and Japanese series have demonstrated that adenocarcinoma in situ (AIS) and minimally invasive adenocarcinoma (MIA), which can be identified preoperatively by a high GGO-to-solid ratio on CT, represents an entity with improved survival and reduced rates of lymph node involvement and distant metastatic spread (30–32). The selection of medically fit patients with very favorable tumors based on peripheral location, small size, and a high GGO-to-solid ratio for intentional sublobar resection is gaining acceptance in the international community. Reviews by Yamada, Yamato, and Wantanabe have each reported 100% survival and no evidence of recurrence when intentional sublobar resection was used in patients with pure GGOs less than 3 cm in size (33–36).

A prospective, randomized multi-institutional phase III trial is being conducted by the Alliance Cooperative Group (CALGB 140503) to determine the effectiveness of an intentional sublobar resection protocol for small (<2 cm) peripheral tumors. A similar trial recently completed accrual in Japan (JCOG0802/WJOG4607). Both trials are similar in design to the LCSG trial, with lobectomy being compared to sublobar resection (wedge resection or segmentectomy), but with a smaller tumor size requirement and use of modern staging studies. Results of these studies will hopefully provide important insights into the role of lung-sparing resections for small, peripheral stage IA tumors.

ADJUVANT THERAPY

Platinum-Based Adjuvant Therapy

Despite complete resection, disease recurrence remains a significant problem for patients with early stage NSCLC, especially within the first 5 years after surgery. Cisplatin-based adjuvant chemotherapy is the standard-of-care following surgery for patients with stage II, III, and high-risk stage IB NSCLC (37). The goal of adjuvant therapy is to eliminate occult metastatic disease, thereby decreasing the recurrence rate and improving survival.

Several large, randomized clinical trials have demonstrated a survival benefit, ranging from approximately 5% to 15%, for adjuvant chemotherapy (38–40). These studies used cisplatin-based, two-drug regimens and enrolled mostly patients with stage IB-IIIA NSCLC. The lung adjuvant cisplatin evaluation (LACE) meta-analysis (7) evaluated pooled data of five large, randomized, controlled adjuvant chemotherapy trials that were performed since 1995: Adjuvant Navelbine International Trialist Association (ANITA) (38), Intergroup trial JRB.10 (39), International Adjuvant Lung Trial (IALT) (40), Big Lung Trial (BLT) (41), and Adjuvant Lung Project Italy (ALPI) (42). These studies accrued a total of 4,585 patients who had undergone complete resection for stage I (7% stage IA, 31% stage IB), stage II (35%), and stage III (27%). With a mean follow-up of 5.2 years, adjuvant chemotherapy resulted in a 5.4% increase in overall survival (HR 0.89). The advantage of adjuvant chemotherapy was not seen in all stages and appeared to be detrimental in patients with stage IA disease. Of note, some of these studies allowed the use of postoperative radiation (PORT), which has been shown to have a negative impact on outcomes in patients with early stage NSCLC, particularly those with N0 disease (43).

A more comprehensive review of trials evaluating the role of adjuvant chemotherapy in early stage NSCLC again demonstrated an absolute survival benefit of 4% at 5 years (44). This meta-analysis included 26 randomized trials that compared outcomes of surgery with or without adjuvant chemotherapy, and 12 trials that compared surgery and radiation with or without adjuvant chemotherapy. Again, a survival advantage was not seen for patients with stage IA disease, and data remains controversial for stage IB. Based on subset analyses of two adjuvant chemotherapy trials, it appears that adjuvant chemotherapy may be beneficial for patients with larger stage IB tumors ≥4 cm (39,45).

The current standard treatment for patients with completely resected high-risk stage IB (≥4 cm), II, or IIIA NSCLC is a cisplatin-based, two-drug regimen for 12 weeks. Preexisting comorbidities, performance status, and time since surgery should be taken into account in the decision to pursue adjuvant chemotherapy. The combination of cisplatin plus vinorelbine was used in the majority of the positive adjuvant trials, but is associated with a relatively high rate of severe toxicities. The National Comprehensive Cancer Network (NCCN) guidelines for adjuvant chemotherapy now include other platinum-based, two-drug regimens that contain pemetrexed, docetaxel, or gemcitabine based on studies in advanced NSCLC that demonstrate equivalent efficacy with less toxicity (46). Since all of the positive adjuvant trials utilized cisplatin-based regimens, this agent should be favored, but carboplatin may be substituted in patients in whom cisplatin is contraindicated or poorly tolerated.

Targeted Adjuvant Therapy

Recently, efforts have focused on the potential role of newer targeted therapies and immunotherapy in the adjuvant setting. Clinical trials are currently underway to evaluate the role of these novel strategies in search of options that are more effective and less toxic than standard chemotherapy. The phase III Eastern Cooperative Oncology Group (ECOG) 1505 study evaluated chemotherapy with or without bevacizumab, a monoclonal antibody targeting vascular endothelial growth factor (VEGF), in the adjuvant setting (47). In this trial, patients with completely resected stage IB, II, or IIIA NSCLC were randomized to cisplatin-based chemotherapy with or without bevacizumab, and there were no significant differences in overall survival (HR 0.99) or disease-free survival (HR 0.98) between the two groups.

Studies evaluating the use of epidermal growth factor receptor (EGFR) tyrosine kinase inhibitors (TKI) in the adjuvant setting have suggested a trend in the improvement of disease-free survival, but no advantage in overall survival, so their use as adjuvant therapy remains controversial. The phase III RADIANT trial randomized patients with completely resected NSCLC, regardless of *EGFR* mutation status, to adjuvant erlotinib versus placebo and found no statistically significant differences in disease-free or overall survival (48). However, among the subgroup of patients whose tumors harbored sensitizing *EGFR* mutations, there was a nonsignificant trend toward improved disease-free survival in the erlotinib group (HR 0.61). Further studies are currently evaluating adjuvant EGFR TKIs in patients with *EGFR*-mutated NSCLC.

The Adjuvant Lung Cancer Enrichment Marker Identification and Sequencing Trial (ALCHEMIST) is an ongoing randomized, phase III study that is evaluating the role of individualized, genotype-directed therapy in the adjuvant setting. Patients with completely resected stage IB, II, or IIIA NSCLC undergo tumor analysis for *EGFR* mutation and *ALK* gene arrangement. If either of these driver-mutations is identified, then the patient can be randomized to receive appropriate targeted therapy (erlotinib or crizotinib, respectively) or placebo for 2 years following completion of standard adjuvant chemotherapy. In light of the recent Food and Drug Administration (FDA) approval of immune checkpoint inhibitors targeting the PD-1/PD-L1 pathway in patients with advanced-stage NSCLC, a third arm has been added to the ALCHEMIST study in which patients whose tumors are *EGFR* and *ALK* wild-type are randomized to receive nivolumab, an anti-PD-1 monoclonal antibody, or undergo standard surveillance without further therapy. As our understanding of the genomic heterogeneity and complexity of NSCLC advances, further definition of which patients are more likely to benefit from these novel adjuvant therapy strategies should follow.

NONSURGICAL THERAPY

Stereotactic Body Radiation Therapy

Many lung cancer patients are considered medically inoperable due to cardiovascular, pulmonary, or other comorbidities. Historically, conventionally fractionated radiation therapy (RT) was used for patients too frail to tolerate surgery. Unfortunately, this approach had high rates of local and regional failure, as well as treatment-related toxicity. Over the past two decades, several nonsurgical modalities have been developed for the treatment of early stage NSCLC, including SBRT, a strategy that employs very large (ablative) doses of radiation delivered in one to five fractions using highly conformal techniques. SBRT requires the use of computerized treatment planning, precise tumor tracking, and noncolinear and noncoplanar beams which allow for a steep decrease of the radiation dose outside of the treatment volume. The earliest reports on the use of SBRT for the treatment of NSCLC appeared in the mid-1990s from Sweden and Japan (49–51), and included patients with early stage NSCLC and pulmonary metastases that were medically unfit for pulmonary resection. The first series examining SBRT for stage I NSCLC exclusively reported a 94% local control rate in 50 patients treated with 50 to 60 Gy in five to ten fractions with minimal toxicity (51).

Interest in this technology grew dramatically in 2004 following a retrospective review of 245 patients with stage I NSCLC treated with SBRT at 14 Japanese centers (52). Treatment schedules varied significantly and the report included both medically operable and inoperable patients. The overall 2-year local control rate was 86%, but was higher in patients receiving a biologically effective dose (BED) greater than 100 Gy than in those receiving BED less than

100 Gy (92% vs. 73%). The overall survival rate was 56% at 3 years and 47% at 5 years, and was significantly better in medically fit patients. The overall survival rate for medically fit patients with stage IA NSCLC treated with BED greater than 100 Gy was 90% at 3 years (52).

Between 2002 and 2008, more than 25 single institution, prospective, phase I and II trials reported results on the use of SBRT for medically inoperable patients with stage I NSCLC. Local control rates ranged from 70% to 100% and were better with doses greater than 48 Gy. Follow-up was less than 3 years in almost all series, but overall survival rates ranged from 47% to 91% at 1 year, with much of the mortality attributed to medical comorbidities. Adverse events occurred in 0% to 20% of patients in most series, with cough, dyspnea, fatigue, musculoskeletal pain, and pneumonitis being the most frequent (53–55).

In 2010, the Radiation Therapy Oncology Group (RTOG) reported the first prospective multicenter, cooperative group study of SBRT for early stage peripheral NSCLC (RTOG 0236). In this phase II trial, medically inoperable patients received 54 Gy in three fractions. Eligible patients had peripheral (≥2 cm from the central trachea-bronchial tree), biopsy-proven NSCLC ≤5 cm in maximum diameter. In 55 evaluable patients with a median follow-up of 34.4 months, the 3-year primary tumor control rate was 97.6% and the overall survival rate was 55.8% (56). The high local control rate was felt to be responsible for the study's high survival rate compared to historic reports of conventional RT techniques.

Since publication of RTOG 0236, grouped data from multiple trials have also reported 3-year local tumor control rates greater than 90% following SBRT for peripheral NSCLC (57). SBRT has emerged as the standard-of-care for medically inoperable patients with peripheral, early stage NSCLC. However, significant practice variations exist for the treatment of large, multifocal, recurrent, or centrally located tumors, and for patients who are medically operable or lack tissue confirmation.

Toxicity of SBRT

SBRT of peripheral tumors can result in toxicity to the skin, soft tissue, and bone of the chest wall. Neuropathic pain and rib fractures occur in 10% to 15% of patients with tumors abutting the chest wall (58). There were initial concerns that lung SBRT would carry a significant risk for lung toxicity in patients with limited pulmonary reserve, but grade 3–4 pulmonary complications were reported in only 16% of patients treated on RTOG 0236 (59). On further review, most of these were prespecified changes in PFT values as opposed to symptomatic lung injury (60). Several subsequent studies have demonstrated minimal PFT changes after SBRT for peripheral lesions (61, 62). Poor pulmonary function and low FEV_1 are predictors of poor survival, but do not correlate with increased treatment-related toxicity (53). Lung toxicity correlates more strongly with tumor size and location. SBRT is a safe treatment modality for stage I NSCLC in fragile, high-risk populations and poor pulmonary function should not exclude patients from SBRT.

Percutaneous Ablative Therapy

Percutaneous ablation is another area of evolving technology for the treatment of thoracic malignancies. Three major modalities are within this realm: RFA, MWA, and cryotherapy. All are typically performed with sedation under CT guidance, and are best suited for small tumors without nodal metastases. RFA and MWA rely on tumor cell coagulation necrosis resulting from temperatures greater than 60°C, while CRYO causes cell death as a result of freezing and thawing.

Radiofrequency Ablation

Of the three modalities, RFA has undergone the greatest amount of clinical evaluation in NSCLC. RFA is recognized for its ease of use, single-setting treatment, tolerability, and cost effectiveness, but, to date, the majority of the data supporting its use in the lung has come from retrospective, single-institution reports that have combined early stage NSCLC with lung metastases with a focus on extremely short-term outcomes. Numerous case series have demonstrated that RFA is safe and feasible for the treatment of medically inoperable patients with early stage NSCLC. The first multi-institutional, prospective evaluation of RFA for such patients was reported by Dupuy et al. in 2015 (63). Fifty-one patients with biopsy-proven T1N0 NSCLC were treated with RFA at 16 institutions; all were deemed medically inoperable by a thoracic surgeon and had clinical follow-up through 2 years. In this frail patient population, RFA demonstrated an excellent safety profile, tolerability, and preservation of pulmonary function. Local recurrences occurred in 40% at 2 years, a figure that is consistent with other series using RFA for early stage NSCLC (64,65). Local control was better for tumors less than 2 cm, but was still not equivalent to that reported for SBRT or sublobar resection. Thermal ablative technologies for NSCLC are limited by tumor size and proximity to bronchovascular structures, the esophagus, pericardium, or trachea. RFA must be used cautiously in lesions greater than 3 cm or within 1 cm of hilar structures because of the risk of incomplete ablation and damage to central structures.

Microwave Ablation

MWA is a thermal-based ablative system which generates heat and coagulation via electromagnetic waves. The theoretical advantage of MWA over RFA is that it generates higher temperatures with a steeper tissue drop off, which allows for shorter treatment times and less of a heat-sink effect. The technology is far less established than RFA and there are only scant reports of its safety and efficacy for pulmonary tumors (66).

Cryotherapy

Cryotherapy is also performed percutaneously under CT guidance, but uses an argon-based freezing system. A unique aspect of cryotherapy is that the formation of an ice ball can be followed with CT. Multiple probes and multiple freeze-thaw cycles are typically required for tumors greater than 2 cm. As with RFA, there can be an incomplete treatment effect in peripheral zones of the tumor, so a 3 to 5 mm margin is recommended. A unique advantage of cryotherapy is the ability to use it for treatment of central tumors, because it preserves collagenous structures.

Radiographic Follow-Up Postablation

All percutaneous ablative therapies result in predictable, posttreatment CT changes. Immediately following ablation, the tumor typically increases in size and takes on a ground-glass appearance with "bubble lucencies" (67). These changes resolve over the first month and by 3 months, the lesion should decrease in size and become denser. An increase in size after 3 months is suspicious for persistent or recurrent disease. Tumors adjacent to segmental bronchi have a tendency to cavitate, while those in the periphery of the lung become linear or wedge shaped with pleural tags and pleural thickening (67). One recent report also noted reversible regional lymph node enlargement with moderate increases in FDG-PET activity following RFA as a result of treatment-related inflammation (68). Close surveillance without further intervention is recommended for typical CT changes for at least 6 months after treatment.

SUMMARY

The management of NSCLC is no longer a "one treatment fits all" scenario. Novel approaches to treatment are far more personalized and take advantage of the unique characteristics of each tumor and each individual patient. For early stage disease, in which surgery can cure 50% to 80% of patients, the development of safer, less invasive strategies is essential. VATS is now recognized as having oncologic equivalence to open procedures, and investigators are reevaluating the use of sublobar resections as a means of preserving pulmonary function. The increased accuracy of CT and FDG-PET have allowed for the emergence of nonsurgical, CT-guided ablative therapies as safe and effective therapeutic options for early stage, lymph node-negative NSCLC. While still experimental for medically fit populations, these techniques are quickly gaining wide acceptance for use in compromised, high-risk populations.

KEY POINTS

- Surgical resection is the primary curative treatment for patients with stage I or II NSCLC who have adequate pulmonary and cardiac reserve.
- Lobectomy or greater plus mediastinal lymph node sampling is the standard procedure for most patients with early stage NSCLC.
- Video-assisted thoracoscopic or robotic-assisted lobectomy appears to yield equivalent oncologic outcomes as lobectomy via open thoracotomy with decreased perioperative morbidity.
- Sublobar resections (wedge resection; segmentectomy) are being explored for treatment of patients with small, peripheral NSCLCs with favorable histologies.
- Adjuvant chemotherapy with platinum-based, two-drug regimens improves overall survival after complete resection of stage II and III NSCLC. Patients with high-risk stage IB tumors (≥4 cm) may also benefit from adjuvant chemotherapy.
- Postoperative RT is detrimental in patients with resected stage I or II NSCLC, but may offer a survival benefit in selected patients with resected stage IIIA-N2 disease.
- SBRT provides effective local control of stage I NSCLC in patients who are medically inoperable or who decline surgical intervention.
- Radiofrequency ablation and cryotherapy are percutaneous ablative techniques that can provide local control in medically inoperable patients with stage I NSCLC.

REFERENCES

1. Edge S, Byrd DR, Compton CC, et al. *AJCC Cancer Staging Handbook*. New York, NY: Springer; 2010:303.
2. Brunelli A, Kim AW, Berger KI, Addrizzo-Harris DJ. Physiologic evaluation of the patient with lung cancer being considered for resectional surgery: diagnosis and management of lung cancer, 3rd ed: American College of Chest Physicians evidence-based clinical practice guidelines. *Chest*. 2013;143:e166S-e190S.
3. Brunelli A, Varela G, Salati M, et al. Recalibration of the revised cardiac risk index in lung resection candidates. *Ann Thorac Surg*. 2010;90:199-203.
4. Darling GE, Allen MS, Decker PA, et al. Randomized trial of mediastinal lymph node sampling versus complete lymphadenectomy during pulmonary resection in the patient with N0 or N1 (less than hilar) non-small cell carcinoma: results of the American College of Surgery Oncology Group Z0030 Trial. *J Thorac Cardiovasc Surg*. 2011;141:662-670.
5. Allen MS, Darling GE, Pechet TT, et al. Morbidity and mortality of major pulmonary resections in patients with early-stage lung cancer: initial results of the randomized, prospective ACOSOG Z0030 trial. *Ann Thorac Surg*. 2006;81:1013-1019; discussion 9-20.
6. Ginsberg RJ, Hill LD, Eagan RT, et al. Modern thirty-day operative mortality for surgical resections in lung cancer. *J Thorac Cardiovasc Surg*. 1983;86:654-658.
7. Pignon JP, Tribodet TH, Scagliotti G, et al. Lung adjuvant cisplatin evaluation: a pooled analysis by the LACE Collaborative Group. *J Clin Oncol*. 2008;26:3552-3559.
8. Rocco G, Internullo E, Cassivi SD, et al. The variability of practice in minimally invasive thoracic surgery for pulmonary resections. *Thorac Surg Clin*. 2008;18:235-247.
9. Jacobaeus H. Ueber die Zystotskopie bei Untersuchung seroser hohlungen Anzuqwnden. *Munich Med Wochenschr*. 1910;57:2090-2092.
10. Kirby TJ, Mack MJ, Landreneau RJ, Rice TW. Initial experience with video-assisted thoracoscopic lobectomy. *Ann Thorac Surg*. 1993;56:1248-1252; discussion 52-53.
11. Kohno T, Murakami T, Wakabayashi A. Anatomic lobectomy of the lung by means of thoracoscopy. An experimental study. *J Thorac Cardiovasc Surg*. 1993;105:729-731.
12. Landreneau RJ, Hazelrigg SR, Mack MJ, et al. Postoperative pain-related morbidity: video-assisted thoracic surgery versus thoracotomy. *Ann Thorac Surg*. 1993;56:1285-1289.
13. Walker WS, Carnochan FM, Pugh GC. Thoracoscopic pulmonary lobectomy. Early operative experience and preliminary clinical results. *J Thorac Cardiovasc Surg*. 1993;106:1111-1117.
14. Ali MK, Mountain CF, Ewer MS, et al. Predicting loss of pulmonary function after pulmonary resection for bronchogenic carcinoma. *Chest*. 1980;77(3):337-342.

15. McKenna RJ Jr., Houck W, Fuller CB. Video-assisted thoracic surgery lobectomy: experience with 1,100 cases. *Ann Thorac Surg*. 2006;81: 421-425; discussion 5-6.
16. Onaitis MW, Petersen RP, Balderson SS, et al. Thoracoscopic lobectomy is a safe and versatile procedure: experience with 500 consecutive patients. *Ann Surg*. 2006;244:420-425.
17. Shaw JP, Dembitzer FR, Wisnivesky JP, et al. Video-assisted thoracoscopic lobectomy: state of the art and future directions. *Ann Thorac Surg*. 2008;85:S705-S709.
18. Swanson SJ, Herndon JE 2nd, D'Amico TA, et al. Video-assisted thoracic surgery lobectomy: report of CALGB 39802—a prospective, multi-institution feasibility study. *J Clin Oncol*. 2007;25:4993-4997.
19. Jones RO, Casali G, Walker WS. Does failed video-assisted lobectomy for lung cancer prejudice immediate and long-term outcomes? *Ann Thorac Surg*. 2008;86:235-239.
20. Ceppa DP, Kosinski AS, Berry MF, et al. Thoracoscopic lobectomy has increasing benefit in patients with poor pulmonary function: a Society of Thoracic Surgeons Database analysis. *Ann Surg*. 2012;256:487-493.
21. Burt BM, Kosinski AS, Shrager JB, et al. Thoracoscopic lobectomy is associated with acceptable morbidity and mortality in patients with predicted postoperative forced expiratory volume in 1 second or diffusing capacity for carbon monoxide less than 40% of normal. *J Thorac Cardiovasc Surg*. 2014;148(1):19-28.
22. Boffa DJ, Kosinski AS, Paul S, et al. Lymph node evaluation by open or video-assisted approaches in 11,500 anatomic lung cancer resections. *Ann Thorac Surg*. 2012;94:347-353; discussion 53.
23. Dylewski MR, Ohaeto AC, Pereira JF. Pulmonary resection using a total endoscopic robotic video-assisted approach. *Semin Thorac Cardiovasc Surg*. 2011;23:36-42.
24. Gharagozloo F, Margolis M, Tempesta B. Robot-assisted thoracoscopic lobectomy for early-stage lung cancer. *Ann Thorac Surg*. 2008;85: 1880-1885; discussion 5-6.
25. Cerfolio RJ, Bryant AS, Skylizard L, et al. Initial consecutive experience of completely portal robotic pulmonary resection with 4 arms. *J Thorac Cardiovasc Surg*. 2011;142:740-746.
26. Giulianotti PC, Buchs NC, Caravaglios G, et al. Robot-assisted lung resection: outcomes and technical details. *Interact Cardiovasc Thorac Surg*. 2010;11:388-392.
27. Park BJ, Melfi A, Mussi A, et al. Robotic lobectomy for non-small cell lung cancer (NSCLC): long-term oncologic results. *J Thorac Cardiovasc Surg*. 2012;143:383-389.
28. Park BJ, Flores RM. Cost comparison of robotic, video-assisted thoracic surgery and thoracotomy approaches to pulmonary lobectomy. *Thorac Surg Clin*. 2008;18:297-300.
29. Ginsberg RJ, Rubinstein LV. Randomized trial of lobectomy versus limited resection for T1 N0 non-small cell lung cancer. Lung Cancer Study Group. *Ann Thorac Surg*. 1995;60:615-622; discussion 22-23.

30. Koike T, Togashi K, Shirato T, et al. Limited resection for noninvasive bronchioloalveolar carcinoma diagnosed by intraoperative pathologic examination. *Ann Thorac Surg*. 2009;88:1106-1111.
31. Suzuki K, Kusumoto M, Watanabe S, et al. Radiologic classification of small adenocarcinoma of the lung: radiologic-pathologic correlation and its prognostic impact. *Ann Thorac Surg*. 2006;81:413-419.
32. Ishiwa N, Ogawa N, Shoji A, et al. Correlation between lymph node micrometastasis and histologic classification of small lung adenocarcinomas, in considering the indication of limited surgery. *Lung Cancer*. 2003;39:159-164.
33. Yamada S, Kohno T. Video-assisted thoracic surgery for pure ground-glass opacities 2 cm or less in diameter. *Ann Thorac Surg*. 2004;77:1911-1915.
34. Yamato Y, Tsuchida M, Watanabe T, et al. Early results of a prospective study of limited resection for bronchioloalveolar adenocarcinoma of the lung. *Ann Thorac Surg*. 2001;71:971-974.
35. Watanabe S, Watanabe T, Arai K, et al. Results of wedge resection for focal bronchioloalveolar carcinoma showing pure ground-glass attenuation on computed tomography. *Ann Thorac Surg*. 2002;73:1071-1075.
36. Watanabe T, Okada A, Imakiire T, et al. Intentional limited resection for small peripheral lung cancer based on intraoperative pathologic exploration. *Jpn J Thorac Cardiovasc Surg*. 2005;53:29-35.
37. Howington JA, Blum MG, Chang AC, et al. Treatment of stage I and II non-small cell lung cancer: diagnosis and management of lung cancer, 3rd ed: American College of Chest Physicians evidence-based clinical practice guidelines. *Chest*. 2013;143:e278S-e313S.
38. Douillard JY, Rosell R, De Lena M, et al. Adjuvant vinorelbine plus cisplatin versus observation in patients with completely resected stage IB-IIIA non-small-cell lung cancer (Adjuvant Navelbine International Trialist Association [ANITA]): a randomised controlled trial. *Lancet Oncol*. 2006;7:719-727.
39. Winton T, Livingston R, Johnson D, et al. Vinorelbine plus cisplatin vs. observation in resected non-small-cell lung cancer. *N Engl J Med*. 2005;352:2589-2597.
40. Arriagada R, Bergman B, Dunant A, et al. Cisplatin-based adjuvant chemotherapy in patients with completely resected non-small-cell lung cancer. *N Engl J Med*. 2004;350:351-360.
41. Waller D, Peake MD, Stephens RJ, et al. Chemotherapy for patients with non-small cell lung cancer: the surgical setting of the Big Lung Trial. *Eur J Cardiothorac Surg*. 2004;26:173-182.
42. Cheng D, Downey RJ, Kernstine K, et al. Video-assisted thoracic surgery in lung cancer resection: a meta-analysis and systematic review of controlled trials. *Innovations (Phila)*. 2007;2:261-292.
43. Lally BE, Zelterman D, Colasanto JM, et al. Postoperative radiotherapy for stage II or III non-small-cell lung cancer using the surveillance, epidemiology, and end results database. *J Clin Oncol*. 2006;24:2998-3006.

44. Burdett S, Pignon JP, Tierney J, et al. Adjuvant chemotherapy for resected early-stage non-small cell lung cancer. *Cochrane Database Syst Rev*. 2015:CD011430.
45. Strauss GM, Herndon JE 2nd, Maddaus MA, et al. Adjuvant paclitaxel plus carboplatin compared with observation in stage IB non-small-cell lung cancer: CALGB 9633 with the Cancer and Leukemia Group B, Radiation Therapy Oncology Group, and North Central Cancer Treatment Group Study Groups. *J Clin Oncol*. 2008;26:5043-5051.
46. National Comprehensive Cancer Network. NCCN guidelines: non-small cell lung cancer. https://www.nccn.org/professionals/physician_gls/f_guidelines_nojava.asp
47. Wakelee HA, Dahlberg SE, Brahmer JR, et al. Differential effect of age on survival in advanced NSCLC in women versus men: analysis of recent Eastern Cooperative Oncology Group (ECOG) studies, with and without bevacizumab. *Lung Cancer*. 2012;76:410-415.
48. Kelly K, Altorki NK, Eberhardt WE, et al. Adjuvant erlotinib versus placebo in patients with stage IB-IIIA non-small-cell lung cancer (RADIANT): a randomized, double-blind, phase III trial. *J Clin Oncol*. 2015;33:4007-4014.
49. Blomgren H, Lax I, Naslund I, Svanstrom R. Stereotactic high dose fraction radiation therapy of extracranial tumors using an accelerator. Clinical experience of the first thirty-one patients. *Acta Oncol*. 1995;34:861-870.
50. Nagata Y, Negoro Y, Aoki T, et al. Clinical outcomes of 3D conformal hypofractionated single high-dose radiotherapy for one or two lung tumors using a stereotactic body frame. *Int J Radiat Oncol Biol Phys*. 2002;52:1041-1046.
51. Uematsu M, Shioda A, Suda A, et al. Computed tomography-guided frameless stereotactic radiotherapy for stage I non-small cell lung cancer: a 5-year experience. *Int J Radiat Oncol Biol Phys*. 2001;51:666-670.
52. Onishi H, Araki T, Shirato H, et al. Stereotactic hypofractionated high-dose irradiation for stage I nonsmall cell lung carcinoma: clinical outcomes in 245 subjects in a Japanese multiinstitutional study. *Cancer*. 2004;101:1623-1631.
53. Henderson M, McGarry R, Yiannoutsos C, et al. Baseline pulmonary function as a predictor for survival and decline in pulmonary function over time in patients undergoing stereotactic body radiotherapy for the treatment of stage I non-small-cell lung cancer. *Int J Radiat Oncol Biol Phys*. 2008;72:404-409.
54. Timmerman R, McGarry R, Yiannoutsos C, et al. Excessive toxicity when treating central tumors in a phase II study of stereotactic body radiation therapy for medically inoperable early-stage lung cancer. *J Clin Oncol*. 2006;24:4833-4839.
55. Paludan M, Traberg Hansen A, Petersen J, et al. Aggravation of dyspnea in stage I non-small cell lung cancer patients following stereotactic body radiotherapy: is there a dose-volume dependency? *Acta Oncol*. 2006;45:818-822.

56. Timmerman R, Paulus R, Galvin J, et al. Stereotactic body radiation therapy for inoperable early stage lung cancer. *JAMA*. 2010;303:1070-1076.
57. Chi A, Liao Z, Nguyen NP, et al. Systemic review of the patterns of failure following stereotactic body radiation therapy in early-stage non-small-cell lung cancer: clinical implications. *Radiother Oncol*. 2010;94:1-11.
58. Hoppe BS, Laser B, Kowalski AV, et al. Acute skin toxicity following stereotactic body radiation therapy for stage I non-small-cell lung cancer: who's at risk? *Int J Radiat Oncol Biol Phys*. 2008;72:1283-1286.
59. Timmerman R, Paulus R, Galvin J, et al. Stereotactic body radiation therapy for inoperable early stage lung cancer. *JAMA*. 2010;303:1070-1076.
60. Stanic S, Paulus R, Timmerman RD, et al. No clinically significant changes in pulmonary function following stereotactic body radiation therapy for early-stage peripheral non-small cell lung cancer: an analysis of RTOG 0236. *Int J Radiat Oncol Biol Phys*. 2014;88:1092-1099.
61. Takeda A, Enomoto T, Sanuki N, et al. Reassessment of declines in pulmonary function ≥1 year after stereotactic body radiotherapy. *Chest*. 2013;143:130-137.
62. Stephans KL, Djemil T, Reddy CA, et al. Comprehensive analysis of pulmonary function test (PFT) changes after stereotactic body radiotherapy (SBRT) for stage I lung cancer in medically inoperable patients. *J Thorac Oncol*. 2009;4:838-844.
63. Dupuy DE, Fernando HC, Hillman S, et al. Radiofrequency ablation of stage IA non-small cell lung cancer in medically inoperable patients: results from the American College of Surgeons Oncology Group Z4033 (Alliance) trial. *Cancer*. 2015;121:3491-3498.
64. Lanuti M, Sharma A, Digumarthy SR, et al. Radiofrequency ablation for treatment of medically inoperable stage I non-small cell lung cancer. *J Thorac Cardiovasc Surg*. 2009;137:160-166.
65. Simon CJ, Dupuy DE, DiPetrillo TA, et al. Pulmonary radiofrequency ablation: long-term safety and efficacy in 153 patients. *Radiology*. 2007;243:268-275.
66. Wolf FJ, Grand DJ, Machan JT, et al. Microwave ablation of lung malignancies: effectiveness, CT findings, and safety in 50 patients. *Radiology*. 2008;247:871-879.
67. Bojarski JD, Dupuy DE, Mayo-Smith WW. CT imaging findings of pulmonary neoplasms after treatment with radiofrequency ablation: results in 32 tumors. *AJR Am J Roentgenol*. 2005;185:466-471.
68. Sharma A, Digumarthy SR, Kalra MK, et al. Reversible locoregional lymph node enlargement after radiofrequency ablation of lung tumors. *AJR Am J Roentgenol*. 2010;194:1250-1256.

7 Management of Locally Advanced Non–Small-Cell Lung Cancer

Smitha P. Menon and Elizabeth M. Gore

Locally advanced non–small-cell lung cancer (LA-NSCLC) refers to disease that is unresectable or not curable with surgery alone. This currently includes stages IIIA (T4 N0 M0; T3-4 N1 M0; T1-3 N2 M0) and IIIB (T4 N2 M0; T1-4 N3 M0). In the upcoming revision of the TNM staging criteria (AJCC, eighth edition), patients with more extensive T3-T4 N3 M0 disease will be reclassified as stage IIIC, with a similar prognosis as patients with stage IVA disease (1). Selected patients with limited-extent stage IIIA NSCLC may be treated surgically, whereas patients with more advanced, unresectable disease or those who are medically inoperable are primarily treated with concurrent chemotherapy and radiation (2). Radiation therapy (RT) alone or sequential chemoradiotherapy is appropriate for patients who are not expected to tolerate concurrent chemoradiotherapy due to poor performance status, multiple or severe comorbid conditions, excessive weight loss, or large volume disease (2).

MEDICALLY INOPERABLE OR UNRESECTABLE LA-NSCLC

The majority of patients with LA-NSCLC have unresectable disease. This includes patients with T4 disease due to invasion of local structures, N3 disease, or multilevel or bulky (>3 cm) N2 lymph node involvement. Medically inoperable patients have potentially resectable disease, but have poor cardiopulmonary function (e.g., FEV_1 < 2.0 L/sec or predicted postoperative functional lung volume <800 mL) or other comorbid conditions that may preclude surgery. In addition to resectable stage IIIA disease, this population may also include medically inoperable patients with stage II disease (primary tumor >5 cm and/or N1 disease).

For patients who are not fit for surgery or have unresectable disease, local-regional disease control and long-term survival are best achieved with concurrent chemotherapy and radiation. Concurrent chemotherapy augments the activity of radiation to improve local-regional control, while also decreasing the risk of distant metastases. The standard radiation dose is 60 Gy delivered in 2 Gy per fraction prescribed to a volume that encompasses the primary tumor and involved regional lymph nodes. RT is generally delivered concurrently with a platinum-based, two-drug chemotherapy regimen.

Patient Selection

Historically, RT alone was prescribed for patients with unresectable lung cancer. Clinical trials to improve local control and decrease distant failures have focused on increasing the intensity of both local and systemic therapies through the use of sequential chemotherapy, concurrent chemoradiotherapy, escalated dose RT, and altered RT fractionation. Trials evaluating aggressive multimodality therapy for unresectable lung cancer have usually included only patients with a favorable Karnofsky performance status (KPS ≥ 70) and limited weight loss, generally defined as greater than 10% in the month prior to diagnosis. A general guideline for baseline pulmonary function that would allow for definitive RT is FEV_1 greater than 1.2 L/s or ≥ 50% predicted. However, treatment eligibility should be individualized based on disease volume and the volume of lung that will be included in the RT portals. Although age is not usually a specific eligibility criterion, the majority of patients enrolled on multimodality trials have been less than 70 years old. Older patients on these trials tend to do as well as younger patients, likely due to careful selection of only the fittest elderly patients with limited comorbidities. Although data are inconsistent, increased esophageal, pulmonary, and hematologic toxicity has been reported in older patients (3, 4). Additionally, older patients tend to have less physical and psychosocial reserve, do not tolerate the side effects of therapy as well, and frequently need more supportive care than younger patients. Careful patient selection, aggressive supportive care, and conservative RT dose parameters for normal tissues should be considered for elderly patients or patients with poor performance status.

Radiation Therapy

The standard RT dose is based on the outcomes of a phase III trial published in 1980 that randomized patients to receive either 40 Gy split–course RT or 40 Gy, 50 Gy, or 60 Gy continuous RT (5). The median survival with RT alone was 12 months with improved survival in the higher dose arm. RT-based strategies to improve local-regional control and survival rates have included dose escalation, altered fractionation, and the addition of concurrent or sequential chemotherapy.

Hyperfractionated RT

Hyperfractionated RT is the delivery of radiation at a lower than standard dose per fraction with more than one fraction per day. The lower dose per fraction decreases the risk of late radiation complications and allows for a higher total dose of RT to the target without increasing toxicity. Radiation Therapy Oncology Group (RTOG) 8311, a phase I/II trial, randomized patients to 60 Gy, 64.8 Gy, 69.6 Gy, 74.4, or 79.2 Gy delivered at 1.2 Gy per fraction given twice daily. Overall, there was no difference in acute or late toxicity among the five arms. In a subset of patients with KPS ≥70 and weight loss of less than 6%, survival was significantly better with 69.6 Gy than with the lower doses ($P = .02$). However, there was no survival advantage for doses higher than 69.6 Gy (6). Based on these results, 69.6 Gy at 1.2 Gy per fraction twice daily was used in RTOG 8808, an Intergroup phase III study comparing hyperfractionated RT alone, standard fractionation RT alone and standard RT with neoadjuvant chemotherapy (discussed in the following section).

Sequential Chemoradiotherapy

A randomized phase III trial conducted by Cancer and Leukemia Group B (CALGB 8433) compared induction chemotherapy followed by standard RT to RT alone (7). Patients were randomized to receive cisplatin plus vinblastine followed by RT (60 Gy at 2.0 Gy per fraction) or the same RT alone. Median survival for the sequential chemotherapy plus RT group was 13.7 months compared to 9.6 months for the RT alone group ($P = .012$). RTOG 8808 confirmed these results while also evaluating hyperfractionated RT (8). Patients were randomized to cisplatin plus vinblastine followed by standard once-daily RT (60 Gy at 2.0 Gy per fraction), standard once-daily RT alone, or hyperfractionated, twice-daily RT alone (69.6 Gy at 1.2 Gy per fraction). Median survival with standard RT alone was 11.4 months; with sequential chemotherapy plus standard RT, 13.2 months; and with hyperfractionated RT, 12 months.

Concurrent Chemoradiotherapy

The follow-up study to RTOG 8808 was RTOG 9410, a phase III trial comparing concurrent chemotherapy plus either standard or hyperfractionated RT to sequential chemotherapy plus standard RT (9). Patients were randomized to either sequential cisplatin plus vinblastine with standard RT beginning after chemotherapy, cisplatin plus vinblastine with standard RT beginning on day 1 of chemotherapy, or cisplatin plus oral etoposide with hyperfractionated RT beginning on day 1 of chemotherapy. Median survival favored concurrent chemotherapy with once-daily RT to 60 Gy (17 months vs. 14.6 months with sequential therapy [*P* = .046] vs. 15.6 months with concurrent hyperfractionated RT [*P* = .46]).

High-Dose RT With Concurrent Chemotherapy

Three single-arm studies that evaluated dose escalation of standard fractionation RT with concurrent chemotherapy reported that 74 Gy was safe and resulted in a median overall survival of 24 to 37 months (10–12). These findings compared favorably to the historical median overall survival of 16.5 to 17 months reported with concurrent chemotherapy and standard dose (60 Gy) RT (9,13).

RTOG 0617 was designed to compare concurrent chemotherapy to standard RT 60 Gy to concurrent chemotherapy plus RT 74 Gy in addition to evaluating the potential benefit of concurrent cetuximab, an anti-epidermal growth factor receptor (EGFR) monoclonal antibody. All patients were to receive consolidative chemotherapy. This two-by-two factorial, phase III trial randomly assigned patients to receive concurrent chemotherapy plus either RT 60 Gy in 30 daily fractions, RT 74 Gy in 37 daily fractions, RT 60 Gy plus cetuximab, or RT 74 Gy plus cetuximab. The study did not show improved survival with 74 Gy and, in fact, suggested that high-dose RT might be detrimental (14). Median overall survival for the standard RT dose group was 28.7 months and for the high-dose group was 20.3 months (*P* = .008). On multivariate analysis, factors predicting overall survival were RT dose (60 Gy), maximum esophagitis grade, planning target volume (PTV), heart V5 (volume of heart receiving 5 Gy or more), and heart V30. The addition of cetuximab to concurrent chemoradiotherapy provided no overall survival benefit.

The median overall survival of 28 months reported in RTOG 0617 with concurrent chemoradiotherapy set a new benchmark (14) when compared to 17 months achieved in RTOG 9410 with the use of a similar regimen. This improvement is likely due to several factors, including stage migration with the incorporation of PET into the staging evaluation, advances in radiation technology, more careful patient selection, and an increased focus on supportive care. Advances in RT delivery include motion management, multimodality imaging for tumor definition, consistent use of three-dimensional conformal radiation therapy (3D-CRT) planning, intensity modulated radiotherapy (IMRT), and image guided radiation therapy (IGRT).

Impaired Patients

For patients who may not tolerate concurrent therapy or who have large volume disease that cannot be treated without exceeding normal tissue RT tolerance, sequential induction chemotherapy followed by definitive RT is a reasonable option with an expected median survival of 13 to 15 months (8,9,13). Induction chemotherapy may decrease disease volume, allowing for more focused delivery of RT to gross tumor with avoidance of normal tissue and less acute radiation toxicity.

For patients who cannot tolerate or refuse chemotherapy, RT alone can be used with an expected median survival of 11 to 18 months (8,15). Hypofractionated therapy regimens deliver a higher dose per fraction of RT to a lower total dose, allowing for a shorter course of therapy with an RT dose that is biologically equivalent to standard treatment. The shorter treatment course decreases the burden of therapy from 6 weeks of RT to 3 weeks, and 45 Gy in 15 3 Gy fractions has been shown to be effective in phase II prospective trials and institutional reviews (16–18).

Radiation Therapy Techniques

RT Dose

The generally accepted standard dose of RT for patients with LA-NSCLC is 60 Gy in 30 fractions delivered at 2 Gy per fraction, once a day, 5 days per week with concurrent chemotherapy. With such treatment, expected median survival is 28.7 months and the 2-year overall survival rate is 57.6% for patients with PET-staged stage III disease, performance status 0 to 1, weight loss less than 10% in 1 month, $FEV_1 \geq 1.2$ L/s, and no contralateral hilar or supraclavicular lymph nodes (10). For patients with poor performance status, extensive weight loss, or other co-morbidities precluding aggressive multimodality therapy, hypofractionated RT to 45 Gy at 3 Gy per fraction should be considered.

RT Simulation

CT simulations should be performed with the patient in a reproducible treatment position with appropriate immobilization. IV contrast is recommended and is particularly useful for target definition of centrally located disease. The use of PET/CT for treatment planning has been shown to improve target accuracy and local control (19). Assessment of three dimensional (3D) tumor and organ motion during simulation is essential for optimal treatment planning. Acceptable methods for motion assessment include fluoroscopy, CT at inhalation and exhalation, slow CT scan, and 4D-CT. It is important to note that respiratory motion changes over time, so reassessment during treatment is required. Motion control methods, including abdominal compression, breath hold, and gating, can be used to decrease the treatment volume needed to cover disease throughout the respiratory cycle. The American Association of Physics in Medicine (AAPM) Task Force 76 report on the management of respiratory motion in radiation oncology is recommended for guidelines on treatment planning and delivery (20).

RT Planning

Gross tumor volume (GTV) consists of all disease that is visible on imaging studies, including the primary tumor and all lymph nodes that are PET positive (SUV >3.0), biopsy-proven, or greater than 1 cm on short axis. The GTV is then expanded to include suspected subclinical disease to create the clinical target volume (CTV). Although the CTV expansion is typically 0.5 cm in lung parenchyma, it should also include involved nodal regions and be confined by normal anatomic boundaries with exclusion of tissues that are clearly not involved with disease, such as vertebral bodies, heart, and great vessels. Uninvolved nodal regions should not be included. The internal target volume (ITV) is technically defined by further expansion of the CTV to account for internal motion due to breathing and heart movement. This expansion ensures that all disease is included in the treatment field throughout the breathing cycle. The PTV is a final expansion, generally 3 to 5 mm that accounts for variations in daily treatment set up. The radiation dose is prescribed to the PTV with a minimum of 95% coverage. Any variations in coverage should be confined to regions of the PTV adjacent to critical structures. The maximum dose should be within the PTV and less than 110% of the prescribed dose.

Maximum acceptable doses to organs at risk (OAR) are listed in Table 7.1. Dose constraints should be tailored to the individual patient. Consideration should be given to factors that may influence the ability to tolerate therapy, such as comorbidities, prior weight loss, and age. Efforts should be made to confine the RT dose to the involved lobes of the ipsilateral lung in patients being treated preoperatively.

Three-Dimensional Conformal Radiation Therapy

3D-CRT uses individualized 3D digital data sets of a patient's tumor and normal adjacent anatomy to develop a radiation plan that typically uses greater than three beams or fields. Each field

Table 7.1 Maximum acceptable doses to organs at risk

Organ at risk	Maximum dose		Mean dose		Dose/volume	
	2 Gy/Fx	3 Gy/Fx	2 Gy/Fx	3 Gy/Fx	2 Gy/Fx	3 Gy/Fx
Lung	N/A	N/A	≤20 Gy	≤18 Gy	V20 < 35% V5 < 65%	V20 < 30%
Heart	≤70 Gy	≤50 Gy	Unknown	Unknown	V30 < 35% V35 < 35%	V30 < 35% V35 < 35%
Spinal cord	≤45 Gy	≤ 36 Gy	N/A	N/A	N/A	N/A
Esophagus	≤70 Gy	≤50 Gy	≤34 Gy	≤30 Gy	V35 < 50%	V30 < 50%
Brachial plexus	≤63 Gy	≤50 Gy	N/A	N/A	N/A	N/A

N/A, not applicable.

is individually shaped and directed to create a conformal dose distribution to the PTV, while sparing surrounding normal structures.

Intensity Modulated Radiation Therapy

Intensity modulated radiation therapy (IMRT) uses a similar data set to create the RT plan. The goal is to conform the dose to the disease and avoid normal tissues, similar to 3D-CRT, although the radiation intensity of each IMRT beam is divided into small segments and modulated throughout the treatment by the multileaf collimator (MLC) attached to the linear accelerator. With multiple modulated radiation segments, IMRT plans are much more conformal and typically result in better sparing of normal tissues.

IMRT usually provides dosimetric and clinical advantages for patients with LA-NSCLC being treated with curative intent RT. IMRT is particularly useful for tumor coverage of disease in close proximity to critical structures and in patients with large treatment volumes due to bulky disease or multilevel or contralateral lymph node involvement. IMRT plans typically will improve the ability to spare normal tissue, thereby minimizing toxicity and improving quality-of-life. In one study comparing IMRT to 3D-CRT, fewer patients who received IMRT had a clinically meaningful decline in quality-of-life 12 months after treatment (21% vs. 46%; *P* = .003) (21). Liao et al. showed an improvement in overall survival in 2 cohorts of patients treated with IMRT versus 3D-CRT; however, the patients treated with IMRT also had four dimensional CT (4D-CT) planning and quite possibly had better tumor coverage (22). Many insurance companies will not approve IMRT for lung cancer if published normal tissue dose constraints can be met with a 3D-CRT plan. Careful target volume definition utilizing CT and PET data with compensation for motion and set up variation and minimization of normal tissue doses with conformal RT fields with or without IMRT is critical for optimizing local-regional tumor control, overall survival, and quality-of-life.

Chemotherapy

Concurrent chemotherapy and RT is preferred over sequential and induction approaches. A meta-analysis of six trials including 1,024 patients demonstrated a 10% absolute overall survival benefit at 2 years with concurrent chemoradiotherapy when compared to sequential chemoradiotherapy (23). Induction chemotherapy, defined as two cycles of full-dose chemotherapy before concurrent chemoradiotherapy, is also not a recommended strategy. In CALGB 39801, 366 patients were assigned to either two doses of carboplatin plus paclitaxel (CP) followed by concurrent weekly CP plus RT or concurrent weekly CP plus RT without induction therapy. There was no significant improvement in survival with induction therapy (median, 14 vs. 12 months; *P* = .3), but toxicity was greater in the induction arm (24).

Selection of Chemotherapy Regimen

When choosing a chemotherapy regimen to combine with RT, agents that enhance the effects of radiation and provide effective systemic therapy without excessive toxicity are preferred. Toxicities that are unique to concurrent thoracic chemoradiotherapy include esophagitis and pneumonitis, so drugs that specifically increase pulmonary toxicity, such as gemcitabine, should be avoided. Common chemotherapy regimens that are utilized concurrently with RT are listed in Table 7.2. Although few clinical trials have directly compared chemotherapy regimens in patients with stage III NSCLC, the efficacy of each of these regimens appears to be similar. Therefore, the selection of an appropriate chemotherapy regimen should be guided by an individual patient's comorbidities, organ function, risk for specific toxicities, and clinician comfort level with the regimen.

Table 7.2 Recent data with concurrent chemoradiotherapy regimens

Study	Regimen	N	Response rate (%)	Overall survival Median (mo)	Overall survival 3-year (%)
Steuer et al. (26) (retrospective)	Cisplatin + pemetrexed	3,789	56	18.4	25
	Cisplatin + etoposide	3,194	65*	19.8*	31*
PROCLAIM (29) (prospective, phase III)	Cisplatin + pemetrexed	301	36	26.8	40
	Cisplatin + etoposide	297	33*	25.0*	37*
Choy et al. (30) (prospective, phase II)	Carboplatin + pemetrexed	46	52	18.7	45†
	Cisplatin + pemetrexed	52	46	27.0	58†

*Not statistically significant.
†2-year overall survival rate.

The two regimens that are used most frequently with concurrent RT are cisplatin plus etoposide (EP) and weekly CP (2). While there are no high-quality randomized trials comparing EP to CP, retrospective and pooled analyses suggest equivalent survival outcomes, but increased toxicity with EP. A retrospective analysis of a Veterans' Administration (VA) database reported on 1,842 patients with stage III NSCLC who underwent concurrent therapy, 27% of whom received EP and 73% CP. Survival was comparable between the two treatments, but EP was associated with increased incidence of hospitalization, infection, acute kidney injury, mucositis, and esophagitis (25). A more comprehensive pooled analysis compared data from 32 studies (3,194 patients) utilizing EP and 51 studies (3,789 patients) utilizing CP along with RT for patients with stage III NSCLC. Response rates (65% vs. 56%, $P = .6$), progression-free survival (11.5 vs. 9.3 months, $P = .2$), and overall survival (19.8 vs. 18.4 months, $P = .48$) were similar in EP and CP treated patients, respectively. Selected toxicities, including cytopenias, nausea, and vomiting, were more common with EP, but both regimens resulted in equivalent rates of esophagitis and pneumonitis (26). Median overall survival in this pooled analysis was less than 24 months for both regimens.

Other Chemotherapy Regimens

Cispaltin plus pemetrexed (PC) is a well-tolerated and effective first-line regimen for treatment of metastatic non-squamous NSCLC (27), and pemetrexed has been shown to be an effective radiosensitizer (28). In the phase III PROCLAIM study, RT plus concurrent PC followed by consolidation therapy with single-agent pemetrexed was compared to RT plus concurrent EP followed by consolidation with a nonpemetrexed containing regimen in patients with stage III non-squamous NSCLC (29). An interim analysis showed that the overall survival in the PC arm was not superior to that in the EP arm (median, 26.8 vs. 25 months, $P = .83$), so the study was discontinued for futility. PC had a more favorable toxicity profile with a lower incidence of grade 3 to 4 adverse events (64% vs. 76.8%, $P = .001$). The only exception was a higher rate of pneumonitis in the CP arm (17% vs. 11%, $P = .37$), but the incidence of severe pneumonitis remained low in both arms (<3%). Phase II studies evaluating carboplatin plus pemetrexed (PCb) given concurrently with RT have also shown an acceptable toxicity profile with a 2-year overall survival rate of 48% (30), offering another option for patients with non-squamous NSCLC who cannot tolerate cisplatin.

Consolidation Chemotherapy

Consolidation chemotherapy with docetaxel after EP is not recommended. A Hoosier Oncology Group study (LUN 01-24) reported that concurrent EP plus RT followed by consolidation docetaxel did not improve survival over concurrent EP plus RT alone. However, consolidation docetaxel was associated with high rates of pneumonitis (9.7%), hospitalization (29%), and treatment-related mortality (5.5%) (31).

In another randomized trial, consolidation cisplatin plus docetaxel after concurrent RT and weekly cisplatin plus docetaxel was compared to the same concurrent chemoradiotherapy regimen without consolidation. Both progression-free survival (median, 9.1 vs. 8.1 months, $P = .36$) and overall survival (21.8 vs. 20.6 months, $P = .44$) were similar in both arms of the study (32). However, cisplatin plus docetaxel is not a commonly used regimen and it is unclear if these results can be extrapolated to the more popular weekly CP regimen.

A pooled analysis of 41 studies including 3,400 patients suggested no benefit from consolidation chemotherapy, but was limited by the heterogeneity of study regimens and patient populations (33). Although supporting data are scarce, for patients receiving low-dose, "radiosensitizing" chemotherapy, such as weekly CP, consolidation chemotherapy may offer some benefit by providing higher-dose systemic therapy (34).

Targeted Therapy

Cetuximab, a monoclonal antibody targeting EGFR, was assessed in combination with concurrent CP and RT in RTOG 0617, and did not improve overall survival when compared to chemoradiotherapy alone (25 vs. 24 months, $P = .29$). However, cetuximab did increase grade 3 or higher toxicity (86% vs. 70%, $P < .0001$) (14). Gefitinib, an EGFR tyrosine kinase inhibitor, was tested against placebo as a maintenance strategy in patients with stage III NSCLC who completed concurrent EP plus RT followed by consolidation docetaxel. Importantly, patients were not selected for EGFR mutational status. Gefitinib had a negative impact on survival when compared to placebo (23 vs. 35 months, $P = .013$), mainly due to recurrent lung cancer (35).

In studies in both NSCLC and SCLC, the addition of bevacizumab, an antiangiogenic monoclonal antibody targeting vascular endothelial growth factor (VEGF), to concurrent chemoradiotherapy greatly increased the risk of tracheaesophageal fistula formation, and such combinations should be avoided (36).

RESECTABLE LA-NSCLC

Primary surgical resection is considered the standard treatment option for patients with stage IIIA—T3N1 NSCLC. The role of surgical resection for patients with more advanced LA-NSCLC remains controversial, but continues to be discussed due to the local failure rate of 30% to 40% for patients treated with standard concurrent chemoradiotherapy (15). When surgery is employed, it is generally preceded by neoadjuvant chemoradiotherapy or chemotherapy alone with or without postoperative RT. Neoadjuvant therapy followed by resection is most often considered in patients with minimal N2 disease involving nonbulky (<3 cm) lymph nodes in 1 to 2 nodal stations.

Patient Selection

Determination of the role of surgery in a patient with N2 lymph node involvement should be made prior to the initiation of any therapy by a multidisciplinary team including a board-certified thoracic surgeon with expertise in thoracic oncology (37). Appropriate patients should have technically resectable disease with low-volume lymph node involvement before the initiation of any therapy. Attempts to convert an unresectable cancer into a resectable cancer with neoadjuvant therapy are rarely successful and should be discouraged.

N2 Disease Burden

Predictors of a favorable outcome with surgery for patients with N2 lymph node involvement include low-volume N2 disease (<3 cm), single-station N2 disease, and nodal down-staging with preoperative therapy. A nonsurgical, combined-modality approach is recommended for patients with a high N2 disease burden.

Occult vs. clinical: Occult or "minimal" N2 disease refers to pathological involvement of the mediastinal lymph nodes found at resection in patients with negative radiographic and pathologic preoperative staging. Clinical N2 disease refers to patients with mediastinal lymph nodes that are enlarged by CT criteria (>1 cm in short axis), metabolically active by PET, and/or biopsy-proven during preoperative staging. The 5-year survival rate after primary surgical resection is 25% to 40% for patients with minimal N2 disease, but only 3% to 10% for those with clinical N2 disease (38–40). Therefore, primary surgical resection is not optimal therapy for patients with clinical N2 lymph node involvement. Patients with a high probability of N2 disease due to a central primary tumor or hilar lymph node involvement (N1) should undergo adequate mediastinal staging prior to resection. If N2 disease is detected, then appropriate treatment would be either definitive chemoradiotherapy or neoadjuvant therapy depending on the N2 disease burden.

Multistation N2 disease: Multistation nodal disease prior to therapy is a poor prognostic factor with a 5-year survival rate of 11% to 17% compared to 34% to 39% for single-station involvement (39–41). The number of lymph node stations involved is a key prognostic factor for both occult and clinical N2 disease. In a study of 702 patients with resected N2-positive NSCLC, the 5-year overall survival rate ranged from 3% in multistation disease to 8% with single-station involvement in patients with clinical N2 involvement compared to 11% and 34%, respectively, in the occult N2 group (40). Isolated N2 disease without N1 involvement, called skip N2, refers to a unique subset of patients with a favorable prognosis similar to those with only N1 involvement (42). In addition to the number of nodal stations involved, the absolute number of lymph nodes with metastatic foci also correlates with prognosis (43).

Location of nodes: Depending on the primary tumor location, a distinct pattern of regional spread to mediastinal nodes has been described (44). Nonregional spread is associated with a poorer prognosis (45). For example, left upper lobe tumors commonly spread to the aortopulmonary lymph nodes and patients with left upper lobe tumors and isolated spread to these nodes have a better prognosis with a 5-year survival rate of about 30% after resection compared to patients with subcarinal lymph node involvement who did not survive beyond 3 years from resection (46).

Mediastinal Staging

Mediastinal staging at diagnosis is important, not only for confirming suspicious nodal disease found on CT and PET, but also for evaluating for occult N3 and multistation N2 disease. Many surgeons have adopted the strategy of invasive mediastinal restaging after neoadjuvant therapy followed by resection only for patients who have been down-staged. Postinduction therapy mediastinal staging by CT, PET, endoscopic ultrasound (EUS), endobronchial ultrasound (EBUS), or repeat mediastinoscopy has a false-negative rate of 20% to 30% (47–50). Repeat mediastinoscopy is a technically difficult procedure, so initial, pretreatment mediastinal staging should be performed with EBUS and/or EUS, reserving mediastinoscopy for restaging after neoadjuvant therapy (51).

Pneumonectomy

Many studies have shown a high early mortality rate after pneumonectomy done following neoadjuvant therapy due to acute respiratory distress syndrome (ARDS) and other factors (52). This risk is higher in patients requiring a right pneumonectomy (53). The risk of surgery after concurrent chemoradiotherapy can be minimized with careful attention to radiotherapeutic and surgical technique, and optimal supportive care. Although pneumonectomy poses a higher risk, the potential need for a pneumonectomy is not an absolute contraindication to preoperative chemoradiotherapy for appropriately selected patients in experienced hands (54,55).

Preoperative Chemotherapy

Two small, landmark phase III trials from the 1990s that compared surgery alone to chemotherapy followed by surgery in patients with stage III NSCLC demonstrated a significant overall survival advantage with induction chemotherapy (median, 26–64 vs. 8–11 months) (56,57). Both studies closed early at interim analysis due to improved survival with chemotherapy. However, as noted earlier, surgery alone is inadequate therapy for most patients with stage III disease, and randomized trials comparing neoadjuvant chemotherapy to chemotherapy plus RT have not been performed. A recent meta-analysis showed a 13% reduction in the relative risk of death with preoperative chemotherapy in patients with stage I to III NSCLC (58).

While early neoadjuvant trials used obsolete, three-drug chemotherapy regimens, more recent studies have typically used standard, platinum-based, two-drug regimens for three cycles. With such regimens, response rates have ranged from 44% to 70% and pathologic compete response rates from 12% to 16%, with only 10% to 14% of patients having disease progression (59–61). A meta-analysis has shown that neoadjuvant chemotherapy provides an overall survival benefit that is comparable to that achieved by adjuvant chemotherapy (62). If induction chemotherapy is to be used, current clinical guidelines recommend a cisplatin-based, two-drug regimen similar to those used in the adjuvant setting with carboplatin substitution for patients who cannot tolerate cisplatin (2).

Preoperative Chemoradiotherapy

Pathologic complete response (pCR) and mediastinal down-staging after preoperative therapy are associated with improved survival (41,59). The addition of RT to chemotherapy in phase II trials increases the rate of mediastinal down-staging when compared to historical results with chemotherapy alone (63). Although phase III trials have shown an advantage for preoperative chemotherapy over surgery alone, concurrent chemoradiotherapy has not been adequately compared to chemotherapy alone in the preoperative setting. Recently, Pless et al. randomized 232 patients with resectable stage IIIA NSCLC to induction chemotherapy with cisplatin plus docetaxel followed by RT versus chemotherapy alone followed by resection and demonstrated no significant difference in event-free survival (12.8 vs. 11.6 months, $P = .67$) or overall survival (61). However, in this study, chemotherapy and RT were given sequentially rather than concurrently and the RT dose was 44 Gy delivered over 3 weeks.

The North American Intergroup trial 0139 is the largest phase III study that has prospectively addressed whether or not survival is improved with surgery after induction chemoradiotherapy for patients with stage IIIA (T1-3 pN2 M0) resectable NSCLC (64). All patients received concurrent chemoradiotherapy with EP and RT to 45 Gy. In the absence of progression, patients were randomized to undergo surgery or continuation of RT to 61 Gy. Both groups received consolidation chemotherapy with two cycles of EP. Mediastinal nodal clearance was noted in 46% of patients and pCR in 18%. Treatment-related mortality was higher in the surgery arm (7% vs. 1.6%). Most postoperative deaths were due to ARDS, predominantly after pneumonectomy. Disease-free survival was significantly prolonged in the surgery arm (14.0 vs. 11.7 months, $P < .02$), but overall survival was similar in both arms (22.2 vs. 23.6 months, $P = .24$). In an exploratory analysis, overall survival was improved with surgery in patients undergoing a lobectomy, but not in those undergoing pneumonectomy.

It is unlikely that another prospective trial will be completed that directly compares definitive chemoradiotherapy to trimodality therapy. Appropriate patients should be counselled about the potential risks and benefits of definitive chemoradiotherapy with and without a surgical resection (preferably by lobectomy). Additionally, INT 0139 emphasized the need for meticulous RT planning, surgical technique, and postoperative care in patients undergoing aggressive trimodality therapy.

The appropriate dose of preoperative RT is currently being reevaluated. Excellent outcomes have been reported in a single-institution trial that utilized neoadjuvant concurrent chemotherapy plus standard-dose RT (>59 Gy) followed by resection incorporating vascularized muscle flaps to cover the bronchial stump, limitation of intraoperative fluids, and avoidance of postoperative barotrauma (65). RTOG 0229 was a multicenter phase II trial that evaluated full-dose RT plus concurrent chemotherapy followed by surgical resection (63). Clearance of mediastinal lymph nodes was noted in an impressive 63% of patients after full-dose chemoradiotherapy, meeting the study endpoint, and the incidence of grade 3 postoperative pulmonary complications was only 14%.

Although mediastinal clearance and pCR rates appear to be improved with standard-dose RT and concurrent chemotherapy, the appropriate dose of RT remains clear. If preoperative chemotherapy plus RT to 45 Gy is planned, it is imperative that surgical evaluation occur rapidly so as not to delay the continuation of RT to a definitive dose if surgery is not possible. An alternative strategy is to use preoperative chemotherapy alone with postoperative RT provided for residual N2 disease or positive surgical margins. If RT is to be delivered, full dose RT (60 Gy) is preferred if surgeons are experienced with resection after high-dose RT.

Adjuvant Therapy for Primarily Resected Occult LA-NSCLC

In surgical series, about 20% of patients who are clinically staged as node-negative are found to have ipsilateral mediastinal lymph node involvement (N2) on pathologic evaluation of the surgical sample (66). These patients have varying prognoses depending on their burden of N2 disease and T stage (40). Randomized trials have shown that adjuvant chemotherapy can improve long-term overall survival in this setting, while retrospective analyses suggest that postoperative RT (PORT) may also favorably impact long-term outcome.

Adjuvant Chemotherapy

Adjuvant chemotherapy is indicated for patients with completely resected stage II and III NSCLC. Three landmark randomized trials, JBR-10, International Adjuvant Lung Cancer Trial (IALT), and Adjuvant Navelbine International Trialist

Association (ANITA), showed improvements in overall survival, ranging from 4% to 15%, with adjuvant chemotherapy, as summarized in Table 7.3 (67–69). The Lung Adjuvant Cisplatin Evaluation (LACE) meta-analysis included five large, randomized trials published after 1995 that randomized 4,584 patients who underwent complete resection of stage I to III NSCLC to cisplatin-based, two-drug chemotherapy versus no chemotherapy. LACE demonstrated a 5.3% absolute benefit in overall survival with adjuvant chemotherapy (HR 0.89, 95% CI 0.82–0.96). The significant benefit was confined to patients with stage II (HR 0.83, 95% CI 0.73–0.95) and stage III (HR 0.83, 95% CI 0.72–0.94) disease, with potential detriment in stage IA (HR 1.4, 95% CI 0.95–2.06) and no significant benefit in stage IB (HR 0.93, 95% CI 0.78–1.10) (70). This benefit was validated by a larger meta-analysis including 26 trials with 8,447 patients which showed an absolute overall survival benefit of 4% at 5 years, (HR 0.86, 95% CI 0.81–0.92) P <.0001 (71). Appropriate patients for adjuvant chemotherapy should have good performance status and an uncomplicated recovery from surgery.

Adjuvant chemotherapy regimens: In a planned subset analysis of the LACE database, patients receiving cisplatin plus vinorelbine (PVb) had an absolute 5-year survival benefit of

Table 7.3 Positive adjuvant chemotherapy trials in NSCLC

Trial	*N*	Stage	Regimen	RT	5-year overall survival: Chemotherapy	5-year overall survival: Observation	*P* value
IALT (56)	1,867	I, II, III	Cisplatin + etoposide, vinorelbine, vindesine, or vinblastine × three–four cycles	±	44%	40%z	.03
ANITA (57)	840	IB, II, IIIA	Cisplatin + vinorelbine × four cycles	±	51%	43%	.013
JBR-10 (55)	482	IB, II	Cisplatin + vinorelbine × four cycles	–	69%	54%	.002

NSCLC, non–small-cell lung cancer.

8.9% compared to observation, which appeared to be indirectly superior to the benefit derived from other cisplatin-based combinations (72). However, PVb is associated with significant toxicity and compliance to therapy is poor compared to newer regimens such as cisplatin plus pemetrexed (CP). This was demonstrated in the TREAT study, where 132 patients with resected non-squamous NSCLC were randomized to receive adjuvant CP or PVb with a primary endpoint of clinical feasibility, which was defined as no grade 4 cytopenia, no grade 3 to 4 febrile neutropenia or non-hematological toxicity, and absence of death or premature study withdrawal. The clinical feasibility rate with CP was superior to that with PVb (96% vs. 75%, P = .001) (73). Current guidelines recommend four cycles of a cisplatin-based, two-drug regimen for eligible patients and carboplatin-based, two-drug regimens for patients who cannot tolerate cisplatin (2). In the recently concluded trial E1505, which evaluated the role of adjuvant bevacizumab in 1,501 patients, oncologists were allowed to choose between four adjuvant chemotherapy regimens, 25% of patients received CVb, 19% cisplatin plus gemcitabine, 23% cisplatin plus docetaxel, and 33% CP (74). Bevacizumab was not found to be beneficial in the adjuvant setting. However, pooled analysis showed that within the squamous and non-squamous subgroups, disease-free and overall survival were similar with each of the chemotherapy regimens. In the non-squamous cohort, there was significantly less grade 3 to 5 toxicity in the CP arm, with increased neutropenia and thrombocytopenia in the CVb and cisplatin plus gemcitabine arms, respectively (74).

Timing of chemotherapy: Most adjuvant chemotherapy studies mandated that patients start treatment within 60 days of surgery, and no randomized trials have addressed the question of delayed adjuvant therapy. A retrospective analysis of the Ontario Cancer Registry showed that delayed initiation of adjuvant chemotherapy, defined as chemotherapy given between 10 and 16 weeks after resection, occurred in one-third of patients and was still associated with a positive effect on survival (75). If both adjuvant chemotherapy and PORT are planned, then they should be delivered in a sequential manner with chemotherapy given first in order to avoid unnecessary treatment delays and interruptions that might be caused by poor tolerance of concurrent therapy.

Elderly patients: Patients over 70 years old accounted for only 9% of those in the LACE database, while patients over 75 years old accounted for only 1.3%. An age-specific pooled analysis showed that elderly patients seemed to derive benefit from adjuvant chemotherapy despite receiving lower doses and fewer cycles of therapy (76). Data in octogenarians is quite limited, but there is some evidence that adjuvant chemotherapy may be detrimental (77). The use of adjuvant chemotherapy in older patients must be individualized with consideration of each patient's potential risks and benefits.

Postoperative RT

The role of postoperative RT (PORT) in patients with completely resected NSCLC remains controversial, but the American Society for Radiation Oncology's (ASTRO) evidence-based clinical practice guidelines state that PORT can be used to optimize local control in patients with positive surgical margins, gross residual disease, or mediastinal lymph node involvement (78).

Incomplete resection: In an evaluation of over 100,000 patients undergoing lung cancer resection, surgical margins were positive in 4.7% and this was associated with a worse 5-year overall survival (59% vs. 34%) (79). An incomplete resection adversely affected prognosis irrespective of the stage and the magnitude of this effect was comparable to shifting the patient to the next higher stage of disease. Factors associated with positive margins include higher stage, advanced tumor grade, squamous cell histology (probably due a central location), tumor involving multiple lobes, and lower socioeconomic status (79). Repeat resection is recommended when feasible, but in the absence of resection with negative margins, PORT is indicated to improve local-regional control.

pN2 disease: The PORT meta-analysis published in 1998 included nine studies, with 2,128 patients, in which surgery followed by PORT was compared to surgery alone. This meta-analysis concluded that PORT produced a significant detrimental effect on survival (80). However, this detrimental effect was confined to patients with pN0 and pN1 disease. Despite antiquated RT techniques, there was a nonsignificant trend toward improved survival with PORT in patients with stage IIIA-pN2 disease. A more recent retrospective analysis of the Surveillance Epidemiology and End Results (SEER) database included 5,600 patients who underwent complete resection of NSCLC and reported a lower overall survival for patients with pN0 or pN1 disease who received PORT. However, the pN2 subgroup of patients had a significant 3-year overall survival benefit (81).

In the ANITA adjuvant chemotherapy trial, the use of postoperative RT for patients with stage III-pN2 NSCLC was determined by individual institutions before initiating the study. If given, PORT (45–60 Gy in 2 Gy fractions) was administered within 2 weeks of completion of chemotherapy or surgery depending on the treatment arm. Overall survival was improved in patients with pN2 disease who received PORT, both in the chemotherapy arm (median, 47 vs. 24 months) and the observation arm (median, 23 vs. 13 months) (82). A retrospective review of the National Cancer Database evaluated the impact of modern PORT (≥45 GY) in 4,483 patients with stage III-N2 NSCLC treated between 2006 and 2010 with surgery and adjuvant chemotherapy. The use of PORT was associated with an increase in median and 5-year overall survival compared with no PORT (median, 45 vs. 41 months; 5-year, 39% vs. 35%; *P* = .014) (83).

CONCLUSION

LA-NSCLC is a heterogeneous disease consisting of subsets of patients ranging from those with resectable or minimal N2 disease with a relatively good prognosis to those with unresectable, bulky, extensive intrathoracic disease with a poor prognosis similar to that of stage IVA patients. Patients with LA-NSCLC are ideally managed by a multidisciplinary team of thoracic surgeons, radiation oncologists, and medical oncologists who can individualize therapy based on each patient's clinical and pathological characteristics.

KEY POINTS

- Locally advanced NSCLC includes stage IIIA (T4 N0; T3–4 N1; T1–T3 N2) and stage IIIB (T4 N2; T1–T4 N3).
- Increasing T and N stage and the extent of mediastinal lymph node involvement (N2 disease) adversely affect prognosis.
- Definitive radiotherapy with concurrent chemotherapy is recommended for patients with unresectable disease.
- Sequential chemoradiotherapy should be considered for patients who are not candidates for concurrent chemoradiotherapy.
- Selected patients with minimal N2 disease can be considered for neoadjuvant chemotherapy or chemoradiotherapy followed by resection.
- Definitive RT should be considered for patients who cannot tolerate chemotherapy.
- Adjuvant chemotherapy is recommended for patients with primarily resected, stage III-N2 disease. Postoperative radiotherapy can also be considered in these patients and in those with positive resection margins.
- Multidisciplinary evaluation is mandatory for patients with locally advanced NSCLC.

REFERENCES

1. Goldstraw, P, Chansky K, Crowley J, et al., The IASLC Lung Cancer Staging Project: proposals for revision of the TNM stage groupings in the forthcoming (eighth) edition of the TNM Classification for Lung Cancer. *J Thorac Oncol*. 2016;11:39-51.
2. National Comprehensive Cancer Network. NCCN guidelines for non–small cell lung cancer Version 4.2016. http://www.nccn.org/professionals/physician_gls/pdf/nscl.pdf
3. Gore E, Movsas B, Santana-Davila R, Langer C. Evaluation and management of elderly patients with lung cancer. *Semin Radiat Oncol*. 2013;22:304-310.
4. Langer C, Hsu C, Curran W, et al. Do elderly patients with locally advanced non–small cell lung cancer benefit from combined modality therapy? A secondary analysis of RTOG 9410. *Int J Radiat Oncol Biol Phys*. 2001;51(suppl 1):20-21.
5. Perez CA, Stanley K, Rubin P, et al. A prospective randomized study of various irradiation doses and fractionation schedules in the treatment of inoperable non-oat cell carcinoma of the lung: Preliminary report by the RT Oncology Group. *Cancer*. 1980;45:2744-2753.
6. Cox JD, Azarnia N, Byhardt RW, et al. A randomized phase I/II trial of hyperfractionated radiation therapy with total doses of 60.0 Gy to 79.2 Gy: possible survival benefit with greater than or equal to 69.6 Gy in favorable patients with RT Oncology Group stage III non–small cell lung carcinoma; report of RT Oncology Group 83.11. *J Clin Oncol*. 1990;8:1543-1555.
7. Dillman RO, Herndon J, Seagren SL, et al. Improved survival in stage III non–small-cell lung cancer: seven-year follow-up of cancer and leukemia group B (CALGB) 8433 trial. *J Natl Cancer Inst*. 1996;88:1210-1215.
8. Sause W, Kolesar P, Taylor S, et al. Final results of phase III trial in regionally advanced unresectable non–small cell lung cancer: Radiation Therapy Oncology Group, Eastern Cooperative Oncology Group, and Southwest Oncology Group. *Chest*. 2000;117:358-364.
9. Curran WJ, Paulus R, Langer CJ, et al. Sequential vs. concurrent chemoradiation for stage III non–small cell lung cancer: randomized phase III trial RTOG 9410. *J Natl Cancer Inst*. 2011;103:1452-1460.
10. Bradley J, Graham M, Swann S, et al. Phase I results of RTOG 0117; a phase I/II dose intensification study using 3DCRT and concurrent chemotherapy for patients with inoperable non–small cell lung cancer. *Proc Am Soc Clin Oncol*. 2005;24:636s.
11. Blackstock A, Socinski MA, Bogart J, et al. Induction plus concurrent chemotherapy with high-dose (74 Gy) 3 dimensional (3-D) thoracic radiotherapy in stage III non–small cell lung cancer: preliminary report of CALGB 30105. *Proc Am Soc Clin Oncol*. 2006;24:374s.
12. Lee C, Socinski MA, Lin L, et al. High-dose 3D chemoradiotherapy in stage III non–small cell lung cancer (NSCLC) at the University of North Carolina: long-term follow up and late complications. *Proc Am Soc Clin Oncol*. 2006;24:400s.

13. Furuse K, Fukuoka M, Kawahara M, et al. Phase III study of concurrent versus sequential thoracic radiotherapy in combination with mitomycin, vindesine, and cisplatin in unresectable stage III non–small cell lung cancer. *J Clin Oncol*. 1999;17:2692-2699.

14. Bradley JD, Paulus R, Komaki R, et al., Standard-dose versus high-dose conformal radiotherapy with concurrent and consolidation carboplatin plus paclitaxel with or without cetuximab for patients with stage IIIA or IIIB non–small-cell lung cancer (RTOG 0617): a randomised, two-by-two factorial phase 3 study. *Lancet Oncol*. 2015;16:187-199.

15. Joo JH, Song SY, Kim SS, et al. Definitive radiotherapy alone over 60 Gy for patients unfit for combined treatment to stage II–III non–small cell lung cancer: retrospective analysis. *Radiat Oncol*. 2015;10:250.

16. Nguyen LN, Komaki R, Allen P, et al. Effectiveness of accelerated radiotherapy for patients with inoperable non-small cell lung cancer (NSCLC) and borderline prognostic factors without distant metastasis: a retrospective review. *Int J Rad Oncol Biol Phys*. 1999;44:1053-1056.

17. Gore E, Bae K, Langer C, et al. PhaseI/II trial of a COX-2 inhibitor with limited field radiation for intermediate prognosis patient who have locally advanced non-small cell lung cancer: Radiation Therapy Oncology Group 0213. *Clin Lung Cancer*. 2011;12:125-130.

18. Amini A, Lin SH, Wei C, et al. Accelerated hypofractionated radiation therapy compared to conventionally fractionated radiation therapy for the treatment of inoperable non–small cell lung cancer. *Radiat Oncol*. 2012;7:33.

19. Ung YC, Gu C-S, Cline K, et al. An Ontario Clinical Oncology Group (OCOG) randomized trial (PET START) of FDG PET/CT in patients with stage 3 non-small cell lung cancer (NSCLC): impact of PET on radiation treatment volumes. *J Thorac Oncol*. 2011;6:S428.

20. Keall PJ, Mageras GS, Balter JM, et al. The management of respiratory motion in radiation oncology report of AAPM Task Group 76. *Med Phys*. 2006;33:3874-3900.

21. Movsas B, Hu C, Sloan J, et al. Quality of life analysis of a radiation dose-escalation study of patients with non-small-cell lung cancer: a secondary analysis of the Radiation Therapy Oncology Group 0617 randomized clinical trial. *JAMA Oncol*. 2015;25:1-9.

22. Liao ZX, Komaki RR, Thames HD Jr, et al. Influence of technologic advances on outcomes in patients with unresectable, locally advanced non-small-cell lung cancer receiving concomitant chemoradiotherapy. *Int J Radiat Oncol Biol Phys*. 2010;76:775-781.

23. O'Rourke N, Roqué I, Figuls M, et al. Concurrent chemoradiotherapy in non-small cell lung cancer. *Cochrane Database Syst Rev*. 2010;6:Article No. CD002140. doi:10.1002/14651858.CD002140.pub3

24. Vokes EE, Herndon JE, Kelley MJ, et al. Induction chemotherapy followed by chemoradiotherapy compared with chemoradiotherapy alone for regionally advanced unresectable stage III non-small-cell lung cancer: Cancer and Leukemia Group B 39801. *J Clin Oncol*. 2007;25:1698-1704.

25. Santana-Davila R, Devisetty K, Szabo A, et al. Cisplatin and etoposide versus carboplatin and paclitaxel with concurrent radiotherapy for stage III non–small-cell lung cancer: an analysis of Veterans Health Administration data. *J Clin Oncol*. 2015;33:567-574.
26. Steuer C, Behera M, Higgins KA, et al. A systematic review of carboplatin-paclitaxel versus cisplatin-etoposide concurrent with thoracic radiation for stage III NSCLC patients. *J Thorac Oncol*. 2015;10(suppl 2):S212.
27. Scagliotti GV, Parikh P, von Pawel J, et al. Phase III study comparing cisplatin plus gemcitabine with cisplatin plus pemetrexed in chemotherapy-naive patients with advanced-stage non-small-cell lung cancer. *J Clin Oncol*. 2008;26:3543-3551.
28. Bischof M, Weber KJ, Blatter J, et al. Interaction of pemetrexed disodium and irradiation in vitro. *Int J Radiat Oncol Biol Phys*. 2002;52:1381-1388.
29. Senan S, Brade A, Wang LH, et al. PROCLAIM: randomized phase III trial of pemetrexed-cisplatin or etoposide–cisplatin plus thoracic radiation therapy followed by consolidation chemotherapy in locally advanced non-squamous non-small-cell lung cancer. *J Clin Oncol*. 2016;34:953-962.
30. Choy H, Schwartzberg LS, Dakhil SR, et al. Phase 2 study of pemetrexed plus carboplatin, or pemetrexed plus cisplatin with concurrent radiation therapy followed by pemetrexed consolidation in patients with favorable-prognosis inoperable stage IIIA/B non-small-cell lung cancer. *J Thorac Oncol*. 2013;8:1308-1316.
31. Hanna N, Neubauer M, Yiannoutsos C, et al. Phase III study of cisplatin, etoposide, and concurrent chest radiation with or without consolidation docetaxel in patients with inoperable stage III non-small-cell lung cancer: the Hoosier Oncology Group and U.S. Oncology. *J Clin Oncol*. 2008;26:5755.
32. Ahn JS, Ahn YC, Kim JH, et al. Multinational randomized phase III trial with or without consolidation chemotherapy using docetaxel and cisplatin after concurrent chemoradiation in inoperable stage III non-small-cell lung cancer: KCSG-LU05-04. *J Clin Oncol*. 2015;33:2660-2666.
33. Tsujino K, Kurata T, Yamamoto S, et al. Is consolidation chemotherapy after concurrent chemo-radiotherapy beneficial for patients with locally advanced non-small-cell lung cancer? A pooled analysis of the literature. *J Thorac Oncol*. 2013;8:1181-1189.
34. Curran WJ Jr. Consolidation chemotherapy after chemoradiation? Not the right answer to not the right question? *J Thorac Oncol*. 2013;8:1116-1117.
35. Kelly K, Chansky K, Gaspar LE, et al. Phase III trial of maintenance gefitinib or placebo after concurrent chemoradiotherapy and docetaxel consolidation in inoperable stage III non-small-cell lung cancer: SWOG S0023. *J Clin Oncol*. 2008;26:2450-2456.
36. Spigel DR, Hainsworth JD, Yardley DA, et al. Tracheoesophageal fistula formation in patients with lung cancer treated with chemoradiation and bevacizumab. *J Clin Oncol*. 2010;28:43-48.

37. Farjah F, Flum DR, VargheseTK, et al. Surgeon specialty and long-term survival after pulmonary resection for lung cancer. *Ann Thorac Surg*. 2009;87:995-1006.
38. Farray D, Mirkovic N, Albain KS, et al. Multimodality therapy for stage III non-small-cell lung cancer. *J Clin Oncol*. 2005;23:3257-3269.
39. Decaluwé H, De Leyn P, Vansteenkiste J, et al. Surgical multimodality treatment for baseline resectable stage IIIA-N2 non-small cell lung cancer: degree of mediastinal lymph node involvement and impact on survival. *Eur J Cardiothorac Surg*. 2009;36:433-439.
40. Andre F, Grunenwald D, Pignon JP, et al., Survival of patients with resected N2 non-small-cell lung cancer: evidence for a subclassification and implications. *J Clin Oncol*. 2000;18:2981-2989.
41. Betticher DC, Schmitz SF, Totsch M, et al. Prognostic factors affecting long-term outcomes in patients with resected stage IIIA pN2 non-small-cell lung cancer: 5-year follow-up of a phase II study. *Br J Cancer*. 2006;94:1099-1106.
42. Asamura H, Chansky K, Crowley J, et al., The International Association for the Study of Lung Cancer Lung Cancer Staging Project: proposals for the revision of the N descriptors in the forthcoming 8th edition of the TNM classification for lung cancer. *J Thorac Oncol*. 10:1675-1684.
43. Wei S, Asamura H, Kawachi R, et al. Which is the better prognostic factor for resected non-small cell lung cancer: the number of metastatic lymph nodes or the currently used nodal stage classification? *J Thorac Oncol*. 2011;6:310-318.
44. Rami-Porta R, Wittekind C, Goldstraw P; International Association for the Study of Lung Cancer (IASLC) Staging Committee. Complete resection in lung cancer surgery: proposed definition. *Lung Cancer*. 2005;49:25-33.
45. Asamura H, Nakayama H, Kondo H, et al. Lobe-specific extent of systematic lymph node dissection for non-small cell lung carcinomas according to a retrospective study of metastasis and prognosis. *J Thorac Cardiovasc Surg*. 117:1102-1111.
46. Citak N, Sayar A, Metin M, et al., The prognostic significance of metastasis to lymph nodes in aortopulmonary zone (stations 5 and 6) in completely resected left upper lobe tumors. *Thorac Cardiovasc Surg*. 2015;63:568-576.
47. De Leyn P, Stroobants S, De Wever W, et al. Prospective comparative study of integrated positron emission tomography–computed tomography scan compared with re-mediastinoscopy in the assessment of residual mediastinal lymph node disease after induction chemotherapy for mediastinoscopy-proven stage IIIA-N2 non–small-cell lung cancer: a Leuven Lung Cancer Group Study. *J Clin Oncol*. 2006;24:3333-3339.
48. Call S, Rami-Porta R, Obiois C, et al., Repeat mediastinoscopy in all its indications: experience with 96 patients and 101 procedures. *Eur J Cardiothorac Surg*. 2011;39:1022-1027.

49. Herth FJF, Annema JT, Eberhardt R, et al. Endobronchial ultrasound with transbronchial needle aspiration for restaging the mediastinum in lung cancer. *J Clin Oncol*. 2008;26:3346-3350.
50. Szlubowski A, Zielinski M, Soja J, et al., Accurate and safe mediastinal restaging by combined endobronchial and endoscopic ultrasound-guided needle aspiration performed by single ultrasound bronchoscope. *Eur J Cardiothorac Surg*. 2014;46:262-266.
51. de Cabanyes Candela S, Detterbeck FC. A systematic review of restaging after induction therapy for stage IIIA lung cancer: prediction of pathologic stage. *J Thorac Oncol*. 2010;5:389-398.
52. Albain KS, Swann RS, Rusch VW, et al. Radiotherapy plus chemotherapy with or without surgical resection for stage III non-small-cell lung cancer: a phase III randomised controlled trial. *Lancet*. 2009;374:379-386.
53. Mansour Z, Kochetkova EA, Santelmo N, et al. Risk factors for early mortality and morbidity after pneumonectomy: a reappraisal. *Ann Thorac Surg*. 2009;88:1737-1743.
54. Sonett JR, Suntharalingam M, Edelman MJ, et al. Pulmonary resection after curative intent radiotherapy (>59 Gy) and concurrent chemotherapy in non–small-cell lung cancer. *Ann Thorac Surg*. 2004;78:1200-1205.
55. Weder W, Collaus D, Eberhardt WE, et al. Pneumonectomy is a valuable treatment option after neoadjuvant therapy for stage III non-small-cell lung cancer. *J Thorac Cardiovasc Surg*. 2010;139:1424-1430.
56. Roth JA, Atkinson E, Fossella F, et al. A randomized trial comparing perioperative chemotherapy and surgery with surgery alone in resectable stage IIIA non-small-cell lung cancer. *J Natl Cancer Inst*. 1994;86:673-680.
57. Rosell R, Gomez-Codina J, Kamps C, et al. A randomized trial comparing preoperative chemotherapy plus surgery with surgery alone in patients with non-small-cell lung cancer. *N Engl J Med*. 1994;330:153-158.
58. NSCLC Meta-analysis Collaborative Group. Preoperative chemotherapy for non-small-cell lung cancer: a systematic review and meta-analysis of individual participant data. *Lancet*. 2014;383:1561-1571.
59. Betticher DC, Schmitz SH, Totsch M, et al. Mediastinal lymph node clearance after docetaxel-cisplatin neoadjuvant chemotherapy is prognostic of survival in patients with stage IIIA pN2 non-small-cell lung cancer: a multicenter phase II trial. *J Clin Oncol*. 2003;21:1752-1759.
60. Pless M, Stupp R, Ris HB, et al. Induction chemoradiation in stage IIIA/N2 non-small-cell lung cancer: a phase 3 randomised trial. *Lancet*. 2015;386:1049-1056.
61. Van Zandwijk N, Smit EF, Kramer GW, et al. Gemcitabine and cisplatin as induction regimen for patients with biopsy-proven stage IIIA N2 non-small-cell lung cancer: a phase II study of the European Organization for Research and Treatment of Cancer Lung Cancer Cooperative Group (EORTC 08955). *J Clin Oncol*. 2000;18:2658-2664.

62. Lim E, Harris G, Patel A, et al. Preoperative versus postoperative chemotherapy in patients with resectable non-small cell lung cancer: systematic review and indirect comparison meta-analysis of randomized trials. *J Thorac Oncol.* 2009;4:1380-1388.
63. Suntharalingam M, Paulus R, Edelman MJ, et al. Radiation Therapy Oncology Group protocol 02-29: a phase II trial of neoadjuvant therapy with concurrent chemotherapy and full-dose radiation therapy followed by surgical resection and consolidative therapy for locally advanced non-small cell carcinoma of the lung. *Int J Radiat Oncol Biol Phys.* 2012;84:456-463.
64. Albain KS, Swann RS, Rusch VW, et al., Radiotherapy plus chemotherapy with or without surgical resection for stage III non-small-cell lung cancer: a phase III randomised controlled trial. *Lancet.* 2009;374:379-386.
65. Sonett JR, Suntharalingam M, Edelman MJ, et al. Pulmonary resection after curative intent radiotherapy (>59 Gy) and concurrent chemotherapy in non–small-cell lung cancer. Ann Thorac Surg. 2004;78:1200-1205.
66. Graham ANJ, et al. Systematic nodal dissection in the intrathoracic staging of patients with non-small cell lung cancer. *J Thorac Cardiovasc Surg.* 1999;117:246-251.
67. Winton T, Livingston R, Johnson D, et al. Vinorelbine plus cisplatin vs. observation in resected non-small-cell lung cancer. *N Engl J Med.* 2005;352:2589-2597.
68. Arriagada R, Bergman B, Dunant A, et al. Cisplatin-based adjuvant chemotherapy in patients with completely resected non-small-cell lung cancer. *N Engl J Med.* 2004;350:351.
69. Douillard JY, Rosell R, De Lena M, et al. Adjuvant vinorelbine plus cisplatin versus observation in patients with completely resected stage IB-IIIA non-small-cell lung cancer (Adjuvant Navelbine International Trialist Association [ANITA]): a randomised controlled trial. *Lancet Oncol.* 2006;7:719.
70. Pignon JP, Tribodet H, Scagliotti GV, et al. Lung Adjuvant Cisplatin Evaluation: a pooled analysis by the LACE Collaborative Group. *J Clin Oncol.* 2008;26:3552-3559.
71. Burdett S, Pignon JP, Tierney J, et al. Adjuvant chemotherapy for resected early-stage non-small cell lung cancer. *Cochrane Database Syst Rev.* 2015;3:CD011430.
72. Douillard JY, Tribodet H, Aubert D, et al. Adjuvant cisplatin and vinorelbine for completely resected non-small cell lung cancer: subgroup analysis of the Lung Adjuvant Cisplatin Evaluation. *J Thorac Oncol.* 2010;5:220-228.
73. Kreuter M, Vansteenkiste J, Fischer JR, et al. Randomized phase 2 trial on refinement of early-stage NSCLC adjuvant chemotherapy with cisplatin and pemetrexed versus cisplatin and vinorelbine: the TREAT study. *Ann Oncol.* 2013;24:986-992.

74. Wakelee HA, Dahlberg SE, Keller SM, et al. Randomized phase III trial of adjuvant chemotherapy with or without bevacizumab in resected non-small cell lung cancer (NSCLC): results of E1505. *J Clin Oncol*. 2016;34(15S):436s.

75. Booth CM, Shepherd FA, Peng Y, et al. Time to adjuvant chemotherapy and survival in non-small cell lung cancer: a population based study. *Cancer*. 2013;119:1243-1250.

76. Fruh M, Rolland E, Pignon JP, et al. Pooled analysis of the effect of age on adjuvant cisplatin-based chemotherapy for completely resected non-small-cell lung cancer. *J Clin Oncol*. 2008;26:3573-3581.

77. Wisnivesky JP, Smith CB, Packer S, et al. Survival and risk of adverse events in older patients receiving postoperative adjuvant chemotherapy for resected stages II–IIIA lung cancer: observational cohort study. *BMJ*. 2011;343:d4013. doi:10.1136/bmj.d4013.

78. Rodriques G, Choy H, Bradley J, et al. Adjuvant radiation therapy in locally advanced non-small cell lung cancer: executive summary of an American Society for Radiation Oncology (ASTRO) evidence-based clinical practice guideline. *Pract Radiat Oncol* 2015;5:149-155.

79. Osarogiagbon RU, Lin CC, Smeltzer MP, et al. Prevalence, prognostic implications, and survival modulators of incompletely resected non–small cell lung cancer in the U.S. National Cancer Database. *J Thorac Oncol*. 2016;11:e5-e16.

80. PORT Meta-analysis Trialists Group. Postoperative radiotherapy in non-small-cell lung cancer: systematic review and meta-analysis of individual patient data from nine randomised controlled trials. *Lancet*. 1998;352:257-263.

81. Lally BE, Zelterman D, Colasanto JM, et al. Postoperative radiotherapy for stage II or III non-small cell lung cancer using the Surveillance, Epidemiology and End Results database. *J Clin Oncol*. 2006;24:2998-3006.

82. Douillard J, Rosell R, De Lena M, et al. Impact of postoperative radiation therapy on survival in patients with complete resection and stage I, II, or IIIA non-small-cell Lung cancer treated with adjuvant chemotherapy: the Adjuvant Navelbine International Trialist Association (ANITA) randomized trial. *Int J Radiat Oncol Biol Phys*. 2008;72:695-701.

83. Robinson CG, Patel AP, Bradley JD, et al. Post-operative radiotherapy for pathologic N2 non–small-cell lung cancer treated with adjuvant chemotherapy: a review of the National Cancer Database. *J Clin Oncol*. 2015;33:870-876.

Management of Advanced-Stage Non–Small-Cell Lung Cancer

8

Conor E. Steuer and Suresh S. Ramalingam

INTRODUCTION

At least 50% of patients with non–small-cell lung cancer (NSCLC) have advanced stage IV disease at the time of diagnosis. Advanced-stage NSCLC includes patients with distant metastatic disease, contralateral pulmonary involvement, and/or malignant pleural or pericardial effusions. Systemic therapy is the primary treatment modality for patients with stage IV NSCLC. Systemic therapy options now include cytotoxic chemotherapy, molecularly targeted therapy, and immunotherapy. The main goal of systemic therapy for stage IV disease is to palliate symptoms and improve survival. In many patients, radiotherapy may be given to improve symptoms such as hemoptysis, pain, or dyspnea. The armamentarium of systemic agents has increased rapidly for patients for advanced NSCLC, highlighted by the fact that the U.S. Food and Drug Administration (FDA) approved six new drugs for lung cancer in 2015. The choice of therapy in an individual patient is based on many factors, including histology, genomic status, performance status, toxicity, cost, and patient preference.

BIOMARKER TESTING

Important discoveries in the molecular biology of NSCLC have allowed for the identification of several oncogenic drivers important in tumor pathogenesis, such as mutations in the epidermal growth factor receptor (*EGFR*) gene, or rearrangement of the *ALK* and *ROS1* genes. This has led to the development of targeted therapies for patients with NSCLC that harbors these genetic biomarkers, bringing precision medicine to the clinic. Therefore, it is important that the first step in the care for a patient with newly diagnosed metastatic NSCLC is consideration for biomarker analysis.

Thus far, driver mutations are recognized as therapeutic targets only in lung adenocarcinomas. Therefore, squamous cell carcinomas (SqCC) are not typically tested (1). However, SqCCs in nonsmokers and mixed-histology tumors with an adenocarcinoma component should be considered for molecular testing. Biomarker analysis consists of mutation testing by multiplex genotyping and molecular FISH analysis. While testing of *EGFR*, *ALK*, and *ROS-1* can be considered the current minimal standard-of-care, more extensive testing is often being performed as new potential targets are rapidly being identified. Molecular testing has been shown to be feasible on a large scale, and aids clinicians with decisions on therapy (2). Finally, if available tumor biopsies are insufficient for molecular testing and obtaining another biopsy is not feasible, then plasma cell-free DNA testing might provide another avenue to ascertain the presence of driver mutations (3).

CHEMOTHERAPY

The role of chemotherapy in advanced NSCLC was clearly established in multiple randomized studies. Comparisons of platinum-based therapy to supportive care alone resulted in modest improvements in survival and quality of life (4). A meta-analysis published in 1995 demonstrated an absolute improvement in the 1-year overall survival rate of approximately 10% with platinum-based chemotherapy over supportive care alone (5). These data ushered in the era of systemic therapy for patients with advanced-stage NSCLC. Subsequently, several newer agents with a variety of mechanisms of action were demonstrated to be active in NSCLC, including: paclitaxel and docetaxel (microtubule-stabilizing agents); vinorelbine (vinca alkaloid); gemcitabine (ribonucleotide reductase inhibitor); irinotecan (topoisomerase I inhibitor); and pemetrexed (multitargeted antifolate). Each of these agents is associated with a single-agent response rate of 10% to 30% in patients with advanced NSCLC. Combination of these third-generation agents with cisplatin or carboplatin results in an incremental improvement in response rates and overall survival over monotherapy. Therefore, a number of combination regimens are now available for the treatment of patients with advanced-stage NSCLC.

Combination Regimens

The ECOG1594 study demonstrated comparable efficacy of four different platinum-based, two-drug chemotherapy regimens (cisplatin plus paclitaxel; carboplatin plus paclitaxel; cisplatin plus docetaxel; cisplatin plus gemcitabine) in 1,207 patients with a good performance status and advanced NSCLC, yielding response rates of 17% to 22%, median overall survival of 7.9 months, and 1-year survival rates of 30% to 40%. Despite a mild increase in progression-free survival (PFS) with cisplatin plus gemcitabine over the other regimens (median, 4.2 vs. 3.1–3.7 months), there were no significant differences in overall survival (6). Other contemporary studies demonstrated similar results and provided evidence of comparable efficacy among various two-drug combination regimens. From these observations, it was concluded that a therapeutic plateau had been reached for chemotherapy in advanced NSCLC.

- SWOG 9509 reported comparable efficacy between cisplatin plus vinorelbine versus carboplatin plus paclitaxel (response rate, 28% vs. 25%; median overall survival, 8 months in both arms) (7).
- Belani et al. found comparable efficacy between cisplatin plus etoposide (ORR 15%) versus carboplatin plus paclitaxel (response rates, 15% vs. 23%, P = .061; median PFS, 3.7 vs. 4.0 months, P = .877; overall survival, no significant difference) (8).
- Ohe et al., in a randomized four-arm trial, noted no significant differences in response rate or median overall survival between cisplatin plus irinotecan (31%; 13.9 months), carboplatin plus paclitaxel (32%; 12.3 months), cisplatin plus gemcitabine (30%; 14 months), and cisplatin plus vinorelbine (33%; 11.4 months) (9).

Many studies have demonstrated that the addition of a third cytotoxic agent results in increased toxicity without an improvement in survival. Therefore, such regimens are not recommended for patients with advanced NSCLC. A large systematic review of 65 randomized trials comparing a two-drug regimen to either a single-agent or a three-drug regimen for patients with advanced NSCLC demonstrated that adding a second drug increased both the response rate (26% vs. 13%, $P < .001$) and overall survival (1-year, 35% vs. 30%, $P < .001$) over single-agent therapy. However, adding a third drug only increased toxicity, primarily infections, myelosuppression, and mucositis, without improving overall survival (1-year, OR 1.01, P = .88) (10).

Nonplatinum regimens have been extensively studied as alternatives to platinum-based chemotherapy, but have not provided added value (11). For example, a phase III study found that cisplatin plus docetaxel was equivalent to gemcitabine plus docetaxel (response rate, 32% vs. 30%; median PFS, 8 vs. 9 months; overall survival, 10 vs. 9.5 months) (12). Similarly, a three-arm study found comparable activity between cisplatin plus paclitaxel, cisplatin plus gemcitabine, and gemcitabine plus paclitaxel (response rate, 32% vs. 37% vs. 28%; median overall survival, 8.1 vs. 8.9 vs. 6.7 months) (13). In addition, there were no salient differences in toxicity, so it appears that nonplatinum, two-drug regimens do not provide any advantage over platinum-based regimens.

Non-Squamous NSCLC

Until recently, all histological sub-types of NSCLC were treated with the same platinum-based regimens. The role of histology in differential sensitivity to chemotherapy was first demonstrated in a randomized phase III study that compared cisplatin plus pemetrexed to cisplatin plus gemcitabine in patients with advanced NSCLC of any histology. In the overall study population, the efficacy of both regimens was comparable (median overall survival, 10.3 months in both arms), but cisplatin plus pemetrexed was superior in the subset of patients with non-squamous histology (median overall survival, 11.8 vs. 10.4 months, $P = .005$). Conversely, in patients with SqCC, cisplatin plus pemetrexed resulted in less favorable outcomes (median overall survival, 9.4 vs. 10.8 months, $P = .05$) (14). Based on these data, cisplatin plus pemetrexed is approved for use only in patients with non-squamous NSCLC.

Two other studies that compared a pemetrexed-based regimen to a taxane-based regimen in patients with non-squamous NSCLC demonstrated comparable efficacy (15,16). A phase III study comparing carboplatin, paclitaxel, and bevacizumab to carboplatin, pemetrexed, and bevacizumab reported no difference in overall survival (median, 13.4 vs. 12.6 months, HR 1.0, $P = .949$), with only slight differences in toxicity between the two regimens. Similarly, an Asian study demonstrated similar efficacy between cisplatin plus docetaxel versus cisplatin plus pemetrexed (median PFS, 4.7 vs. 4.6 months) (17). Therefore, platinum-based regimens with either pemetrexed or one of the taxanes are deemed appropriate for the treatment of patients with non-squamous NSCLC.

Anti-Angiogenic Therapy

Bevacizumab is a humanized, monoclonal antibody that targets vascular endothelial growth factor A. The benefit of bevacizumab in NSCLC was shown in two phase III randomized clinical trials. E4599 examined carboplatin plus paclitaxel versus carboplatin, paclitaxel, and bevacizumab 15 mg/kg followed by maintenance bevacizumab in patients with advanced NSCLC patients. The addition of bevacizumab improved overall survival (median, 12.3 vs. 10.3 months, $P = .003$), PFS (median, 6.3 vs. 4.8 months), and response rate (35% vs. 15%) (18). The AVAiL study evaluated cisplatin plus gemcitabine alone or with bevacizumab at two doses (7.5 mg/kg or 15 mg/kg) and documented a minor improvement in PFS with bevacizumab (6.7 vs. 6.1 months, $P = .003$), but this did not translate to an overall survival benefit (19). The main toxicities associated with bevacizumab include hypertension, proteinuria, and bleeding. Of note, patients with SqCC were excluded from these studies based on a significantly increased rate of pulmonary hemorrhage in those treated with bevacizumab in a previous phase II study (20). Bevacizumab at 15 mg/kg is now an FDA-approved option in combination with a platinum-based, two-drug regimen in patients with advanced non-squamous NSCLC. Salient exclusion factors for the use of bevacizumab are hemoptysis, cavitary lung lesions, older patients (>75 years old), and recent mediastinal radiation therapy (RT). Unfortunately, there are presently no proven biomarkers for the selection of patients who are most likely to benefit from bevacizumab. For patients who have continued control of disease after receiving a maximum of six cycles of chemotherapy plus bevacizumab, bevacizumab can be continued as maintenance therapy until progression of disease. The role of continuation of bevacizumab beyond progression after first-line therapy is unproven and is therefore not recommended. The modest success achieved with bevacizumab led to the evaluation of several VEGF-receptor inhibitors in NSCLC, but clinical trials with these agents have failed to demonstrate an improvement in efficacy in the first-line setting.

Squamous Cell Carcinoma

Necitumumab

While pemetrexed and bevacizumab are not used in SqCC, necitumumab, an anti-*EGFR* monoclonal antibody, has recently been approved by the FDA in combination with chemotherapy for first-line treatment. In a large, phase III clinical trial, patients with SqCC were randomized to receive cisplatin plus gemcitabine with or without necitumumab. The addition of necitumumab resulted in a modest improvement in overall survival (median, 11.5 vs. 9.9 months, HR 0.84, $P = .01$), although both response rate and PFS were not significantly improved. The main side effects associated with necitumumab include rash and hypomagnesemia. The incidence of thromboembolic events was also higher with necitumumab (21). Although the level of EGFR protein expression by immunohistochemistry was not predictive of benefit with necitumumab, high *EGFR* gene copy number was associated with a better outcome with necitumumab in a subset analysis and warrants prospective evaluation in future clinical trials.

Nab-Paclitaxel

Nab-paclitaxel was developed in an effort to improve the safety profile of standard-formulation paclitaxel and to obviate the need for steroid premedication. Comparative studies of carboplatin plus nab-paclitaxel versus carboplatin plus paclitaxel have demonstrated a modest increment in response rate (33% vs. 25%,

$P = .005$) and a more favorable toxicity profile. The improvement in response rate was more pronounced in patients with SqCC versus non-squamous histologies (41% vs. 24%, $P < .001$), though there was no difference in overall survival (12.1 vs. 11.2 months, $P = .271$) (22).

Biomarkers in SqCC

While biomarker testing is not as well defined in SqCC as in adenocarcinoma, investigations are underway to define predictive biomarkers for targeted therapy for these patients. One example is the LUNG-MAP multi-cooperative group umbrella trial, which tests SqCC tumors for derangements of biomarkers such as *CCND1*, *PIK3CA*, and *FGFR* and pairs patients with such abnormalities with investigational targeted agents (23). This design is intended to expedite the development of new drugs for the SqCC patient population.

Cisplatin Versus Carboplatin

Both cisplatin and carboplatin have been extensively studied in combination regimens for the treatment of advanced NSCLC, with the higher toxicity associated with cisplatin driving the interest in carboplatin-based regimens. Initial studies that compared cisplatin-based regimens directly to carboplatin-based regimens yielded mixed results. Subsequently, a meta-analysis of such randomized studies noted comparable survival between cisplatin and carboplatin-based regimens, when given in combination with a third-generation cytotoxic agent (median overall survival, 9.1 vs. 8.4 months, $P = .1$) with a slight advantage in response rate for cisplatin-based regimens (30% vs. 24%, $P < .001$) (24). In the United States, carboplatin-based regimens are used commonly for patients with advanced NSCLC. Given that the primary goal of treatment is palliation, the modest potential advantage in activity of cisplatin over carboplatin is counterbalanced by the lower toxicity of the later. In recent years, improvements in antiemetic therapy have lessened some of the toxicity of cisplatin-based regimens, but ototoxicity, neurotoxicity, and nephrotoxicity remain significance concerns. For younger patients with good renal function, cisplatin-based regimens may be used, but in general, carboplatin seems to be the more reasonable choice in a palliative setting. The recommended dose of cisplatin is 75 mg/m^2 given every 3 weeks, since higher doses do not result in improved efficacy, but add considerable toxicity.

Table 8.1 provides a list of commonly used chemotherapy regimens for patients with advanced NSCLC. The choice of the second agent added to cisplatin or carboplatin should be

Table 8.1 Common chemotherapy regimens for advanced NSCLC

Adenocarcinoma	Squamous cell carcinoma
Carboplatin/cisplatin + pemetrexed ± bevacizumab	Carboplatin/cisplatin + gemcitabine
Carboplatin + paclitaxel ± bevacizumab	Carboplatin + paclitaxel
Carboplatin/cisplatin + docetaxel	Carboplatin + nab-paclitaxel
Carboplatin/cisplatin + vinorelbine	Carboplatin/cisplatin + docetaxel
Carboplatin/cisplatin + gemcitabine	Carboplatin/cisplatin + vinorelbine
	Cisplatin + gemcitabine + necitumumab

individualized based on histology (non-squamous vs. squamous), preference for infusion schedule (e.g., every 3 weeks with pemetrexed or paclitaxel vs. multiweek infusions for gemcitabine), and toxicity. For example, severe renal insufficiency would exclude pemetrexed, while a preexisting neuropathy would make paclitaxel a less favorable choice.

Duration of Combination Chemotherapy

The optimal number of cycles of primary chemotherapy for the treatment of metastatic NSCLC has been established in a series of randomized clinical trials.

- Socinski et al. compared carboplatin plus paclitaxel × four cycles to the same regimen given until progression of disease with no differences reported in response rate (22% vs. 24%, P = .8), overall survival (median, 6.6 vs. 8.5 months, P = .63), or quality of life. There was a higher rate of neuropathy in patients who received the longer course of treatment (25).
- Park et al. evaluated four versus six cycles of various platinum doublets. While there was a statistically significant increase in time to progression for patients who received six cycles of therapy (median, 6.2 vs. 4.6 months, P = .001), this did not translate into increased overall survival (median, 14.9 vs. 15.9 months, P = .461) (26).

Therefore, four cycles is the accepted standard duration for first-line platinum-based chemotherapy in advanced NSCLC, with a consideration of two additional cycles if response is ongoing after four cycles. However, the consideration for continuing combination chemotherapy beyond four cycles must be balanced against the cumulative toxicity of such regimens.

Maintenance Therapy

Maintenance therapy has been evaluated as a strategy to improve survival without undue toxicity in patients who benefit from first-line therapy. There are two main strategies for maintenance therapy: switch maintenance and continuation maintenance. Switch maintenance utilizes an agent not used in the first-line platinum-based chemotherapy regimen in an effort to prevent resistance, while continuation maintenance continues one or more of the agents used in the first-line regimen. The potential benefits of continuation maintenance are that the drug was already known to be part of an effective regimen for the patient, so maintenance therapy could presumably prolong that benefit. Switch maintenance was developed to delay resistance and progression by adding a different systemic agent. In both situations, maintenance therapy is started immediately after completion of the first-line course of treatment in patients with response or stability and good performance status.

Bevacizumab

In the E4599 trial discussed earlier, patients who received carboplatin, paclitaxel, and bevacizumab followed by bevacizumab maintenance therapy did better than those getting carboplatin plus paclitaxel alone. These results made continuation maintenance with bevacizumab a viable option, although the specific contribution of the maintenance therapy was not examined (18). For patients who are treated with chemotherapy plus bevacizumab as first-line treatment, continuation maintenance with bevacizumab is an appropriate option.

Pemetrexed

Pemetrexed has been studied in the maintenance setting. In the JMEN phase III trial of switch maintenance, patients with advanced NSCLC that had not progressed after platinum-based, two-drug therapy were randomized to switch maintenance with pemetrexed versus placebo until disease progression. Pemetrexed maintenance significantly improved both PFS (median, 4.3 vs. 2.6 months, HR 0.50, $P < .0001$) and overall survival (median, 13.4 vs. 10.6 months, HR 0.79, $P = .012$), and was well tolerated (27). In the PARAMOUNT phase III, continuation maintenance study, patients with advanced non-squamous NSCLC were initially treated with cisplatin plus pemetrexed and those without progression were then randomized to receive either supportive care or continuation of pemetrexed therapy. Again, pemetrexed was associated with improvements in PFS (median, 4.1 vs. 2.8 months, $P = .0001$) and overall survival (median, 13.9 vs. 11.0 months, $P = .0195$), while preserving quality of life (28–30). Based on these two trials, pemetrexed was approved by the FDA for both switch and continuation maintenance therapy.

Pemetrexed Plus Bevacizumab

The AVAPERL trial provided further insight into the validity of continuation maintenance therapy with both pemetrexed and bevacizumab in advanced NSCLC. In this trial, all patients received cisplatin, pemetrexed, and bevacizumab followed by maintenance with either pemetrexed plus bevacizumab or bevacizumab alone. While PFS was significantly improved with pemetrexed plus bevacizumab maintenance (median, 7.4 vs. 3.7 months, HR 0.48, $P < .001$), there was no significant difference in overall survival (median, 17.1 vs. 13.2 months, $P = .29$) (15,31). The question of whether pemetrexed, bevacizumab, or the combination of the two is the best maintenance treatment for advanced lung adenocarcinoma is currently unknown, and will be answered in the ongoing clinical trial, E5508 (NCT01107626).

Erlotinib

Erlotinib has been approved by the FDA for maintenance therapy based on the results of the SATURN trial, in which patients with advanced NSCLC were treated with platinum-based chemotherapy × four cycles and then randomized to receive either placebo or erlotinib until progression. While there was a modest, but statistically significant, improvement in PFS with erlotinib (12.3 vs. 11.1 weeks, $P < .0001$), the clinical significance of this finding is unclear (32). In addition, the relevance of this trial has now declined given the high prevalence of upfront *EGFR* mutation testing and the use of first-line targeted therapy for patients with a sensitizing *EGFR* mutation. For patients with wild-type *EGFR*, the efficacy of erlotinib is relatively modest with limited potential to improve outcomes.

Recommendations for Maintenance Therapy

- Maintenance therapy can be considered for patients who achieve a response or have stable disease with platinum-based combination regimens.
- The decision on whether or not to initiate maintenance therapy should be based on performance status, disease-related symptoms, and tolerance of prior chemotherapy, disease burden, and patient preference.

- Pemetrexed is approved as both switch and continuation maintenance therapy in patients with non-squamous NSCLC, while bevacizumab can be used as continuation maintenance in these patients.
- Erlotinib is approved for switch maintenance therapy in patients with any histology based on a very modest improvement in outcome.
- Patients who do not receive maintenance therapy should undergo close radiographic surveillance every 2 to 3 months with initiation of second-line therapy upon evidence of progressive disease.

TARGETED THERAPY

EGFR-Mutated NSCLC

The discovery of oncogenic driver mutations in NSCLC and the subsequent development of targeted therapy have resulted in a major paradigm shift in the treatment of patients with NSCLC. *EGFR*-mutated NSCLC has emerged at the forefront of precision medicine. Prior to the discovery of *EGFR* mutations, the EGFR signaling pathway was known to be up-regulated in NSCLC and was believed to play an important role in pathogenesis and disease progression (33,34). Therefore, specific EGFR tyrosine kinase inhibitors (TKI), such as erlotinib and gefitinib, were developed and evaluated in NSCLC (35–37).

Erlotinib first received FDA approval based on the BR.21 trial, which reported an overall survival benefit with erlotinib over placebo in unselected patients with previously treated advanced NSCLC (median, 7.0 vs. 4.7 months, HR 0.70, $P < .001$) (38). Several groups subsequently identified mutations in the *EGFR* gene that predicted response to EGFR TKIs (39–41). Specifically, deletions in exon 19, the exon 21 L858R point mutation, and the less frequent deletions in exon 18 were shown to be predictive biomarkers. Sensitizing *EGFR* mutations are found in 10% to 15% of lung adenocarcinomas in the U.S. population (2). With this new information, development of EGFR TKIs focused on the selection of patients with sensitizing *EGFR* mutations. While EGFR mutations are found more commonly in patient subgroups with specific clinical features (i.e., women, adenocarcinoma histology, never-smokers, East Asian ethnicity), patient selection for first-line use of EGFR TKIs should not be based on these parameters since they have a greater chance of having wild-type *EGFR* than an *EGFR* mutation and chemotherapy is superior to EGFR TKIs in patients with wild-type *EGFR*. Therefore, molecular testing for identification of *EGFR* mutations should be performed in all patients with stage IV lung adenocarcinoma, and an EGFR TKI should be used as first-line therapy for patients with a known sensitizing mutation.

Gefitinib and erlotinib are first-generation EGFR TKIs, and afatinib is considered a second-generation agent. Erlotinib and gefitinib are reversible inhibitors of the EGFR kinase domain, while afatanib is an irreversible inhibitor of several ErbB family members. Clinical trials that compared an EGFR TKI to chemotherapy in patients with sensitizing EGFR mutations have consistently demonstrated superior response rates (55%–65%) and PFS (9–13 months) with targeted therapy (Table 8.2). The PFS benefit did not generally translate into an improvement in overall survival in these studies due to the high prevalence of cross over from chemotherapy to an EGFR inhibitor upon disease progression. However, a pooled subset analysis of two afatinib versus chemotherapy trials did demonstrate improved overall survival with afatinib in patients with exon 19 deletions, but not in those with L858R mutations.

A recent study compared gefitinib 250 mg/day to afatinib 40 mg/day as front-line therapy in patients with *EGFR*-mutated NSCLC, and demonstrated an improved response rate (70% vs. 56%, $P = .008$) and PFS (median, 11 vs. 10.9 months, HR = 0.73, $P = .016$) with afatinib (42). This modest clinical benefit should be balanced with the higher incidence of skin and mucosal toxicity with afatinib when selecting therapy for patients with a sensitizing *EGFR* mutation, since nearly 40% of patients treated with afatinib required a dose–reduction to 30 mg/day.

Treatment with an EGFR TKI should be continued until clinically significant progression of disease. If progression is limited to one or two sites, the use of local therapy, such as RT, followed by continuation of the EGFR TKI is a reasonable approach. Similarly, for patients who develop progression only in the brain, the EGFR TKI can be continued after appropriate local therapy.

The most common side effects seen with EGFR TKIs are rash, nail changes/paronychia, diarrhea, and increased liver enzymes. Skin toxicities are typically managed with a combination of topical steroids and topical or oral antibiotics based on severity. Diarrhea usually responds to antidiarrheal medications. Dose–reductions may also be used in conjunction with appropriate supportive care measures to improve quality of life and tolerance of therapy.

Resistance

Despite the impressive responses seen with EGFR TKIs in patients with sensitizing mutations, the typical time to progression is only 9 to 13 months (43,44). Research into the mechanisms

Table 8.2 Randomized trials of EGFR TKI versus chemotherapy as first-line therapy in *EGFR*-mutated NSCLC

					Response rate (%)		Median progression-free survival (mo)		Median overall survival (mo)	
Study	Location	*N*	EGFR TKI	Chemo regimen	TKI	Chemo	TKI	Chemo	TKI	Chemo
IPASS* (76, 77)	East Asia	437	G	CbP	71.2	47.3	9.5	6.3	21.6	21.9
WJTOG3405 (78, 79)	Japan	177	G	CDDP-D	62.1	32.2	9.2	6.3	34.8	37.3
NEJ002 (44)	Japan	230	G	CbP	73.7	30.7	10.8	5.4	30.5	23.6
OPTIMAL (80, 81)	China	165	E	CbG	83	36	13.1	4.6	22.7	28.9
EURTAC (43)	Europe	173	E	Pl-2D	64	18	9.7	5.2	19.3	19.5
LUX-Lung 3 (82, 83)	Global	345	A	CDDP-Pe	56	23	11.1	6.9	28.2	28.2
LUX-Lung 6 (82, 84)	Asia	364	A	CDDP-G	66.9	23	11	5.6	23.1	23.5

A, afatinib; CbG, carboplatin plus gemcitabine; CbP, carboplatin plus paclitaxel; CDDP-D, cisplatin plus docetaxel; CDDP-G, cisplatin plus gemcitabine; CDDP-Pe, cisplatin plus pemetrexed; E, erlotinib; G, gefitinib; Pl-2D, platinum-based, two-drug regimen.
*Data extracted from patients in whom EGFR mutational status was assessed.

of resistance to the first- and second-generation EGFR TKIs revealed that approximately 60% of patients develop a secondary exon 20 T790M mutation, which adds a bulky methionine residue within the tyrosine kinase domain, thereby inhibiting EGFR TKI binding (45). Additional mechanisms of resistance include *MET* amplification, epithelial-to-mesenchymal transition, activation of the PI3K pathway, and histological transformation to small cell carcinoma (2%–5%) (45,46). Patients who progress on a first-line EGFR TKI should undergo repeat biopsy for evaluation for the T790M mutation since third-generation EGFR TKIs with activity against this mutation are now available.

Third-Generation EGFR TKIs

The third-generation EGFR TKIs have been developed specifically to target the T790M resistance mutation. Osimertinib is an orally administered, irreversible, mutation-specific EGFR inhibitor that was recently approved by the FDA for patients with T790M-mediated resistance to first-line TKI therapy. In a phase I study, osimertinib demonstrated a response rate of 64% in patients with tumors harboring a T790M mutation, with a median PFS of 10 to 13 months. Due to greater selectivity for the mutant receptor relative to the wild-type receptor, osimertinib is associated with considerably less skin and GI toxicity than first-generation EGFR TKIs (47). Other T790M-selective inhibitors are in clinical development. For patients with T790M-negative recurrence, chemotherapy utilizing a standard first-line regimen remains a reasonable option.

Recommendations for EGFR-Mutated NSCLC

- Molecular testing should be conducted for all patients with stage IV lung adenocarcinoma and for never-smokers with any histologic subtype.
- For patients with *EGFR* exon 19 deletions or L858R mutations, a first or second generation TKI is recommended as first-line therapy (erlotinib 150 mg/day, gefitinib 250 mg/day, afatinib 40 mg/day).
- A repeat biopsy for T790M testing is recommended for patients who develop acquired resistance to first-line EGFR TKI therapy.
- Osimertinib (80 mg/day) is approved for patients' tumors harboring a T790M mutation.
- Chemotherapy is recommended for patients with T790M-negative tumors after progression on a first-line EGFR TKI.

ALK-Rearranged NSCLC

The *EML4-ALK* rearrangement that occurs in 3% to 6% of patients with NSCLC defines another molecular subset of patients that benefit from targeted therapy (48). Nearly all patients with *ALK*-rearranged NSCLC have adenocarcinoma and are never or light-former smokers. Initially reported in 2007, an inversion within the short arm of chromosome 2 leads to a fusion protein in which the N-terminal domain of the EML4 is joined to the intracellular kinase domain of ALK, leading to an oncogenic, constitutive activation of the ALK signal transduction pathway (49).

Crizotinib

At the time, crizotinib was already in clinical development as a MET inhibitor, so given its known ability to inhibit ALK activity, clinical trials were rapidly designed in this new population. In the expanded phase I study of patients with *ALK*-rearranged NSCLC, crizotinib demonstrated a response rate of 60%, a disease control rate of 90%, and a median PFS of approximately 10 months, resulting in the approval of crizotinib for treatment of patients with *ALK*-rearranged NSCLC. In a phase III study, crizotinib was compared to second-line chemotherapy with docetaxel or pemetrexed in patients with *ALK*-rearranged NSCLC. Both response rate (65% vs. 20%, $P < .001$) and PFS (median, 7.7 vs. 3.0 months, $P < .001$) were superior with crizotinib. Another phase III trial reported the superiority of PFS for crizotinib over platinum-based chemotherapy in the first-line setting for patients with *ALK*-rearranged NSCLC (median, 10.9 vs. 7.0 m, $P < .001$) (50,51). Common toxicities of crizotinib include visual disturbances, increased liver enzymes, and nausea/vomiting. Supportive medications, dose interruptions, and dose–reductions are the typical interventions used to control these side effects.

Second-Generation ALK Inhibitors

Upon progression, many mechanisms of resistance to crizotinib have been identified, including secondary mutations in the *ALK* gene. Common acquired resistance mutations include L1196M, G1269A, C1156Y, L1152R, G1202R, S1206Y, and 1151Tins (52). The second-generation ALK TKIs, ceritinib, and alectinib, have been approved for the treatment of patients who develop resistance to crizotinib. Both of these agents are associated with a response rate of 40% to 55% in this setting with a median PFS of 7 to 9 months. Another important advantage of these second-generation agents is their ability to achieve greater activity against brain metastasis. The main side effects of ceritinib are nausea, vomiting, and diarrhea, while alectinib can induce constipation and fatigue (53,54).

Table 8.3 summaries selected clinical trials of the FDA-approved ALK inhibitors. Many newer ALK inhibitors are in clinical development.

Recommendations for ALK-Rearranged NSCLC

- Crizotinib (250 mg BID) is approved for the treatment of ALK-rearranged NSCLC.
- Ceritinib (750 mg/d) and alectinib (600 mg BID) are preferred options for treatment of acquired resistance to or intolerance of crizotinib.
- Both ceritinib and alectinib have higher level of activity against brain metastasis than crizotinib.

Uncommon Mutations: *BRAF, ROS1, RET, MET*

In addition to *EGFR* mutations and *ALK*-rearrangements, several other driver mutations have been identified in lung adenocarcinoma and rational therapies targeting these pathways are currently undergoing clinical investigation. Randomized data in these patient subsets will be difficult to generate given the rarity of each of these biomarkers. However, promising phase I and II data provide support for the use of targeted agents in the following molecularly defined patient subsets after progression on platinum-based, first-line therapy.

ROS1

ROS1-rearrangements occur in approximately 1% of lung adenocarcinomas. In a phase I trial, crizotinib yielded a response rate of 72% in patients with *ROS1*-rearranged NSCLC with a median PFS of 19 months (55). Recently, the U.S. FDA approved crizotinib for the treatment of patients with *ROS1*-rearranged NSCLC.

MET

Mutations in the *MET* oncogene can result in "skipping" of exon 14 in 2% to 3% of patients with NSCLC (56). They appear to be more common in patients with adenocarcinoma and sarcomatoid carcinoma. Targeting this pathway with MET inhibitors, such as crizotinib, has demonstrated promising clinical responses in select cases, and clinical trials are underway to more fully evaluate this strategy (57).

RET

A *RET* translocation occurs in 1% to 2% of pulmonary adenocarcinomas. Early clinical data have demonstrated responses with the *RET* inhibitor, cabozantinib (58).

Table 8.3 Selected trials of ALK inhibition in *ALK*-rearranged NSCLC

Study	Line of therapy	*N*	ALK TKI	Chemo regimen	Response rate (%)		Median progression-free survival (mo)		Median overall survival (mo)	
					TKI	Chemo	TKI	Chemo	TKI	Chemo
PROFILE 1014 (51)	First	343	Cri	Pl-Pe	74	45	10.9	7	NR	NR
PROFILE 1007 (50)	Second	347	Cri	Pe or D	65	20	7.7	3	20.3	22.8
Shaw et al. (54)	After first	114	Ce	NA	58	NA	7	NA	NR	NA
AF-002JG (53)	Post-Cri	87	A	NA	48	NA	8.1	NA	NR	NA

A, alectinib; Ce, ceritinib; Cri, crizotinib; NA, not applicable; NR, not reported; Pe or D, pemetrexed or docetaxel; Pl-Pe, platinum plus pemetrexed.

BRAF

While best known as a therapeutic target in melanoma, patients NSCLC with a *BRAF* V600 mutation have had a response rate of 42% when treated with vemurafenib (59). In addition, the combination of dabrafenib, a BRAF inhibitor, and trametinib, a MEK inhibitor, resulted in a response rate of 66% with a median PFS of approximately 9 months. The role of these agents in tumors with non-V600 *BRAF* mutations is unclear at this time.

IMMUNOTHERAPY

The discovery of the efficacy of immunotherapy in advanced NSCLC is one of the most impactful recent developments in the field. The immune checkpoint inhibitors have dramatically altered the care for this patient population, and their role in progressive disease is discussed in Chapter 9. Clinical trials are now examining immune checkpoint inhibitors in the first-line setting. Recently, pembrolizumab, an anti-PD1 antibody, was compared to chemotherapy as first-line therapy in patients with advanced NSCLC whose tumors expressed PD-L1 in ≥50% of tumor cells (60). In this selected population (about 30% of patients), pembrolizumab was superior to chemotherapy in terms of PFS (median, 10.3 vs. 6.0 months, $P < .001$), overall survival (HR 0.60, $P = .005$), response rate (45% vs. 28%), and duration of response (not reached vs. 6.3 months). Based on these data, pembrolizumab should soon become the standard first-line treatment option for patients with advanced NSCLC with high PD-L1 expression.

OLIGOMETASTATIC DISEASE

Advanced NSCLC is an incurable disease. However, patients who present with a low burden of metastatic disease deserve further discussion since long-term survival has been seen in those with such oligometastatic disease (61). Oligometastasis is broadly defined as a state of minimal systemic metastatic tumors for which local therapy can be pursued with curative intent (62). However, there is no clear consensus on the number of lesions that would define a patient with "oligometastatic" disease.

CNS Metastasis

One of the most common sites of oligometastatic disease is the brain. It is estimated that approximately 7% of patients with metastatic NSCLC will present with a solitary metastatic brain lesion (63). For patients with widespread disease, treatment of brain metastasis typically consists of corticosteroids and RT, and the prognosis remains poor. However, for patients with disease that is oligometastatic to the brain, aggressive local therapy is often utilized. Multiple retrospective studies have reviewed the role of surgical resection of isolated brain metastases, reporting promising outcomes with aggressive treatment (64). Several older prospective clinical trials have also found that surgery plus whole brain RT prolongs survival and quality of life for patients with solitary brain metastasis (65,66). More recently, stereotactic radiosurgery has become an attractive treatment modality for isolated brain metastasis as a way to spare patients the neurocognitive side effects of whole brain RT (67–72). A randomized trial from Japan assessed stereotactic radiosurgery with or without whole brain RT, and found no difference in overall survival, but patients who did not receive whole brain RT upfront had a higher incidence of intracranial recurrence (67).

Other Oligometastatic Sites

A solitary adrenal metastasis should also be considered for aggressive local therapy, with potential adrenalectomy when feasible, provided it is the sole site of metastatic disease (73,74). Similarly, patients with bilateral lung involvement with solitary lesions in each lung may have two separate primaries or metastatic disease. In this situation, long-term survival has been reported, particularly when there is no involvement of mediastinal lymph nodes (75). When considering aggressive resection of the primary lung tumor and a solitary metastatic lesion elsewhere, it is important to exclude involvement of mediastinal nodes, since N2-positivity portends a poor prognosis in the setting of an aggressive surgical approach.

Finally, for patients with a good response to systemic therapy, residual oligometastatic lesions or sites of localized progression can be treated with local modalities other than surgery, such as RT or radiofrequency ablation. This is particularly true for patients with driver mutations who experience localized progression while on targeted therapy. For patients with oligometastatic NSCLC or localized progression on systemic therapy, a multidisciplinary discussion should be held to assess potential treatment options. The decision to take an aggressive approach for oligometastatic disease should be made carefully, as treatment comes with the risks of more aggressive interventions. However, the potential for long-term disease control is compelling for appropriately selected patients.

CONCLUSION

Significant advances have been made in the treatment of advanced NSCLC. Chemotherapeutic agents with improved tolerability have been developed allowing for disease control with a more favorable therapeutic index. The identification of the molecular drivers of NSCLC, including *EGFR, ALK,* and *ROS1,* has already led to the development of well-tolerated and effective targeted agents. These advances, along with progress in immunotherapy, have now translated into a multitude of treatment options for patients that can improve quality of life and prolong survival.

KEY POINTS

- All newly diagnosed metastatic lung adenocarcinomas should be subjected to molecular testing, at a minimum for *EGFR* mutations, and *ALK* and *ROS1* rearrangement.
- Platinum-based, two-drug chemotherapy is the standard treatment for patients with advanced NSCLC with a good performance status in the absence of a targetable driver mutation.
- Carboplatin or cisplatin can be combined with paclitaxel, docetaxel, nab-paclitaxel, gemcitabine, pemetrexed, or vinorelbine as first-line therapy for advanced NSCLC.
- Platinum-based chemotherapy should be given for a maximum of four to six cycles, with consideration of maintenance therapy in appropriately selected patients.
- Pemetrexed and bevacizumab should only be used in non-squamous NSCLC.
- Erlotinib, gefitinib, or afatinib are the standard, first-line treatments for patients with *EGFR*-mutated NSCLC.
- Progression of *EGFR*-mutated NSCLC on *EGFR* TKI warrants a re-biopsy to evaluate for the T790M mutation. If T790M is found, then treatment should be initiated with a third-generation *EGFR* TKI (e.g., osimertinib).
- Crizotinib is the recommended treatment for *ALK*- or *ROS1*-rearranged metastatic NSCLC. The second-generation *ALK* TKIs, ceritinib, or alectinib, are available for patients with *ALK*-rearranged tumors with disease progression on crizotinib.
- The immune checkpoint inhibitor, pembrolizumab, is superior to chemotherapy as first-line treatment for patients with advanced NSCLC with high PD-L1 expression.

REFERENCES

1. Cancer Genome Atlas Research Network. Comprehensive genomic characterization of squamous cell lung cancers. *Nature*. 2012;489:519-525.
2. Kris MG, Johnson BE, Berry LD, et al. Using multiplexed assays of oncogenic drivers in lung cancers to select targeted drugs. *JAMA*. 2014;311:1998-2006.
3. Maheswaran S, Sequist LV, Nagrath S, et al. Detection of mutations in EGFR in circulating lung-cancer cells. *N Engl J Med*. 2008;359:366-377.
4. Cullen MH, Billingham LJ, Woodroffe CM, et al. Mitomycin, ifosfamide, and cisplatin in unresectable non–small-cell lung cancer: effects on survival and quality of life. *J Clin Oncol*. 1999;17:3188-3194.
5. Alberti W, Anderson G, Bartolucci A, et al. Chemotherapy in non-small cell lung cancer: a meta-analysis using updated data on individual patients from 52 randomized clinical trials. *BMJ*. 1995;311:899-909.
6. Schiller JH, Harrington D, Belani CP, et al. Comparison of four chemotherapy regimens for advanced non-small-cell lung cancer. *N Engl J Med*. 2002;346:92-98.
7. Kelly K, Crowley J, Bunn PA, et al. Randomized phase III trial of paclitaxel plus carboplatin versus vinorelbine plus cisplatin in the treatment of patients with advanced non–small-cell lung cancer: a Southwest Oncology Group trial. *J Clin Oncol*. 2001;19:3210-3218.
8. Belani CP, Lee JS, Socinski MA, et al. Randomized phase III trial comparing cisplatin–etoposide to carboplatin–paclitaxel in advanced or metastatic non-small cell lung cancer. *Ann Oncol*. 2005;16:1069-1075.
9. Ohe Y, Ohashi Y, Kubota K, et al. Randomized phase III study of cisplatin plus irinotecan versus carboplatin plus paclitaxel, cisplatin plus gemcitabine, and cisplatin plus vinorelbine for advanced non-small-cell lung cancer: four-arm cooperative study in Japan. *Ann Oncol*. 2007;18:317-323.
10. Delbaldo C, Michiels S, Rolland E, et al. WITHDRAWN: second or third additional chemotherapy drug for non-small cell lung cancer in patients with advanced disease. *Cochrane Database Syst Rev*. 2012;4:Cd004569.
11. Boni C, Tiseo M, Boni L, et al. Triplets versus doublets, with or without cisplatin, in the first-line treatment of stage IIIB-IV non-small cell lung cancer (NSCLC) patients: a multicenter randomised factorial trial (FAST). *Br J Cancer*. 2012;106:658-665.
12. Georgoulias V, Papadakis E, Alexopoulos A, et al. Platinum-based and non-platinum-based chemotherapy in advanced non-small-cell lung cancer: a randomised multicentre trial. *Lancet*. 2001;357:1478-1484.
13. Smit EF, van Meerbeeck JP, Lianes P, et al. Three-arm randomized study of two cisplatin-based regimens and paclitaxel plus gemcitabine in advanced non-small-cell lung cancer: a phase III trial of the European Organization for Research and Treatment of Cancer Lung Cancer Group–EORTC 08975. *J Clin Oncol*. 2003;21:3909-3917.
14. Scagliotti GV, Parikh P, von Pawel J, et al. Phase III study comparing cisplatin plus gemcitabine with cisplatin plus pemetrexed in

chemotherapy-naive patients with advanced-stage non–small-cell lung cancer. *J Clin Oncol.* 2008;26:3543-3551.

15. Patel JD, Socinski MA, Garon EB, et al. PointBreak: a randomized phase III study of pemetrexed plus carboplatin and bevacizumab followed by maintenance pemetrexed and bevacizumab versus paclitaxel plus carboplatin and bevacizumab followed by maintenance bevacizumab in patients with stage IIIB or IV non-squamous non-small-cell lung cancer. *J Clin Oncol.* 2013;31:4349-4357.
16. Zinner RG, Obasaju CK, Spigel DR, et al. PRONOUNCE: randomized, open-label, phase III study of first-line pemetrexed + carboplatin followed by maintenance pemetrexed versus paclitaxel + carboplatin + bevacizumab followed by maintenance bevacizumab in patients ith advanced non-squamous non-small-cell lung cancer. *J Thorac Oncol.* 2015;10:134-142.
17. Kim Y, Oh I, Kim K, et al. LBA41_PR a randomized phase III study of docetaxel plus cisplatin versus pemetrexed plus cisplatin in first line non-squamous non-small cell lung cancer (NSQ-NSCLC). *Ann Oncol.* 2014;25 (suppl 4).
18. Sandler A, Gray R, Perry MC, et al. Paclitaxel–carboplatin alone or with bevacizumab for non–small-cell lung cancer. *N Engl J Med.* 2006;355:2542-2550.
19. Reck M, von Pawel J, Zatloukal P, et al. Phase III trial of cisplatin plus gemcitabine with either placebo or bevacizumab as first-line therapy for non-squamous non–small-cell lung cancer: AVAiL. *J Clin Oncol.* 2009;27:1227-1234.
20. Johnson DH, Fehrenbacher L, Novotny WF, et al. Randomized phase II trial comparing bevacizumab plus carboplatin and paclitaxel with carboplatin and paclitaxel alone in previously untreated locally advanced or metastatic non-small-cell lung cancer. *J Clin Oncol.* 2004;22:2184-2191.
21. Thatcher N, Hirsch FR, Luft AV, et al. Necitumumab plus gemcitabine and cisplatin versus gemcitabine and cisplatin alone as first-line therapy in patients with stage IV squamous non-small-cell lung cancer (SQUIRE): an open-label, randomised, controlled phase 3 trial. *Lancet Oncol.* 2015;16:763-774.
22. Socinski MA, Bondarenko I, Karaseva NA, et al. Weekly nab-paclitaxel in combination with carboplatin versus solvent-based paclitaxel plus carboplatin as first-line therapy in patients with advanced non-small-cell lung cancer: final results of a phase III trial. *J Clin Oncol.* 2012;30:2055-2062.
23. Available at: http://www.lung-map.org
24. Ardizzoni A, Boni L, Tiseo M, et al. Cisplatin- versus carboplatin-based chemotherapy in first-line treatment of advanced non-small-cell lung cancer: an individual patient data meta-analysis. *J Natl Cancer Inst.* 2007;99:847-857.
25. Socinski MA, Schell MJ, Peterman A, et al. Phase III trial comparing a defined duration of therapy versus continuous therapy followed by

second-line therapy in advanced-stage IIIB/IV non–small-cell lung cancer. *J Clin Oncol*. 2002;20:1335-1343.

26. Park JO, Kim SW, Ahn JS, et al. Phase III trial of two versus four additional cycles in patients who are nonprogressive after two cycles of platinum-based chemotherapy in non small-cell lung cancer. *J Clin Oncol*. 2007;25:5233-5239.
27. Ciuleanu T, Brodowicz T, Zielinski C, et al. Maintenance pemetrexed plus best supportive care versus placebo plus best supportive care for non-small-cell lung cancer: a randomised, double-blind, phase 3 study. *Lancet*. 2009;374:1432-1440.
28. Paz-Ares L, de Marinis F, Dediu M, et al. Maintenance therapy with pemetrexed plus best supportive care versus placebo plus best supportive care after induction therapy with pemetrexed plus cisplatin for advanced non-squamous non-small-cell lung cancer (PARAMOUNT): a double-blind, phase 3, randomised controlled trial. *Lancet Oncol*. 2012;13:247-255.
29. Gridelli C, de Marinis F, Pujol JL, et al. Safety, resource use, and quality of life in paramount: a phase III study of maintenance pemetrexed versus placebo after induction pemetrexed plus cisplatin for advanced non-squamous non-small-cell lung cancer. *J Thorac Oncol*. 2012;7:1713-1721.
30. Paz-Ares LG, de Marinis F, Dediu M, et al. PARAMOUNT: final overall survival results of the phase III study of maintenance pemetrexed versus placebo immediately after induction treatment with pemetrexed plus cisplatin for advanced non-squamous non-small-cell lung cancer. *J Clin Oncol*. 2013;31:2895-2902.
31. Barlesi F, Scherpereel A, Gorbunova V, et al. Maintenance bevacizumab-pemetrexed after first-line cisplatin-pemetrexed-bevacizumab for advanced non-squamous nonsmall-cell lung cancer: updated survival analysis of the AVAPERL (MO22089) randomized phase III trial. *Ann Oncol*. 2014;25:1044-1052.
32. Cappuzzo F, Ciuleanu T, Stelmakh L, et al. Erlotinib as maintenance treatment in advanced non-small-cell lung cancer: a multicentre, randomised, placebo-controlled phase 3 study. *Lancet Oncol*. 2010;11:521-529.
33. Brabender J, Danenberg KD, Metzger R, et al. Epidermal growth factor receptor and HER2-neu mRNA expression in non-small cell lung cancer Is correlated with survival. *Clin Cancer Res*. 2001;7:1850-1855.
34. Rusch V, Klimstra D, Venkatraman E, et al. Overexpression of the epidermal growth factor receptor and its ligand transforming growth factor alpha is frequent in resectable non-small cell lung cancer but does not predict tumor progression. *Clin Cancer Res*. 1997;3:515-522.
35. Fukuoka M, Yano S, Giaccone G, et al. Multi-institutional randomized phase II trial of gefitinib for previously treated patients with advanced non-small-cell lung cancer (The IDEAL 1 Trial) [corrected]. *J Clin Oncol*. 2003;21:2237-2246.
36. Kris MG, Natale RB, Herbst RS, et al. Efficacy of gefitinib, an inhibitor of the epidermal growth factor receptor tyrosine kinase, in symptomatic

patients with non-small cell lung cancer: a randomized trial. *JAMA*. 2003;290:2149-2158.

37. Moyer JD, Barbacci EG, Iwata KK, et al. Induction of apoptosis and cell cycle arrest by CP-358,774, an inhibitor of epidermal growth factor receptor tyrosine kinase. *Cancer Res*. 1997;57:4838-4848.
38. Shepherd FA, Rodrigues Pereira J, Ciuleanu T, et al. Erlotinib in previously treated non-small-cell lung cancer. *N Engl J Med*. 2005;353:123-132.
39. Lynch TJ, Bell DW, Sordella R, et al. Activating mutations in the epidermal growth factor receptor underlying responsiveness of non-small-cell lung cancer to gefitinib. *N Engl J Med*. 2004;350:2129-2139.
40. Paez JG, Janne PA, Lee JC, et al. EGFR mutations in lung cancer: correlation with clinical response to gefitinib therapy. *Science*. 2004;304:1497-1500.
41. Pao W, Miller V, Zakowski M, et al. EGF receptor gene mutations are common in lung cancers from "never smokers" and are associated with sensitivity of tumors to gefitinib and erlotinib. *Proc Natl Acad Sci USA*. 2004;101:13306-13311.
42. Soria JC, Felip E, Lu S, et al. Afatinib versus erlotinib as second-line treatment of patients with advanced squamous cell carcinoma of the lung (LUX-Lung 8): an open-label randomised controlled phase 3 trial. *Lancet Oncol*. 2015;16(8):897–907.
43. Rosell R, Carcereny E, Gervais R, et al. Erlotinib versus standard chemotherapy as first-line treatment for European patients with advanced EGFR mutation-positive non-small-cell lung cancer (EURTAC): a multicentre, open-label, randomised phase 3 trial. *Lancet Oncol*. 2012;13:239-246.
44. Maemondo M, Inoue A, Kobayashi K, et al. Gefitinib or chemotherapy for non-small-cell lung cancer with mutated EGFR. *N Engl J Med*. 2010;362:2380-2388.
45. Sequist LV, Waltman BA, Dias-Santagata D, et al. Genotypic and histological evolution of lung cancers acquiring resistance to EGFR inhibitors. *Sci Transl Med*. 2011;3:75ra26.
46. Engelman JA, Zejnullahu K, Mitsudomi T, et al. MET amplification leads to gefitinib resistance in lung cancer by activating ERBB3 signaling. *Science*. 2007;316:1039-1043.
47. Jänne PA, Yang JC-H, Kim D-W, et al. AZD9291 in EGFR inhibitor–resistant non–small-cell lung cancer. *N Engl J Med*. 2015;372:1689-1699.
48. Steuer CE, Ramalingam SS. ALK-positive non-small cell lung cancer: mechanisms of resistance and emerging treatment options. *Cancer*. 2014;120:2392-2402.
49. Soda M, Choi YL, Enomoto M, et al. Identification of the transforming EML4-ALK fusion gene in non-small-cell lung cancer. *Nature*. 2007;448:561-566.
50. Shaw AT, Kim DW, Nakagawa K, et al. Crizotinib versus chemotherapy in advanced ALK-positive lung cancer. *N Engl J Med*. 2013;368:2385-2394.

51. Solomon BJ, Mok T, Kim D-W, et al. First-line crizotinib versus chemotherapy in ALK-positive lung cancer. *N Engl J Med.* 2014;371:2167-2177.
52. Rolfo C, Passiglia F, Castiglia M, et al. ALK and crizotinib: after the honeymoon ... what else? Resistance mechanisms and new therapies to overcome it. *Transl Lung Cancer Res.* 2014;3:250-261.
53. Gadgeel SM, Gandhi L, Riely GJ, et al. Safety and activity of alectinib against systemic disease and brain metastases in patients with crizotinib-resistant ALK-rearranged non-small-cell lung cancer (AF-002JG): results from the dose-finding portion of a phase 1/2 study. *Lancet Oncol.* 2014;15:1119-1128.
54. Shaw AT, Kim DW, Mehra R, et al. Ceritinib in ALK-rearranged non-small-cell lung cancer. *N Engl J Med.* 2014;370:1189-1197.
55. Shaw AT, Ou S-HI, Bang Y-J, et al. Crizotinib in ROS1-rearranged non–small-cell lung cancer. *N Engl J Med.* 2014;371:1963-1971.
56. Awad MM, Oxnard GR, Jackman DM, et al. MET exon 14 mutations in non-small-cell lung cancer are associated with advanced age and stage-dependent MET genomic amplification and c-Met overexpression. *J Clin Oncol.* 2016;34:721-730.
57. Paik PK, Drilon A, Fan PD, et al. Response to MET inhibitors in patients with stage IV lung adenocarcinomas harboring MET mutations causing exon 14 skipping. *Cancer Discov.* 2015;5:842-849.
58. Drilon A, Wang L, Hasanovic A, et al. Response to Cabozantinib in patients with RET fusion-positive lung adenocarcinomas. *Cancer Discov.* 2013;3:630-635.
59. Hyman DM, Puzanov I, Subbiah V, et al. Vemurafenib in multiple nonmelanoma cancers with BRAF V600 mutations. *N Engl J Med.* 2015;373:726-736.
60. Reck M, Rodriguez-Abreu D, Robinson AG, et al. Pembrolizumab versus chemotherapy for PD-L1-positive non-small-cell lung cancer. *N Engl J Med.* Published online ahead of print on October 8, 2016. doi: 10.1056/NEJMoa1606774.
61. Ashworth A, Rodrigues G, Boldt G, Palma D. Is there an oligometastatic state in non-small cell lung cancer? A systematic review of the literature. *Lung Cancer.* 2013;82:197-203.
62. Kaneda H, Saito Y. Oligometastases: defined by prognosis and evaluated by cure. *Cancer Treat Commun.* 2015;3:1-6.
63. Villaruz LC, Kubicek GJ, Socinski MA. Management of non-small cell lung cancer with oligometastasis. *Curr Oncol Rep.* 2012;14:333-341.
64. Bonnette P, Puyo P, Gabriel C, et al. Surgical management of non-small cell lung cancer with synchronous brain metastases. *Chest.* 2001;119:1469-1475.
65. Patchell RA, Tibbs PA, Walsh JW, et al. A randomized trial of surgery in the treatment of single metastases to the brain. *N Engl J Med.* 1990;322:494-500.

66. Vecht CJ, Haaxma-Reiche H, Noordijk EM, et al. Treatment of single brain metastasis: radiotherapy alone or combined with neurosurgery? *Ann Neurol.* 1993;33:583-590.
67. Aoyama H, Shirato H, Tago M, et al. Stereotactic radiosurgery plus whole-brain radiation therapy vs stereotactic radiosurgery alone for treatment of brain metastases: a randomized controlled trial. *JAMA.* 2006;295:2483-2491.
68. De Ruysscher D, Wanders R, van Baardwijk A, et al. Radical treatment of non-small-cell lung cancer patients with synchronous oligometastases: long-term results of a prospective phase II trial (Nct01282450). *J Thorac Oncol.* 2012;7:1547-1555.
69. Milano MT, Katz AW, Zhang H, Okunieff P. Oligometastases treated with stereotactic body radiotherapy: long-term follow-up of prospective study. *Int J Radiat Oncol Biol Phys.* 2012;83:878-886.
70. Lischalk JW, Oermann E, Collins SP, et al. Five-fraction stereotactic radiosurgery (SRS) for single inoperable high-risk non-small cell lung cancer (NSCLC) brain metastases. *Radiat Oncol.* 2015;10:216.
71. Won YK, Lee JY, Kang YN, et al. Stereotactic radiosurgery for brain metastasis in non-small cell lung cancer. *Radiat Oncol J.* 2015;33: 207-216.
72. Wegner RE, Olson AC, Kondziolka D, et al. Stereotactic radiosurgery for patients with brain metastases from small cell lung cancer. *Int J Radiat Oncol Biol Phys.* 2011;81:e21-e27.
73. Parikh RB, Cronin AM, Kozono DE, et al. Definitive primary therapy in patients presenting with oligometastatic non-small cell lung cancer. *Int J Radiat Oncol Biol Phys.* 2014;89:880-887.
74. Beitler AL, Urschel JD, Velagapudi SR, Takita H. Surgical management of adrenal metastases from lung cancer. *J Surg Oncol.* 1998;69:54-57.
75. Walts AE, Mirocha JM, Leong T, Marchevsky AM. Pathologic staging and survival of patients with synchronous bilateral lung carcinomas. *Am J Clin Pathol.* 2016;45:244-250.
76. Mok TS, Wu YL, Thongprasert S, et al. Gefitinib or carboplatin–paclitaxel in pulmonary adenocarcinoma. *N Engl J Med.* 2009;361: 947-957.
77. Fukuoka M, Wu YL, Thongprasert S, et al. Biomarker analyses and final overall survival results from a phase III, randomized, open-label, first-line study of gefitinib versus carboplatin/paclitaxel in clinically selected patients with advanced non-small-cell lung cancer in Asia (IPASS). *J Clin Oncol.* 2011;29:2866-2874.
78. Mitsudomi T, Morita S, Yatabe Y, et al. Gefitinib versus cisplatin plus docetaxel in patients with non-small-cell lung cancer harbouring mutations of the epidermal growth factor receptor (WJTOG3405): an open label, randomised phase 3 trial. *Lancet Oncol.* 2010;11:121-128.
79. Yoshioka H, Mitsudomi T, Morita S, et al. Final overall survival results of WJTOG 3405, a randomized phase 3 trial comparing gefitinib (G)

with cisplatin plus docetaxel (CD) as the first-line treatment for patients with non-small cell lung cancer (NSCLC) harboring mutations of the epidermal growth factor receptor (EGFR). Poster presented at ASCO Annual Meeting; 2014; Chicago, IL.

80. Zhou C, Wu YL, Chen G, et al. Erlotinib versus chemotherapy as first-line treatment for patients with advanced EGFR mutation-positive non-small-cell lung cancer (OPTIMAL, CTONG-0802): a multicentre, open-label, randomised, phase 3 study. *Lancet Oncol.* 2011;12:735-742.
81. Zhou C, Wu YL, Liu X, et al. Overall survival (OS) results from OPTIMAL (CTONG0802), a phase III trial of erlotinib (E) versus carboplatin plus gemcitabine (GC) as first-line treatment for Chinese patients with EGFR mutation-positive advanced non-small cell lung cancer (NSCLC). Poster presented at ASCO Annual Meeting; 2012; Chicago, IL.
82. Yang JC, Wu YL, Schuler M, et al. Afatinib versus cisplatin-based chemotherapy for EGFR mutation-positive lung adenocarcinoma (LUX-Lung 3 and LUX-Lung 6): analysis of overall survival data from two randomised, phase 3 trials. *Lancet Oncol.* 2015;16:141-151.
83. Sequist LV, Yang JC, Yamamoto N, et al. Phase III study of afatinib or cisplatin plus pemetrexed in patients with metastatic lung adenocarcinoma with EGFR mutations. *J Clin Oncol.* 2013;31:3327-3334.
84. Wu YL, Zhou C, Hu CP, et al. Afatinib versus cisplatin plus gemcitabine for first-line treatment of Asian patients with advanced non-small-cell lung cancer harbouring EGFR mutations (LUX-Lung 6): an open-label, randomised phase 3 trial. *Lancet Oncol.* 2014;15:213-222.

9 Management of Recurrent Non–Small-Cell Lung Cancer

Bryan J. Schneider

INTRODUCTION

The management of recurrent non–small-cell lung cancer (NSCLC) has become more challenging over the past 10 years. Previously, few chemotherapy options were available and all patients were viewed as having the same disease with no discrimination based on tumor histology or genetic biomarkers. Front-line therapeutic options were often toxic and many patients were too ill to consider second-line treatment at the time of cancer progression. With the advent of less toxic therapy and improved symptom management, many patients are now able to receive therapy beyond the front-line regimen.

It is important to be mindful of the goals of therapy when treatment is considered. The majority of patients with recurrent disease will be treated with palliative intent to improve symptoms and maintain quality of life. Rarely, recurrent NSCLC may present in a limited manner with the potential for cure, and these situations should not be missed.

PRESENTATION OF RECURRENCE

NSCLC has a high rate of recurrence regardless of the initial stage and treatment. Stage I–II patients with completely resected disease have a 30% to 60% chance of metastatic spread that often manifests within the first 2 years postresection. Similarly, up to 80% of patients with stage III disease treated with definitive local-regional therapy will recur. Stage IV NSCLC is almost uniformly incurable despite aggressive front-line, platinum-based therapy, or targeted therapy for driver mutation-positive disease. These numbers suggest that 80% of patients with NSCLC will ultimately relapse and may be eligible for subsequent therapy.

Upon evidence of recurrent disease, repeat staging scans and a biopsy to confirm relapse are strongly recommended, especially if oligometastatic disease is identified on imaging and aggressive treatment is considered. For patients with early stage disease, relapse may occur locally at the site of surgical resection or radiation therapy (RT). In addition, regional spread to hilar and/or mediastinal lymph nodes is not uncommon after primary resection. Rarely, patients may present with a metachronous, isolated, metastatic site in the brain, contralateral lung, or adrenal gland. However, the majority of patients develop diffusely metastatic disease. Therapeutic options at the time of relapse are based on the initial treatment received, the location of relapse, tumor burden, tumor histology, presence of actionable genetic biomarkers, and patient performance status (PS).

INTRATHORACIC LOCAL-REGIONAL RECURRENCE

Patients may develop a local recurrence after definitive therapy, such as surgical resection for stage I–II NSCLC or chemoradiotherapy for stage III disease. If the repeat staging work-up fails to identify extrathoracic metastases, further local therapy should be considered since some patients may still be cured. A new, second primary lung malignancy can occur in up to 5% of such patients annually and should be treated with surgical resection or stereotactic body radiation (SBRT) if detected at an early stage. Similarly, patients may present with a regional (e.g., hilar or mediastinal) nodal recurrence after surgical resection for stage I or II disease, and definitive chemoradiotherapy should be strongly considered with intent to cure. Progression of a tumor nodule previously treated with SBRT may be treated with radiofrequency ablation (RFA) with good long-term outcome. It is important to consider these potentially curative treatment options for recurrent disease isolated to the thorax, since systemic therapy alone will only delay disease progression.

OLIGOMETASTATIC RECURRENCE

Adrenal Gland Metastasis

Aggressive local treatment should be considered for NSCLC that metastasizes to an adrenal gland after definitive therapy for early-stage disease. An adrenal gland metastasis identified after surgical resection may also be surgically resected with the possibility for improved long-term outcome (1). A pooled analysis of the published literature reported a 5-year survival rate of 25% after adrenalectomy, although the benefit of this approach is typically limited to patients with previously resected stage I disease who develop an adrenal metastasis months after the primary tumor was removed. The benefit of resection of an isolated adrenal metastasis in resected stage II disease remains unproven, and adrenal metastectomy should not generally be considered in stage III NSCLC given the extremely high likelihood of further metastatic disease.

Brain Metastasis

Metachronous brain metastasis after definitive treatment for localized NSCLC is a relatively common occurrence. Although treatment of brain metastases is beyond the scope of this chapter, surgical resection should be considered for a solitary brain metastasis, especially if the patient has significant neurologic symptoms. One to three metastases may be treated with stereotactic radiosurgery with or without whole brain radiation (WBRT). More than three brain metastases will likely require WBRT, given the high chance of subclinical brain metastases not identified on imaging. A careful discussion between the patient, medical oncologist, and radiation oncologist is required to personalize the treatment approach based on symptoms, comorbidities, treatment preferences, and the extent of extracranial disease. Systemic therapy following definitive local treatment of grossly visible brain metastases has not been shown to improve patient outcome and should be considered on a case-by-case basis.

Other Metastatic Sites

Rarely, NSCLC may present as an isolated metastasis to the liver, bone, or a distant lymph node, or other site. Limited case reports suggest an improved long-term outcome with definitive local therapy, although no high-quality data support this approach. In the absence of other metastatic sites, a definitive treatment approach with RT or resection is an option, especially if the patient has a good PS and has had a prolonged disease-free interval after treatment of early stage disease. This should be discussed in a multidisciplinary forum with input from surgery, radiation oncology, and medical oncology.

SYSTEMIC RECURRENCE

Non–Small-Cell Lung Cancer Without Driver Mutations

Immunotherapy

PD1 inhibitors: nivolumab and pembrolizumab

Agents that enhance the innate antitumor immune response have garnered much interest in oncology, especially in the treatment of lung cancer. Several immune checkpoint-inhibitor antibodies have been developed that target either the programmed death 1 (PD-1) receptor on activated T-cells or its ligand (PD-L1), which is expressed on tumor cells and infiltrating immune cells. The binding of PD-L1 to PD-1 results in the inactivation of T-cells and thus, the protection of tumors from cytotoxic immune surveillance. Monoclonal antibodies to either PD-1 or PD-L1 can interfere with ligand-receptor binding, allowing activated T-cells to attack the tumor. Two PD-1-directed monoclonal antibodies, nivolumab and pembrolizumab, are currently approved for second-line therapy after the failure of initial platinum-based therapy in NSCLC regardless of tumor histology.

Nivolumab (Odivo®) is a fully human IgG4 antibody that targets PD-1. Brahmer et al. randomized 272 patients with relapsed squamous cell NSCLC to nivolumab 3 mg/kg every 2 weeks or docetaxel 75 mg/m^2 every 3 weeks until disease progression (2). The primary endpoint of overall survival favored nivolumab over docetaxel (median, 9.2 vs. 7.3 months, 1 year 42% vs. 24%; HR, 0.59, 95% CI 0.44–0.79; $P < .001$). Response rate (20% vs. 9%) and median progression-free survival (PFS; 3.5 vs. 2.8 months) were also improved with nivolumab compared to docetaxel. In addition, 20% of patients receiving nivolumab remained progression-free 1 year from initiation of treatment, suggesting a prolonged duration of response to therapy. Fewer grades 3 and 4 toxicities, mainly fatigue, decreased appetite, and leukopenia, were identified with nivolumab than with docetaxel (7% vs. 55%), and nivolumab did not cause any treatment-related deaths. The most common grades 1 and 2 toxicities with nivolumab were rash, nausea, diarrhea, and fatigue. Tumor cell PD-L1 expression by immunohistochemistry did not correlate with either prognosis or response to treatment.

Similarly, Borghaei et al. randomized 582 patients with relapsed non-squamous NSCLC to nivolumab 3 mg/kg every 2 weeks or docetaxel 75 mg/m^2 every 3 weeks until disease progression (3). Overall survival, the primary endpoint, again favored nivolumab over docetaxel (median, 12.2 vs. 9.4 months; HR 0.73, 95% CI 0.59–0.89; $P = .002$). Response rate also favored nivolumab (19% vs. 12%), but median PFS favored docetaxel (2.3 vs. 4.2 months). Despite this unexpected finding, 19% of patients receiving nivolumab remained progression-free 1 year from initiation of treatment compared to 8% with docetaxel. Fewer grades 3 and 4 toxicities, mainly fatigue, nausea, and diarrhea, were identified with nivolumab than with docetaxel (10% vs. 54%). Common grades 1 and 2 toxicities with nivolumab included rash (9%), pruritus (8%), diarrhea (8%), and hypothyroidism (7%). One treatment-related death from encephalitis occurred with nivolumab. Contrary to the squamous trial, PD-L1 expression levels had a significant predictive association with all efficacy endpoints. However, this biomarker is not currently indicated to guide the use of nivolumab in routine practice. Nivolumab is now approved as second-line therapy in NSCLC regardless of histology or PD-L1 tumor expression.

Pembrolizumab (Keytruda®) is another monoclonal antibody that binds PD-1 and inhibits the binding of PD-L1 and PD-L2. KEYNOTE-001 was a phase I study of pembrolizumab in several tumor types, including NSCLC, which enrolled 61 patients with previously treated NSCLC with at least 50% of tumor cells with membranous PD-L1 expression (4). Pembrolizumab demonstrated a response rate of 44% and a median PFS of 6.1 months (95% CI 2.9–12.5). The median duration of response was 12.5 months in this selected patient population. Interestingly, pembrolizumab demonstrated a better response rate in current and former smokers than in never smokers (23% vs. 10%), and it is postulated that this is related to a higher tumor mutational burden resulting in greater neoantigen expression in smokers. As with nivolumab, the common side effects of pembrolizumab included fatigue (19%), pruritus (11%), decreased appetite (10%), and rash (9.7%). Pneumonitis was identified in 3.6% of patients, with one death (0.2%) from this complication. Based on an analysis of 1,143 NSCLC patients, 23% of previously treated patients had membranous PD-L1 expression in at least 50% of their tumor cells. According to the Keytruda (pembrolizumab) package insert (October 2015), the current indication for pembrolizumab is, "for the treatment of patients with metastatic non-small cell lung cancer (NSCLC) whose tumors express programmed death ligand 1 (PD-L1) as determined by an FDA-approved test, with disease progression on or after platinum-containing chemotherapy." The need to confirm PD-L1 tumor expression will likely limit the use of pembrolizumab, since nivolumab can be prescribed as second-line therapy without the need for PD-L1 analysis.

PD-L1 inhibitors: atezolizumab and Durvalumab

A second checkpoint-inhibitor strategy targets PD-L1, thereby inhibiting interaction with PD-1. The two anti-PD-L1 monoclonal antibodies that are farthest along in clinical development are atezolizumab (MPDL3280A) and Durvalumab. Over 80 patients \3 weeks until disease progression (5). Although survival data are immature, the response rate was 17% for all evaluable patients and 27% for those with high PD-L1 expression. Fatigue, nausea, and decreased appetite were the most commonly reported toxicities.

A phase I study of Durvalumab included an expansion cohort of 178 patients with relapsed NSCLC treated with 10 mg/kg every 2 weeks (6). The response rate for patients treated with only one prior line of therapy was 19%, and was higher in patients with squamous cell carcinoma than with non-squamous NSCLC (21% vs. 13%). PD-L1-positive patients and current or former smokers had a higher chance of response. Preliminary results also suggest that patients with PD-L1-positive tumors have improved overall survival compared to those with PD-L1-negative tumors. Common side effects of Durvalumab included diarrhea (7%), rash (8%), hyperthyroidism (4%), and hypothyroidism (4%).

Pseudo-progression

Pseudo-progression has complicated the response assessment of immune checkpoint-inhibitors. Early studies, particularly in melanoma, identified a subset of patients whose tumors grew or who developed a new lesion after the initial few weeks of immunotherapy. Although treatment was discontinued, subsequent imaging revealed significant disease regression. In this select group of patients, biopsies of enlarging lesions demonstrated inflammatory cell infiltrates or tumor necrosis. However, this is a relatively rare occurrence in patients with solid tumors, including NSCLC, and reviews of limited trial data suggest that pseudoprogression occurs in less than 5% of patients (7). If early imaging suggests pseudoprogression, but symptoms related to the cancer are improved or controlled, it is reasonable to continue treatment and repeat imaging in 4 to 6 weeks to assess for delayed response. However, progressive disease on imaging accompanied by worsening symptoms, such as weight loss, fatigue, dyspnea, cough, or pain, suggests true progression and immune checkpoint therapy should be discontinued.

Practical use of immunotherapy

Given the improved survival and favorable toxicity profile of immune checkpoint-inhibitors when compared to standard chemotherapy, these agents are commonly the preferred second-line therapy for patients with relapsed NSCLC. Patients with a documented history of autoimmune disease (except vitiligo, Grave's disease, or psoriasis not currently on therapy) or inflammatory bowel disease (i.e., Crohn's disease or ulcerative colitis), or who are on immunosuppressive therapy (i.e., >10 mg of prednisone daily or its equivalent), should not be treated with immune checkpoint therapy.

It is encouraging that approximately 20% of unselected patients with advanced squamous and non-squamous NSCLC will achieve a durable response with anti-PD-1 or anti-PD-L1 antibodies. Unfortunately, clinical benefit is not seen in the majority of patients who receive these agents and rare immune-mediated side effects, such as pneumonitis, hepatitis, nephritis, colitis, and hypophysitis, can be life threatening. Patients must be carefully monitored and prescribers must have a low threshold to discontinue the agent and administer corticosteroid therapy to avoid serious complications. Future studies will focus on the toxicity and efficacy of combining immune checkpoint-inhibitors with RT, chemotherapy, and other immune modulators to enhance the therapeutic benefit of these agents.

Single-Agent Chemotherapy

The vast majority of patients with advanced NSCLC will not have a targetable driver mutation identified and will be treated with front-line, platinum-based chemotherapy. Of note, in patients who received adjuvant chemotherapy for resected, early-stage disease, or chemoradiotherapy for locally advanced disease, retreatment with a platinum-doublet regimen is reasonable if recurrence is identified greater than 6 months from completion of prior therapy. Patients who recur within 6 months of completing adjuvant chemotherapy or definitive chemoradiotherapy should be treated with a second-line agent. With few exceptions, clinical trials have demonstrated that multidrug regimens in the relapsed setting result in increased response rates and modest improvements in PFS, but are uniformly more toxic and have not improved overall survival (8). Patients with non-squamous NSCLC not tested for driver mutations at initial presentation should have the tumor analyzed for *EGFR* mutation and *ALK* and *ROS1* gene rearrangement given the significant impact that therapy targeting these driver mutations can have on outcomes. Figure 9.1 provides an algorithm for managing patients with relapsed NSCLC without a targetable driver mutation.

Docetaxel

Docetaxel is the most extensively studied agent in patients with relapsed or refractory NSCLC. Two randomized, phase III trials have evaluated the efficacy of docetaxel in patients with advanced NSCLC who had progressed after prior chemotherapy (9,10). In the study by Shepherd et al., 204 patients who had been previously treated with a platinum-based regimen were randomized to receive docetaxel 100 mg/m^2 or best supportive care (9). All patients had a PS of 0 to 2 and had not had any prior taxane therapy. Due to excessive toxicity in the first 49 patients assigned to receive docetaxel 100 mg/m^2, including three treatment-related deaths, the dose was reduced to 75 mg/m^2 for the subsequent 55 patients randomized to the treatment arm and no further treatment-related mortality was observed. Patients who received docetaxel 75 mg/m^2 had a response rate of only 5.5%, but demonstrated a significant improvement in median (7.5 vs. 4.6 months) and 1-year overall survival (37% vs. 19%) compared to those assigned to best supportive care.

Fossella et al. conducted a three-arm randomized trial comparing two doses of docetaxel (75 mg/m^2 and 100 mg/m^2) to a control arm of either single-agent vinorelbine or ifosfamide in 373 patients who had progressed after one or more platinum-based regimens (10). Response rates were 6.7% for docetaxel 75 mg/m^2, 10.8% for docetaxel 100 mg/m^2, and 0.8% for control chemotherapy. One-year survival rates for patients on docetaxel 75 mg/m^2, docetaxel 100 mg/m^2, and control chemotherapy were 32%, 21%, and 19%, respectively. Neither response rate nor survival was significantly impacted by prior taxane exposure, suggesting that docetaxel and paclitaxel are not completely cross-resistant.

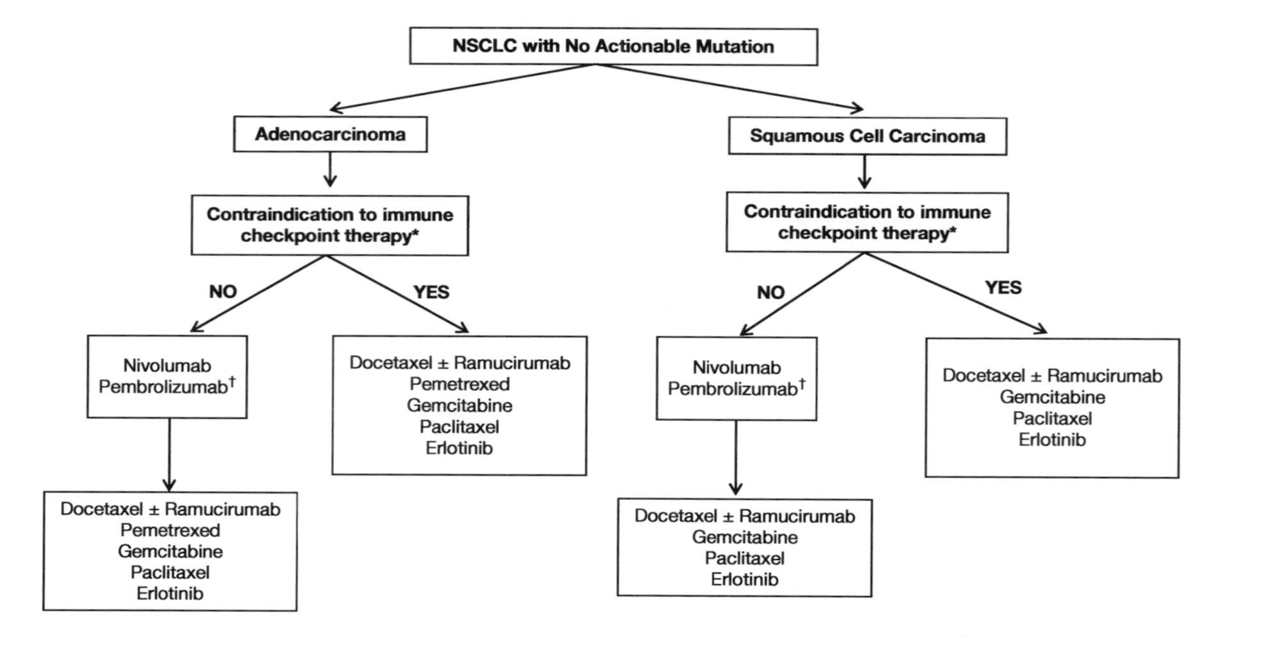

* Active autoimmune disease, corticosteroid therapy (≥10 mg prednisone daily), interstitial lung disease
† Requires PDL1-positive disease by immunohistochemistry

Figure 9.1 **Treatment of Recurrent Non–Small-Cell Lung Cancer (NSCLC) Without Driver Mutations**

Weekly docetaxel appears to have similar efficacy and an improved toxicity profile when compared to the every 3-week dosing schedule. Schuette et al. conducted a randomized phase III trial that enrolled 215 patients with relapsed NSCLC to docetaxel 75 mg/m^2 every 3 weeks or 35 mg/m^2 weekly on days 1, 8, and 15 of a 28-day cycle (11). Median overall survival favored the weekly regimen over the 3-week regimen, but did not reach statistical significance (9.2 vs. 6.3 months; $P = .07$). One-year survival rates also favored weekly docetaxel (40% vs. 27%). Fewer patients with grade 3/4 leucopenia (1% vs. 28%), neutropenia (5% vs. 21%), and anemia (1% vs. 6%) were reported with weekly dosing, although nonhematologic toxicity, including nausea, vomiting, nail changes, and pain, was similar between the groups. An individual patient data meta-analysis of five trials including 865 patients treated with weekly or every 3-week docetaxel further supports the weekly regimen with nearly identical median overall survival (26.1 vs. 27.4 weekly, $P = .24$) (12). There was less febrile neutropenia with weekly dosing although other toxicity rates were similar with either schedule. Based on comparable efficacy and an improved toxicity profile, weekly docetaxel should be strongly considered over the every 3-week schedule, especially in patients with a borderline PS.

Pemetrexed

Pemetrexed (Alimta®) is an option for patients with non-squamous NSCLC initially treated with a taxane-based regimen. Pemetrexed is an antifolate antimetabolite that inhibits multiple enzymes involved in purine and pyrimidine synthesis, including thymidylate synthase, dihydrofolate reductase, and glycinamide ribonucleotide formyltransferase. A phase III trial compared pemetrexed 500 mg/m^2 with vitamin B12 and folate supplementation to docetaxel 75 mg/m^2 in patients with relapsed or refractory NSCLC (13). This trial included 571 patients with a PS of 0 to 2 who had progressed after one prior regimen for advanced NSCLC. Response rates (9.1% vs. 8.8%) and overall survival (median, 8.3 vs. 7.9 months) were similar in the pemetrexed and docetaxel arms, respectively. However, toxicity favored the pemetrexed arm, with significantly less neutropenia (5% vs. 40%), neutropenic fever (2% vs. 13%), and peripheral neuropathy (3% vs. 8%). Subsequent studies demonstrated a lack of response with pemetrexed in patients with squamous cell NSCLC and pemetrexed use is now restricted to patients with non-squamous NSCLC (14). Common side effects of pemetrexed include myelosuppression, fatigue, rash, excessive lacrimation, and elevations of hepatic transaminases.

Gemcitabine

Gemcitabine (Gemzar®) is a nucleotide analog that inhibits ribonucleotide reductase and DNA polymerases, thereby interfering with DNA synthesis and function. In the second-line setting, single-agent gemcitabine has been evaluated in over 300 patients enrolled in phase II trials, primarily using 1,000 mg/m^2 on days 1, 8, and 15 of a 28-day cycle (15,16). Response rates with single-agent gemcitabine ranged from 5% to 21% with median overall survivals of 4.3 to 8.5 months and 1-year survival rates of 16% to 45%. Overall, gemcitabine monotherapy was well tolerated, with a modest degree of myelosuppression, rash, "flu-like" symptoms, and peripheral edema. Quality-of-life assessment that suggested stabilization or improvement in fatigue, cough, hemoptysis, and pain in up to 30% of patients. Despite the lack of phase III data, single-agent gemcitabine is a reasonable option for patients with relapsed or refractory NSCLC regardless of histology after prior platinum and/or taxane therapy. Many clinicians now drop the day 15 dose and treat on days 1 and 8 of a 21-day cycle to avoid excessive dose reductions and treatment delays due to myelosuppression in this heavily pretreated population.

Other single-agents

Many other chemotherapy agents including paclitaxel, vinblastine, mitomycin, and ifosfamide have been evaluated in patients with relapsed NSCLC and most demonstrate response rates similar to the aforementioned agents. Vinorelbine (Navelbine®), a semisynthetic vinca alkaloid derived from vinblastine has been uniformly disappointing in the second-line setting. One single agent, phase II trial demonstrated no objective responses, while a second yielded two partial responses in 10 patients (17). The low efficacy of single-agent vinorelbine raises doubts regarding its utility in the relapsed or refractory setting.

Irinotecan (Camptosar®) is a semisynthetic derivative of camptothecin that potently inhibits topoisomerase I, a nuclear enzyme that plays a critical role in DNA replication and transcription. In the second-line setting, a Japanese study reported no responses among 26 previously treated patients receiving irinotecan monotherapy (19).

Targeted Therapy in Unselected Patients

EGFR Inhibition

Erlotinib (Tarceva®) remains an option for second or third-line therapy regardless of tumor histology. In the BR21 trial, over 700 patients with relapsed NSCLC were randomized to either erlotinib or placebo and the response rate favored erlotinib (8.9% vs. <1%) (20). Median overall survival also favored erlotinib (6.7 vs. 4.7 months; HR 0.70, $P < .001$) in this patient population that was not selected for *EGFR*-mutant disease. Side effects were manageable with mild to moderate rash (76%) and diarrhea (55%) as the main toxicities.

Afatinib (Gilotrif®) is a second-generation EGFR/HER-2 tyrosine-kinase inhibitor (TKI) currently approved as initial therapy for *EGFR*-mutant NSCLC. The LUX-Lung 1 trial randomized 585 patients who progressed on both chemotherapy and a first-generation EGFR-TKI to either afatinib 40 mg orally daily or placebo (21). Patients were required to have at least 12 weeks of demonstrated benefit from a previous EGFR-TKI, so although *EGFR* mutation status was not assessed, the trial was enhanced for patients likely to benefit from further EGFR inhibition. The trial failed to demonstrate improved overall survival with afatinib over placebo (10.8 vs. 12 months), suggesting that afatinib is not a good treatment choice for patients who progress on erlotinib or gefitinib.

In the LUX-Lung 8 study, afatinib was compared to erlotinib in patients with relapsed squamous NSCLC without concern for *EGFR* mutation status (22). Almost 800 patients who had progressed after initial platinum-based chemotherapy received afatinib 40 mg daily or erlotinib 150 mg daily. The primary endpoint of PFS favored afatinib (2.4 vs. 1.9 months; HR 0.82, 95% CI 0.68-1.00; P = .04). More grade 3 diarrhea (10% vs. 2%) and stomatitis (4% vs. 0%) were seen with afatinib and more grade 3 rash (10% vs. 6%) with erlotinib.

Several trials have compared EGFR-TKIs, such as erlotinib and gefitinib, to standard chemotherapy in the second-line setting in patients who were unselected for *EGFR* driver mutations or who had *EGFR* wild-type disease (23,24). These studies have demonstrated either equivalent therapeutic benefit or a modest improvement in overall survival with chemotherapy. Therefore, immunotherapy or single-agent chemotherapy is now the favored approach for unselected or *EGFR* wild-type patients with relapsed NSCLC.

VEGFR Inhibition

Ramucirumab (Cyramza®) is a human IgG1 monoclonal antibody that binds to the VEGFR-2 receptor. Garon et al. randomized 1,253 patients with squamous or non-squamous NSCLC who had progressed after front-line, platinum-based chemotherapy to docetaxel 75 mg/m^2 every 3 weeks plus ramucirumab 10 mg/mg or to docetaxel plus placebo (25). The primary endpoint of overall survival favored docetaxel plus ramucirumab over docetaxel alone (10.5 vs. 9.1 months; HR 0.86, 95% CI 0.75–0.98; P = .023). Both median PFS (4.5 vs. 3.0 months; HR 0.75, 95% CI 0.68–0.86; $P < .0001$) and response rate (23% vs. 14%) also favored combination therapy. However, ramucirumab did increase grade 3 toxicity, including neutropenia (49% vs. 40%), febrile neutropenia (16% vs. 10%), fatigue (14% vs. 10%), and hypertension (6% vs. 3%). Grade 1 and 2 bleeding was also greater with ramucirumab (27% vs. 13%), but there was no increase in grade 3 or greater pulmonary hemorrhage even in patients with squamous cell carcinoma. Although this combination is the only approved two-drug regimen for second-line NSCLC, the addition of ramucirumab substantially increases the cost of therapy, adds toxicity, and offers only a modest clinical benefit, making this combination a less-attractive treatment option for patients with relapsed NSCLC.

NSCLC With Driver Mutations

Molecular profiling of non-squamous NSCLC has become standard practice and a significant minority of patients is found to have a targetable driver mutation at initial presentation. Patients treated with a front-line EGFR-TKI for *EGFR*-mutant disease or an ALK inhibitor for an *ALK*-rearranged tumor will ultimately relapse and present unique challenges in determining optimal subsequent therapy. Providers are often faced with complicated decisions regarding repeat tumor biopsies, continuation of the initial targeted therapy alone or in combination with other treatments, and the use of local therapies. Unfortunately, many of the recommendations in this situation are based on scant prospective data, relying on small studies and retrospective reports.

EGFR-Mutant NSCLC

Despite the initial dramatic responses seen with EGFR-TKIs in *EGFR*-mutant NSCLC, all patients will eventually develop resistance, typically within 12 to 24 months of beginning treatment. With traditional cytotoxic agents, any evidence of cancer progression is viewed as a sign of treatment failure, signaling the need to change therapy. However, due to the relatively indolent nature of *EGFR*-mutant NSCLC, this subset of patients requires a more thoughtful assessment of the type of progression occurring in each patient as it may lead to a markedly different treatment approach. Specifically, progression should be classified as slow progression, oligoprogression, or systemic progression. Figure 9.2 provides an algorithm for managing patients with relapsed *EGFR*-mutant NSCLC.

Slow progression

It is not uncommon to see slow progression of disease on repeat CT imaging at several month intervals. Although there is no formal definition of "slow progression," it is typified by lesions that slightly enlarge over several months without progressive symptoms. This often occurs in patients with multiple, small, asymptomatic, intrapulmonary metastases that grow by a few millimeters every

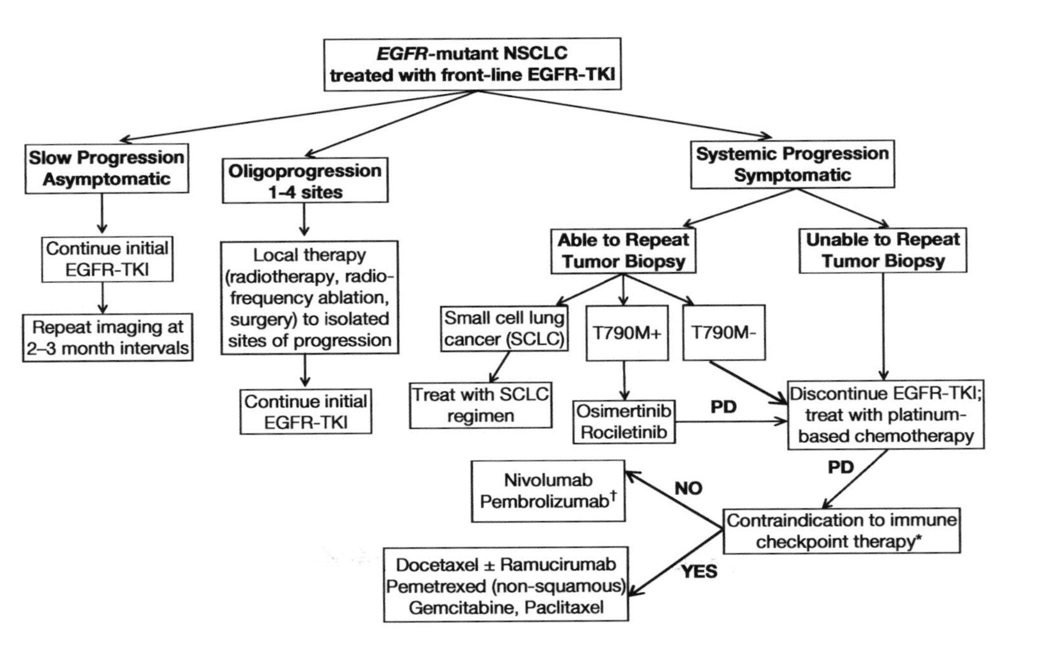

* Active autoimmune disease, corticosteroid therapy (≥10 mg prednisone daily), interstitial lung disease
† Requires PDL1-positive disease by immunohistochemistry

Figure 9.2 Treatment of Recurrent EGFR-Mutant Non–Small-Cell Lung Cancer (NSCLC)

few months. It is important to remember that stage IV NSCLC is an incurable disease and that the goal of treatment is palliation of symptoms to promote quality-of-life and functionality. Since a subset of sensitive tumor clones may still be responding to the EGFR-TKI, the drug may be slowing disease progression. Therefore, an acceptable approach is to continue EGFR-TKI monotherapy despite slowly progressive disease with careful monitoring of symptoms (26–28).

Oligometastatic progression

Another common type of recurrence is loosely defined as oligometastatic progression, where the majority of the cancer remains controlled by the EGFR-TKI, but progression is identified in four or fewer sites. For example, metastatic lung nodules may continue to respond while an adrenal metastasis grows. Retrospective data suggest that aggressive local treatment to the areas of progression with RT, RFA, or surgery, while continuing the EGFR-TKI, may lead to an improved clinical outcome. One study suggested that the targeted agent could be continued for a median of 6 months after local treatment of oligometastatic progression. Another small study demonstrated a median overall survival of 41 months with continuation of the EGFR-TKI after local therapy (29,30). This approach should be limited to select patients with oligometastatic progression who are otherwise deriving benefit from the EGFR-TKI, have a good PS, and can handle the potential toxicity of local therapy.

Symptomatic systemic progression

Unfortunately, many patients eventually develop rapid, systemic, symptomatic progression. Several mechanisms of resistance to initial EGFR-TKI therapy have been identified, including the *EGFR* T790M secondary resistance mutation, amplification of the *MET* oncogene, and histologic transformation to small cell lung cancer. A repeat tumor biopsy at progression to identify the mechanism of resistance is now recommended in light of newer therapeutic options whose use is based on molecular findings.

The addition of chemotherapy to the EGFR-TKI at progression does not appear to improve survival. In the IMPRESS trial, 265 patients with *EGFR*-mutant NSCLC who had progressed on front-line gefitinib were randomized to receive cisplatin and pemetrexed for six cycles plus either continuation of gefitinib or placebo followed by maintenance therapy with gefitinib or placebo (31). Median PFS was 5.4 months in both arms (HR 0.86, 95% CI 0.65–1.13) and although overall survival data were immature, it favored the placebo arm. This trial failed to support the concern for "tumor flare" once the EGFR-TKI is stopped (32).

Therefore, discontinuation of the EGFR-TKI and initiation of platinum-based chemotherapy is the most reasonable treatment option at the time of significant disease progression.

Approximately 50% to 60% of patients who develop resistance to initial EGFR-TKI therapy develop a new *EGFR* T790M mutation. Third-generation, mutation-selective EGFR-TKIs have been developed that can overcome the T790M mutation and have the added benefit of sparing wild-type EGFR, thus reducing the class-specific toxicities of rash and diarrhea that are commonly seen with first and second-generation EGFR-TKIs.

Osimertinib (Tagrisso®) is a third-generation EGFR-TKI approved for the treatment of *EGFR*-mutant NSCLC with the T790M gatekeeper mutation. A large phase I/II trial evaluated osimertinib in 253 patients with acquired resistance to prior EGFR-TKI therapy (33). Patients with T790M-positive disease demonstrated a response rate of 61% and median PFS of 10 months with osimertinib. Patients without the T790M mutation demonstrated a response rate of 21% and median PFS of only 3 months. The approved dose of osimertinib is 80 mg orally once daily with or without food and common side effects include diarrhea, rash, dry skin, and nail changes. Interstitial lung disease/pneumonitis occurred in 3.3% of patients and cardiomyopathy in 1.4%.

Rociletinib is another third-generation, mutation-selective EGFR-TKI that is active in T790M-positive NSCLC. The TIGER-X phase I/II study evaluated rociletinib in 130 patients with *EGFR*-mutant NSCLC who previously received an EGFR-TKI (34). Patients with T790M-positive disease had a response rate of 59% and a median PFS of 13.1 months. Patients without the T790M mutation had a response rate of 29% and a median PFS of 5.6 months. An unanticipated side effect of rociletinib was grades 3 and 4 hyperglycemia in 15% of patients, which required treatment with an oral hypoglycemic agent and is likely due to the accumulation of M502, a metabolite of rociletinib that inhibits insulin-like growth factor 1 receptor (IGF1R). Other side effects included diarrhea (all grade, 25%), rash (1%), and reversible pneumonitis (2%).

ALK-Rearranged NSCLC

Patients who present with *ALK*-rearranged NSCLC are typically treated with the TKI crizotinib with a high response rate and a median PFS of 11 months (35). Resistance to crizotinib occurs via a variety of mechanisms, including the development of *ALK* L1196M or G1269A gatekeeper mutations, *ALK* fusion-gene amplification, or activation of bypass signaling pathways.

Ceritinib (Zykadia®) is an FDA approved second-generation ALK inhibitor. Over 160 patients with *ALK*-rearranged NSCLC with progressive disease on crizotinib were treated with ceritinib and demonstrated a response rate of 55% and median PFS of 6.9 months (95% CI 5.6–8.7 months) (36). Interestingly, a retrospective review of patients with brain metastases revealed an intracranial disease control rate of 65% in patients previously treated with crizotinib, suggesting that ceritinib has significant activity against brain metastases (37). Common side effects of ceritinib at 750 mg/day include diarrhea (84%), nausea (77%), vomiting (57%), fatigue (36%), and increased ALT (36%), and dose modification is required in many patients.

Alectinib has also been approved for patients with *ALK*-rearranged NSCLC resistant to crizotinib. Patients with documented progression on crizotinib were treated with alectinib 600 mg twice daily with a response rate of 44% (38). Interestingly, in 34 patients with measurable CNS metastases the intracranial response rate was 56%, suggesting good CNS activity. Side effects of alectinib include fatigue (41%), constipation (34%), edema (30%), and elevated transaminases (all grades, 34%–50%; grade 3/4, 3%–4%).

MANAGEMENT GUIDELINES

Table 9.1 highlights the trials and results that support treatment of patients with relapsed NSCLC. Many patients with relapsed NSCLC do not have a good PS due to constitutional symptoms related to advanced cancer and residual toxicity from prior treatment. Before considering second-line therapy for patients with marginal PS, one should recall that the major goals of therapy are symptom palliation and maintenance of quality-of-life. In such situations, treatment may often cause more harm than good. It is the oncologist's responsibility to present an honest overview of the potential benefits and risks of available treatment options, including investigational clinical trials and "best supportive care," along with a clear indication that all treatment, including targeted therapy and immune checkpoint inhibitors, is given with palliative intent. Frequently, local therapy, including palliative RT, can be very useful in alleviating symptoms such as pain due to bone metastases or cough and dyspnea due to bronchial obstruction.

For patients with relapsed NSCLC who have maintained a good PS, further systemic treatment remains an option. Immune checkpoint inhibitors are rapidly becoming the preferred treatment approach for relapsed NSCLC without an actionable driver mutation due to improved efficacy and tolerability when compared to second-line docetaxel. Single-agent chemotherapy or erlotinib also remain reasonable alternatives.

Patients with *EGFR*-mutant or *ALK*-rearranged NSCLC have a growing list of options based on the identification of the

Table 9.1 Selected clinical trials for patients with relapsed NSCLC

Agent (ref.)	Dose and schedule	*N*	Histology	Genetic alteration	ORR (%)	MS (mo)	1-Year survival (%)
Docetaxel (9) BSC	100 mg/m² q 3 wk 75 mg/m² q 3 wk –	49 55 100	NSCLC NOS	NR	6.3 5.5 –	5.9 7.5 4.6	19 37 19
Docetaxel weekly (11) Docetaxel q3 wk	35 mg/m² d 1,8,15 q4w 75 mg/m² q 3 wk	105 103	NSCLC NOS	NR	10.5 12.6	9.2 6.3	40 27
Pemetrexed (13) Docetaxel	500 mg/m² q 3 wk 75 mg/m² q 3 wk	283 288	NSCLC NOS	NR	9.1 8.8	8.3 7.9	30 30
Gemcitabine (15)	1,000 mg/m² d 1,8,15 q 4 wk	83	NSCLC NOS	NR	19	8.5	45
Erlotinib (20) BSC	150 mg orally daily –	488 243	NSCLC NOS	NR	9 <1	6.7 4.7	31 22
Afatinib (21) BSC	50 mg orally daily –	390 195	NSCLC NOS	*EGFR* + 67% *EGFR* + 71%	7 <1	10.8 12.0	45 50
Docetaxel/ ramucirumab (25) Docetaxel	75 mg/m² /10 mg/kg q 3 wk 75 mg/m² q 3 wk	628 625	NSCLC NOS	*EGFR* + 2% *EGFR* + 3%	23 14	10.5 9.1	43 38

(continued)

Table 9.1 Selected clinical trials for patients with relapsed NSCLC (*continued*)

Agent (ref.)	Dose and schedule	*N*	Histology	Genetic alteration	ORR (%)	MS (mo)	1-Year survival (%)
Nivolumab (2) Docetaxel	3 mg/kg q 2 wk 75 mg/m² q 3 wk	135 137	Squamous	NR	20 9	9.2 6.0	42 24
Nivolumab (3) Docetaxel	3 mg/kg q 2 wk 75 mg/m² q 3 wk	292 290	Adenocarcinoma	NR	19 12	12.2 9.4	51 39
Pembrolizumab (4)	10 mg/kg q 2 or 3 wk	61	NSCLC PD-L1+	NR	44	NR	60
Osimertinib (33)	80 mg orally daily	138	Adenocarcinoma	*EGFR*+ T790M+	61	13.1[a]	NR
Rociletinib (34)	625 mg orally twice daily	46	Adenocarcinoma	*EGFR*+ T790M+	59	10.4[a]	NR
Ceritinib (37)	750 mg orally daily	163	Adenocarcinoma	*ALK*+	55	6.9[a]	NR
Alectinib (38)	600 mg orally daily	138	Adenocarcinoma	*ALK*+	44	NR	NR

ALK+, anaplastic lymphoma kinase-rearrangement-positive; BSC, best supportive care; *EGFR* +, epidermal growth factor receptor activating mutation-positive; MS, median survival; NOS, not otherwise specified; NR, not reported; NSCLC, non—small-cell lung cancer; ORR, objective response rate; PD-L1+, programmed death 1 receptor ligand-positive; T790M+, *EGFR* T790M resistance mutation-positive.

[a]Progression-free survival.

resistance mechanism and type of progression, as outlined earlier. A repeat biopsy on progression is preferable to guide further therapy. For patients with *EGFR*-mutant disease, the identification of the T790M resistance mutation would allow treatment with a third-generation EGFR-TKI. If a secondary biopsy is not possible, discontinuation of the EGFR-TKI and initiation of platinum-based, front-line chemotherapy is recommended. Due to the modest benefits reported with standard therapy, it is clear that enrollment on clinical trials, including phase I trials, remains a reasonable option for all patients with good PS and relapsed or refractory NSCLC.

KEY POINTS

- Intrathoracic recurrence of NSCLC may still be curative with aggressive local therapy.
- Metachronous adrenal or brain metastases may be treated with surgery and/or radiation therapy with the goal of improved long-term survival.
- Nivolumab and pembrolizumab are approved as second-line therapy for NSCLC regardless of tumor histology. Pembrolizumab requires confirmation of PD-L1-positive disease prior to treatment.
- Less than 5% of patients with NSCLC treated with immunotherapy (e.g., nivolumab or pembrolizumab) will demonstrate pseudoprogression.
- Combination therapy with multiple systemic agents is not recommended for relapsed NSCLC. Sequential, single-agent therapy is recommended.
- Asymptomatic, slow growing, *EGFR*-mutant NSCLC may be treated with an EGFR-TKI alone until the development of symptoms or rapid disease progression.
- Patients with *EGFR*-mutant NSCLC treated with an EGFR-TKI may develop limited sites tumor progression. If the bulk of the cancer is controlled, the few areas of progression should be treated with aggressive local therapy (e.g., surgery, radiation, RFA) and patients should continue the EGFR-TKI.
- After symptomatic progression of *EGFR*-mutant NSCLC, a repeat biopsy should be obtained to assess for the *EGFR* T790M gatekeeper mutation that is sensitive to third-generation EGFR-TKIs (e.g., osimertinib).

- Patients with *EGFR*-mutant NSCLC who progress on a frontline EGFR-TKI and lack the T790M mutation should discontinue the EGFR-TKI and initiate platinum-based chemotherapy.
- Ceritinib and alectinib are available for patients with *ALK*-rearranged NSCLC who progress after treatment with crizotinib. These agents have better activity against brain metastases.

REFERENCES

1. Tanvetyanon T, Robinson LA, Schell MJ, et al. Outcomes of adrenalectomy for isolated synchronous versus metachronous adrenal metastases in non-small-cell lung cancer: a systematic review and pooled analysis. *J Clin Oncol*. 2008;26(7):1142.
2. Brahmer J, Reckamp KL, Baas P, et al. Nivolumab versus docetaxel in advanced squamous-cell non-small-cell lung cancer. *N Engl J Med*. 2015;373(2):123-135.
3. Borghaei H, Paz-Ares L, Horn L, et al. Nivolumab versus docetaxel in advanced non-squamous non-small-cell lung cancer. *N Engl J Med*. 2015;373(17):1627-1639.
4. Garon EB, Rizvi NA, Hui R, et al. Pembrolizumab for the treatment of non-small-cell lung cancer. *N Engl J Med*. 2015;372(21): 2018-2028.
5. Spigel DR, Chaft JE, Gettinger SN, et al. Clinical activity and safety from a phase II study (FIR) of MPDL3280! (anti-PDL1) in PD-L1-selected patients with non-small cell lung cancer (NSCLC). *J Clin Oncol*. 2015;33(suppl; abstr 8028).
6. Rizvi NA, Brahmer JR, Ou SI, et al. Safety and clinical activity of MEDI4736, an anti-programmed cell death-ligand 1 (PD-L1) antibody, in patients with non-small cell lung cancer (NSCLC). *J Clin Oncol*. 33, 2015 (suppl; abstr 8032).
7. Chiou VL, Burotto M. Pseudoprogression and immune-related response in solid tumors. *J Clin Oncol*. 2015;33(31):3541-3543.
8. Di Maio M, Chiodini P, Georgoulias V, et al. Meta-analysis of single-agent chemotherapy compared with combination chemotherapy as second-line treatment of advanced non-small-cell lung cancer. *J Clin Oncol*. 2009;27(11):1836-1843.
9. Shepherd FA, Dancey J, Ramlau R, et al. Prospective randomized trial of docetaxel versus best supportive care in patients with non-small cell lung cancer previously treated with platinum-based chemotherapy. *J Clin Oncol*. 2000;18:2095-2103.
10. Fossella FV, DeVore R, Kerr RN, et al. Randomized phase III trial of docetaxel versus vinorelbine or ifosfamide in patients with advanced

non-small cell lung cancer previously treated with platinum-containing chemotherapy regimens. *J Clin Oncol*. 2000;18:2354-2362.

11. Schuette W, Nagel S, Blankenburg T, et al. Phase III study of second-line chemotherapy for advanced non-small-cell lung cancer with weekly compared with 3-weekly docetaxel. *J Clin Oncol*. 2005;23:8389-8395.
12. Di Maio M, Perrone F, Chiodini P, et al. Individual patient data meta-analysis of docetaxel administered once every 3 weeks compared with once every week second-line treatment of advanced non-small-cell lung cancer. *J Clin Oncol*. 2007;25:1377-1382.
13. Hanna N, Shepherd FA, Fossella FV, et al. Randomized phase III trial of pemetrexed versus docetaxel in patients with non-small-cell lung cancer previously treated with chemotherapy. *J Clin Oncol*. 2004;22(9):1589-1597.
14. Scagliotti GV, Parikh P, von Pawel J, et al. Phase III study comparing cisplatin plus gemcitabine with cisplatin plus pemetrexed in chemotherapy-naïve patients with advanced-stage non-small-cell lung cancer. *J Clin Oncol*. 2008;26(21):3543-3551.
15. Crino L, Mosconi AM, Scagliotti G, et al. Gemcitabine as second-line treatment for advanced non-small cell lung cancer: a phase II trial. *J Clin Oncol*. 1999;17:2081-2085.
16. Gridelli C, Perrone F, Gallo C, et al. Single-agent gemcitabine as second-line treatment in patients with advanced non-small cell lung cancer: a phase II trial. *Anticancer Res*. 1999;19:4535-4538.
17. Pronzato P, Landucci M, Vaira F, et al. Failure of vinorelbine to produce responses in pretreated non-small cell lung cancer patients. *Anticancer Res*. 1994;14:1413-1416.
18. Santoro A, Maiorino L, Santoro M. Second-line with vinorelbine in the weekly monochemotherapy for the treatment of advanced non-small cell lung cancer. *Lung Cancer*. 1994;11:S130.
19. Negoro S, Fukuoka M, Niitani H, et al. A phase II study of CPT-11, a camptothecin derivate, in patients with primary lung cancer. *Jpn J Cancer Chemother*. 1991;18:1013-1019.
20. Shepherd FA, Pereira JR, Ciuleanu T, et al. Erlotinib in previously treated non-small-cell lung cancer. *N Engl J Med*. 2005;353:123-132.
21. Miller VA, Hirsh V, Cadranel J, et al. Afatinib versus placebo for patients with advanced, metastatic non-small-cell lung cancer after failure of erlotinib, gefitinib, or both and one or two lines of chemotherapy (LUX-Lung 1): a phase 2b/3 randomized trial. *Lancet Oncol*. 2012;13:528-538.
22. Soria J-C, Felip E, Cobo M, et al. Afatinib versus erlotinib as second-line treatment of patients with advanced squamous cell carcinoma of the lung (LUX-Lung 8): an open-label randomized controlled phase 3 trial. *Lancet Oncol*. 2015;16:897-907.
23. Kim ES, Hirsh V, Mok T, et al. Gefitinib versus docetaxel in previously treated non-small-cell-lung cancer (INTEREST): a randomized phase III trial. *Lancet*. 2008;372:1809.

24. Garassino MC, Martelli O, Broggini M, et al. Erlotinib versus docetaxel as second-line treatment of patients with advanced non-small-cell lung cancer and wild-type EGFR tumors (TAILOR): a randomized controlled trial. *Lancet Oncol.* 2013;14:981.
25. Garon EB, Ciuleanu TE, Arrieta O, et al. Ramucirumab plus docetaxel versus placebo plus docetaxel for second-line treatment of stage IV non-small-cell lung cancer after disease progression on platinum-based therapy (REVEL): a multicenter, double-blind, randomized phase 3 trial. *Lancet.* 2014;384:665.
26. Oxnard GR, Lo P, Jackman DM, et al. Delay of chemotherapy through use of post-progression erlotinib in patients with EGFR-mutant lung cancer. *J Clin Oncol.* 2012;30 (suppl; abstr 7547).
27. Asami K, Okuma T, Hirashima T, et al. Continued treatment with gefitinib beyond progressive disease benefits patients with activating EGFR mutations. *Lung Cancer.* 2013;79:276-282.
28. Nishie K, Kawaguchi T, Tamiya A, et al. Epidermal growth factor receptor tyrosine kinase inhibitors beyond progressive disease: a retrospective analysis for Japanese patients with activing EGFR mutations. *J Thorac Oncol.* 2012;7:1722-1727.
29. Weickhardt AJ, Scheier B, Burke JM, et al. Local ablative therapy of oligoprogressive disease prolongs disease control by tyrosine kinase inhibitors in oncogene-addicted non-small-cell lung cancer. *J Thorac Oncol.* 2012;7:1807-1814.
30. Yu HA, Sima CS, Huang J, et al. Local therapy with continued EGFR tyrosine kinase inhibitor therapy as a treatment strategy in EGFR-mutant advanced lung cancers that have developed acquired resistance to EGFR tyrosine kinase inhibitors. *J Thorac Oncol.* 2013;8:346-351.
31. Soria J-C, Wu YL, Nakagawa K, et al. Gefitinib plus chemotherapy versus placebo plus chemotherapy in EGFR-mutation-positive non-small-cell lung cancer after progression on first-line gefitinib (IMPRESS): a phase 3 randomised trial. *Lancet Oncol.* 2015;16:990-998.
32. Chaft JE, Oxnard GR, Sima CS, Kris MG, Miller VA, Riely GJ. Disease flare after tyrosine kinase inhibitor discontinuation in patients with EGFR-mutant lung cancer and acquired resistance to erlotinib or gefitinib: implications for clinical trial design. *Clin Cancer Res.* 2011;17(19):6298-6303.
33. Janne PA, Yang JC, Kim DW et al. AZD9291 in EGFR inhibitor-resistant non-small-cell lung cancer. *N Engl J Med.* 2015;372(18);1689.
34. Sequist LV, Soria J-C, Goldman JW, et al. Rociletnib in EGFR-mutated non-small-cell lung cancer. *N Engl J Med.* 2015;372:1700-1709.
35. Solomon BJ, Mok T, Kim DW, et al. First-line crizotinib versus chemotherapy in ALK-positive lung cancer. *N Engl J Med.* 2014;371(23):2167-2177.
36. Kim DW, Mehra R, Tan D, et al. Ceritinib in advanced anaplastic lymphoma kinas (ALK)-rearranged (ALK+) non-small cell lung cancer

(NSCLC): results of the ASCEND-1 trial. *J Clin Oncol.* 2014;32:5s(suppl; abstr 8003).

37. Kim DW, Mehra R, Tan D, et al. Ceritinib treatment of patients (pts) with ALK-rearranged (ALK+) non-small cell lung cancer (NSCLC) and brain metastases: ASCEND-1 trial experience. *Ann Oncol.* 2015;26(suppl 1):i35.
38. Ou S, Ahn JS, De Petris L, et al. Efficacy and safety of the ALK inhibitor alectinib in ALK+ non-small-cell lung cancer (NSCLC) patients who have failed prior crizotinib: an open-label, single-arm, global phase 2 study (NP28673). *J Clin Oncol.* 2015;33(suppl; abstr 8008).

10 Management of Limited-Stage Small Cell Lung Cancer

Michael F. Gensheimer and Billy W. Loo Jr.

INTRODUCTION

Small cell lung cancer (SCLC) is a high-grade neuroendocrine carcinoma of the lung that is prone to early metastatic spread and often responds well to chemotherapy and radiation therapy (RT), but tends to recur after treatment. Around 40% of patients present with limited-stage disease (LS-SCLC), which is potentially curable with RT, chemotherapy, and/or surgery. The remaining 60% of patients present with typically incurable, extensive-stage disease (ES-SCLC) (1). Survival after treatment for LS-SCLC is poor due to frequent disease recurrence. Most patients with LS-SCLC have stage III disease with mediastinal lymph node involvement and a median survival of 12 to 14 months (1). In fit patients, the goal of treatment for LS-SCLC is cure, but treatment can also palliate symptoms.

Initial Evaluation

At a minimum, patients should undergo CT of the chest and abdomen with IV contrast, laboratory tests including complete blood count and serum chemistries, and brain MRI. Fluorodeoxyglucose-PET (FDG-PET)/CT scan is also recommended as it is more sensitive than CT alone, particularly for the detection of distant metastases. In a collection of prospective and retrospective studies, PET scan findings altered initial management in 28% of patients, either due to stage shift or a change in the RT field (2). If conventional imaging or biopsy shows clear evidence of distant metastatic disease, then PET/CT may be omitted. Patients with clinically lymph node-negative disease who are being considered for surgical resection should undergo invasive mediastinal staging (e.g., mediastinoscopy or endobronchial ultrasound-guided biopsy) prior to tumor resection since identification of mediastinal lymph node involvement would change local treatment from surgery to RT.

Stage Classification

Less than 5% of patients with SCLC present with localized disease that is amenable to surgical resection. Most patients have locally advanced or metastatic disease and will be treated most appropriately with either chemotherapy plus RT or chemotherapy alone. Determining which patients are candidates for definitive RT was the rationale for the influential 1973 Veteran's Administration Lung Group (VALG) staging system (3). By this system, LS-SCLC was defined as disease in the ipsilateral hemithorax that can be safely encompassed within a tolerable radiation portal. All other patients were defined as having ES-SCLC. This two-stage system is of historical importance for understanding the SCLC literature, including the many clinical trials that have used the VALG system or minor variations of it. Problems with this system include the lumping together of patients with varied prognoses into the LS-SCLC designation, and the subjectivity of defining a tolerable radiation portal.

More recently, the American Joint Committee on Cancer (AJCC) seventh edition adopted a uniform tumor/node/metastasis (TNM) staging system for both non–small cell and SCLC as it has been shown to be prognostic in both diseases (1). The TNM system should be used because of its more precise therapeutic implications and to permit stage-based analysis of clinical outcomes going forward. By combining the functional nature of the VALG two-stage system with the granularity of the AJCC TNM system, the National Comprehensive Cancer Network (NCCN) Guideline for SCLC defines limited-stage as AJCC stage I to III (T any, N any, M0) that can be safely treated with definitive RT doses, excluding T3-4 due to multiple lung nodules that are too extensive or have tumor/nodal volume that is too large to be encompassed in a tolerable RT plan, and extensive-stage as AJCC stage IV (T any, N any, M1a/b) or T3-4 due to multiple lung nodules that are too extensive or have tumor/nodal volume that is too large to be encompassed in a tolerable RT plan. Figure 10.1 shows PET scans from patients with AJCC stage IIIA/LS-SCLC and AJCC stage IV/ES-SCLC.

TREATMENT OF LS-SCLC

Standard treatment for LS-SCLC involves four to six cycles of chemotherapy with definitive thoracic RT given early during the chemotherapy course. Patients with radiographic response to treatment and without progression after completion of chemotherapy and RT should be considered for prophylactic cranial irradiation (PCI). Rare patients with very limited extent of disease (T1-2, N0, and M0) can be considered for surgery followed by adjuvant chemotherapy instead of concurrent chemoradiotherapy.

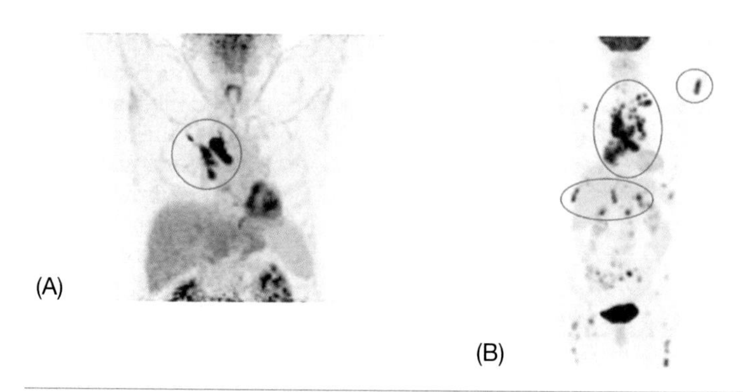

Figure 10.1 PET Images of Two Patients With Small Cell Lung Cancer: (A) AJCC Stage IIIA/VALG Limited-Stage Confined to the Right Lung and Ipsilateral Hilar/Mediastinal Lymph Nodes; (B) AJCC Stage IV/VALG Extensive-Stage With Bone and Extra-Thoracic Lymph Node Metastases

Chemotherapy

SCLC is highly sensitive to chemotherapy and early chemotherapy drugs, such as alkylating agents, showed activity in this disease. Due to improved outcomes with combination regimens over single agents, cyclophosphamide, doxorubicin, and vincristine (CAV) became a standard regimen for SCLC. More recently, the combination of etoposide plus cisplatin (EP) showed less toxicity and similar to improved efficacy when compared to alkylator/anthracycline-based regimens in several randomized trials. A Norwegian Lung Cancer Study Group trial comparing EP to cyclophosphamide, epirubicin, and vincristine included 436 patients with LS-and ES-SCLC (4). Patients with LS-SCLC received thoracic RT with cycle 3 of chemotherapy. Survival was improved in the EP arm (median, 10.2 vs. 7.8 months, $P = .004$), and the survival benefit appeared to be confined to patients with limited-stage disease (median, 14.5 vs. 9.7 months), perhaps because EP was better tolerated in combination with RT. For example, EP avoids synergistic toxicity, particularly cardiac toxicity, between anthracyclines and RT (5).

Cisplatin Versus Carboplatin

Many patients with SCLC are not good candidates for cisplatin, due to comorbidities such as preexisting renal impairment, neuropathy, or hearing loss. Several trials have studied the combination of etoposide plus carboplatin (EC) as an alternative to EP. An early trial from Greece compared six cycles of EC to six cycles of

EP in 147 patients with either LS-SCLC or ES-SCLC (6). Patients with LS-SCLC received thoracic RT with cycle 3. Median survival was not different between the study arms, at around 12 months in each. Severe toxicity was more frequent with EP, including leukopenia, neutropenic fever, nausea, vomiting, and neurotoxicity. A subsequent meta-analysis of a trial that compared cisplatin-based versus carboplatin-based regimens in SCLC also found equivalent survival and response rates (7). Hematologic toxicity was more common with carboplatin, but nonhematologic toxicity was greater with cisplatin. In summary, it is reasonable to substitute carboplatin for cisplatin in combination with etoposide, especially in patients with cisplatin-specific toxicity concerns (8).

Alternate Regimens

Trials evaluating alternative chemotherapy regimens for LS-SCLC have not shown superiority to EP. In a recent Japanese trial, all patients received one cycle of EP concurrently with RT prior to randomization to three more cycles of EP or three cycles of cisplatin plus irinotecan (9). Overall survival was not improved with irinotecan and toxicity was similar between the two arms. Targeted agents and immunotherapy are currently being evaluated in patients with ES-SCLC, and if found to provide survival benefit they would eventually be assessed in LS-SCLC. For instance, in a phase I/II trial in patients with ES-SCLC, the immune checkpoint inhibitor nivolumab, given with or without the CTLA4 inhibitor ipilimumab, induced durable responses lasting up to 11 months (10).

Elderly and Poor Performance Status Patients

Standard therapy for LS-SCLC with platinum-based chemotherapy plus concurrent RT is toxic. For instance, in a recent trial of fit patients (≤70 years old, ECOG performance status 0–1), four cycles of EP plus RT resulted in a 95% rate of neutropenia and a high rate of neutropenic fever (25% during concurrent chemoradiotherapy plus an additional 16% during consolidation chemotherapy) (9). Therefore, it would be helpful to deintensify treatment for LS-SCLC, especially for older patients or those with poor performance status.

Published studies have not shown encouraging results with treatment deintensification for SCLC. One study enrolled 300 patients who were ≤75 years old with either LS-SCLC or ES-SCLC, and randomized them to chemotherapy with cyclophosphamide, vincristine, and etoposide, given either up-front or at time of symptomatic or radiographic progression (11). Median survival was the same in the two arms (36 weeks for up-front and 32 weeks for delayed chemotherapy, $P = .96$). However, the delayed chemotherapy arm had inferior quality-of-life, specifically in the domains of mood, sleep, and general well-being. This suggests that there is value in preemptive palliation, or treatment given before symptoms become severe. In a second trial, patients who were ≥75 years old with any stage of SCLC, or younger patients with ES-SCLC, were randomized to a standard chemotherapy regimen (EP alternating with CAV) versus oral etoposide, which was expected to be better tolerated (12). However, progression-free survival (PFS) was inferior in the oral etoposide arm (median, 3.6 vs. 5.6 months, $P = .001$), with a trend toward inferior overall survival (median, 4.8 vs. 5.9 months, $P = .13$). Quality-of-life was also inferior in the oral etoposide arm, presumably due to symptoms of progressive cancer.

While these two trials do not provide support for delayed or deintensified treatment for LS-SCLC, patients unable to tolerate full-intensity therapy due to comorbidities or performance status were not included in most randomized trials in LS-SCLC and their treatment should be individualized. If there are concerns that an individual patient will not tolerate concurrent chemoradiotherapy, starting treatment with chemotherapy alone is a reasonable option with the addition of RT with a later cycle if the patient tolerates treatment well. Sequential chemotherapy followed by definitive RT could also be considered. For patients with very poor performance status, palliative RT without chemotherapy, or supportive care without active anticancer treatment are appropriate options.

Thoracic RT

Clinical trials reported in the 1970s and 1980s showed that the addition of RT to chemotherapy improved local control in the chest, but some did not demonstrate a significant improvement in overall survival. Two meta-analyses, both published in 1992, helped clarify this issue by reporting an improvement in overall survival with the addition of RT (13, 14). The meta-analysis reported by Pignon et al. analyzed individual data on 2,103 patients with LS-SCLC enrolled in 13 trials that compared chemotherapy with or without RT (13). In some of the trials, RT was delivered concurrently with chemotherapy, while in others it was given after the completion of chemotherapy. The relative risk of death in the combined-therapy group was 0.86, with an increase in 3-year overall survival from 9% to 14%. Most of the benefit was seen in patients younger than 65 years old.

Timing of RT

Once concurrent chemotherapy and thoracic RT had been established as the standard-of-care, the next question to be answered was whether RT should be given early or late in the chemotherapy course. A few influential studies showed that early RT given with the first or second cycle of chemotherapy likely improves outcomes. In a trial performed by the National Cancer Institute of Canada, 308 patients all received six cycles of CAV alternating with EP chemotherapy with randomization to undergo thoracic RT (40 Gy in 15 fractions) with either the first or last cycle of EP (15). In both arms, 83% of patients completed all six cycles of chemotherapy, but more patients on the early thoracic RT arm received RT (96% vs. 87%). Overall survival was improved in the early thoracic RT arm (median, 21 vs. 16 months, $P = .006$), with a sustained separation of the survival curves (5 years, 20% vs. 11%). A subsequent meta-analysis of thoracic RT timing by Fried et al. analyzed 1,524 patients from seven trials, though they did not have access to individual patient data (16). Early RT was defined as beginning with cycle 1 or 2 of chemotherapy and less than 9 weeks after the start of chemotherapy. A small, but statistically significant, benefit in 2-year overall survival was seen in the early RT arm (relative risk of death 0.85, $P = .03$). Finally, another meta-analysis analyzed overall survival according to time from start of any treatment to the end of radiotherapy (SER), and found the best survival when SER was less than 30 days, with a decrease in 5-year survival rate of around 2% per week of extension of SER ($P = .0003$) (17).

In summary, thoracic RT should be started with the first or second cycle of chemotherapy, and the time from initiation of treatment to completion of RT may be a valuable predictor of treatment effectiveness. Although RT should be started with cycle 1 whenever possible, in specific situations it is acceptable to start with cycle 2 or even later. First, if a patient is symptomatic and needs to start treatment urgently, it may be best to start chemotherapy before RT to allow time for careful RT planning. Second, if disease is very bulky, it may be useful to use chemotherapy to downsize the treatment volume and reduce the risks of RT-induced toxicity, such as radiation pneumonitis. A prospective trial demonstrated that targeting RT to the postchemotherapy extent of disease does not compromise disease control (18). In this study, RT was given with cycle 3 of chemotherapy and patients were randomized to RT targeting the pre- or postchemotherapy tumor volume. The rate of isolated out-of-field local-regional recurrence was less than 3% in both arms.

RT Dose and Fractionation

The delivery of thoracic RT for SCLC has evolved over the decades as RT technology and imaging continue to improve, leading to a better understanding of appropriate doses and target volumes. A landmark randomized trial, Intergroup 0096, published by Turrisi et al. in 1999, established accelerated RT as superior to conventionally fractionated RT (19). Tolerable acceleration, or reduction of the overall duration of the treatment course, was achieved by hyperfractionation, or twice-daily administration. In the trial, 417 patients received four cycles of EP, and RT was started with the first cycle of chemotherapy. The hyperfractionated-accelerated arm received 45 Gy in twice-daily 1.5 Gy fractions over 3 weeks and the control arm received the 45 Gy in once-daily 1.8 Gy fractions over 5 weeks. Acute toxicity was higher in the accelerated arm, with 27% versus 11% of patients experiencing grade 3 to 4 esophagitis. As such, 45 Gy was considered the maximum tolerated dose when given on the accelerated schedule. However, the accelerated arm had improved overall survival (median, 23 vs. 19 months; 5-year 26% vs. 16%; P = .04). Finally, accelerated treatment also reduced the rate of local failure from 52% to 36%. The superiority of accelerated RT provides clinical evidence for the radiobiological phenomenon of accelerated repopulation of SCLC, in which rapid tumor cell growth between RT fractions later in the course diminishes the effectiveness of a given total dose of RT with prolonged treatment duration.

Despite the results of this study, accelerated RT has not been widely adopted into clinical practice in the United States. A 2003 patterns of care study showed that fewer than 10% of patients with LS-SCLC received accelerated RT, while more than 80% received once-daily treatment (20). This is likely in part due to the logistical challenge of twice-daily delivery. Furthermore, the true advantage of the hyperfractionated regimen has been questioned because the RT regimen of 45 Gy over 5 weeks used in the control arm of the Intergroup study (19), though promising in contemporaneous trials (21), is now considered suboptimal for definitive therapy, attenuating the impact of the comparison to accelerated RT. A North Central Cancer Treatment Group trial conducted at the same time as the Intergroup trial failed to show an advantage for 48 Gy of twice-daily RT compared to 50.4 Gy of once-daily RT, though a 2.5 week RT break in the twice-daily arm may have allowed accelerated repopulation (22). CALGB 8,837 demonstrated that the maximum tolerated dose when delivered in once-daily fractions of 2 Gy exceeds 70 Gy (23), a dose that is consistent with the definitive dose used for locally advanced NSCLC.

Two ongoing cooperative group trials are now comparing a higher total dose of conventional RT to a lower total dose on an accelerated schedule. The CALGB 30610/RTOG 0538 trial randomizes patients to either 45 Gy twice-daily RT over 3 weeks or 70 Gy once-daily RT over 5 weeks starting with the first or second cycle of EP. The EORTC CONVERT trial is testing a similar RT question, but all patients receive RT starting with the second cycle of chemotherapy.

RT Target Volume

Historically, due to the risk of microscopic regional lymph node involvement, patients were treated with elective nodal irradiation (ENI), which called for large fields that included the mediastinum, bilateral lung hila, and supraclavicular fossae even if these regions were not clearly involved with the cancer. There has been a steady trend toward the use of smaller fields, in an attempt to reduce RT-related toxicity, such as esophagitis and pneumonitis. This trend has converged toward involved-field irradiation (IFI), in which only areas that are clinically involved on PET or CT are targeted (Figure 10.2). Several single-institution studies suggest that IFI is associated with low rates of out-of-field regional recurrence when PET-CT is used to target involved nodes that might be missed by CT alone. In two of these studies, only 3 of 120 patients (2.5%) had isolated out-of-field regional failure (24,25). Current clinical trials, such as CALGB 30,610, have adopted the IFI approach. Of note, with reduced treatment volumes, it is likely that the maximal tolerated dose would exceed 45 Gy, even with an accelerated hyperfractionated schedule, but this issue has not yet been evaluated in a clinical trial.

RT Summary

While still undergoing evolution, expert consensus on standard practice currently recommends IFI treatment volumes using dosing regimens ranging from 45 Gy of accelerated hyperfractionated RT over 3 weeks to 60 to 70 Gy of conventionally fractionated

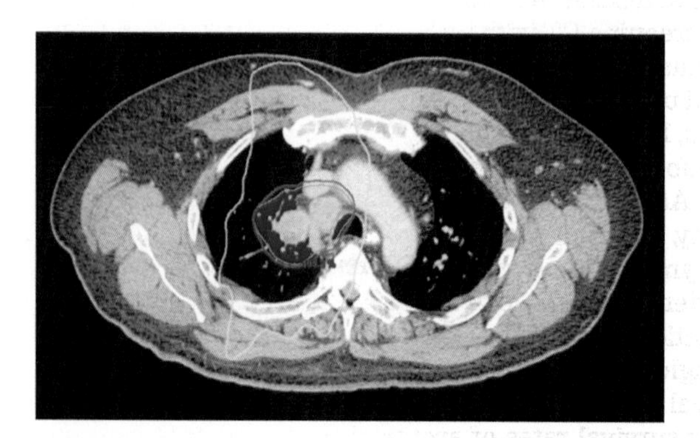

Figure 10.2 Involved-Field Irradiation. Only Areas With Clinically Evident Disease Are Treated Without Elective Irradiation of Other Mediastinal Lymph Node Stations. The Planning Target Volume Is Shaded in Green; The Area Receiving 100% of Prescribed Radiation Dose Is Outlined in Red; and the Area Receiving 50% Dose Is Outlined in Teal

RT over 6 to 7 weeks (8). Expected outcomes with this strategy include a complete radiographic response rate of 50%, median overall survival of around 2 years, a 5-year overall survival rate of 25%, and a local-regional failure rate of 25% to 35% (19,18). The majority of disease recurrences are at distant sites.

RT simulation and treatment planning for SCLC are similar to that for stage III NSCLC. Patients should undergo simulation with IV contrast, and motion management, such as 4D-CT with internal target volume delineation, should be used. For patients receiving accelerated hyperfractionated RT, normal tissue dose limits are stricter than for those receiving once-daily, conventionally fractionated treatment. For instance, the spinal cord should be limited to a maximum point dose of 41 Gy (8). Note that this is higher than the 36 Gy limit used in Intergroup 0096, because in that trial a portion of the RT course was administered using opposed anterior–posterior fields that encompassed entire segments of the spinal cord, whereas modern RT uses a multibeam configuration that spares the cord from the full dose with each fraction.

Surgery

Fewer than 5% of patients with SCLC are treated surgically, due to the sensitivity of the disease to RT and its propensity for spread to regional lymph nodes and distant sites. A randomized trial showed no survival advantage for surgical resection compared to RT in patients with LS-SCLC who also received chemotherapy (26). However, occasionally patients present with a very limited extent of disease, for instance a solitary pulmonary nodule found on a screening CT with no FDG-PET evidence of nodal or distant metastases. If medically fit for surgical resection, such patients should undergo invasive mediastinal staging and those with stage I (T1-2, N0, M0) SCLC should be considered for definitive surgery with lobectomy and mediastinal lymph node dissection or sampling. Adjuvant chemotherapy is generally recommended after surgery, and if patients are unexpectedly found to have mediastinal lymph node involvement, postoperative RT should also be considered (8, 27). However, high-level evidence for these recommendations is lacking.

Single-institution retrospective series have shown promising survival results after surgical resection of early stage SCLC, with 5-year survival rates of around 50% for patients with pathologic stage I disease (27, 28). It is difficult to compare these results to those achieved with chemoradiotherapy since the large majority of patients in chemoradiotherapy trials had stage III disease. Population-based studies using the Surveillance, Epidemiology, and End Results database and other registries also support the use of surgery in early stage SCLC (29). These population-based studies should be interpreted with caution, given the high likelihood of selection bias where patients selected for surgery are likely fitter and have less extensive disease than those receiving primary RT.

Emerging data suggest that stereotactic ablative RT (SABR) followed by chemotherapy may be an alternative to resection for lymph node-negative SCLC. A retrospective, multiinstitutional, Japanese study evaluated 64 patients who received SABR with or without chemotherapy for stage I SCLC (30). Sixty-six percent of patients were medically inoperable and 56% received chemotherapy. The 2-year disease-specific survival rate was 79% and the 2-year local control rate was 89%, results that are roughly comparable to those reported with surgical resection. Open questions for patients with stage I SCLC include whether SABR is as effective as resection, how chemotherapy should be sequenced with SABR, and whether PCI should be considered (31).

Prophylactic Cranial Irradiation

Efficacy

At least 18% of patients with SCLC have brain metastases at diagnosis, and the incidence at 2 years is 80% (32). Among patients with LS-SCLC, at least 50% develop brain metastases within 2 years (33). This has led to interest in PCI with the goal of eradicating micrometastatic disease in the brain and preventing or delaying the onset of symptomatic brain metastases. An individual patient meta-analysis of randomized trials comparing PCI to no PCI established PCI as a standard-of-care for patients with LS-SCLC who had responded well to induction therapy (34). Patients with complete response to chemotherapy and/or RT were eligible, and 86% of patients included had limited-stage disease. The PCI dose ranged from 8 to 40 Gy. PCI dramatically reduced the cumulative incidence of brain metastases (relative risk 0.46; 3-year rate, 33.3% vs. 58.6%; $P < .001$) and the risk of death (relative risk 0.84; 3-year survival rate, 21% vs. 15%; $P = .01$). Some of these patients may not have undergone brain imaging to rule out brain metastases prior to PCI, which could have biased the results to favor PCI. However, individual trials that did require brain imaging also have shown a strong benefit from PCI (35).

Most trials of PCI versus no PCI only included patients with complete response to initial therapy (34, 35). However, PCI likely has a benefit for patients with partial response as well, and consensus guidelines recommend PCI for patients with LS-SCLC who have had a partial or complete response to initial therapy and no contraindications, such as preexisting neurocognitive impairment (2, 8, 36).

Dose and Fractionation

A variety of doses and fractionation schemes have been used in trials of PCI, with treatment times ranging from 1 to 20 days (34). Higher biologically effective doses may produce higher in-brain control rates, but also induce more severe neurocognitive side effects. An Intergroup trial randomized 720 patients with LS-SCLC in complete remission to PCI using low-dose (25 Gy in 10 fractions) or high-dose (36 Gy in once-daily 2 Gy or twice-daily 1.5 Gy fractions) radiation (37). The 2-year incidence of brain metastases was similar in the two groups (29% vs. 23%, respectively; $P = .18$), while the 2-year overall survival rate was actually higher in the low-dose group (42% vs. 37%, $P = .05$), which was attributed to increased cancer-related mortality in the high-dose group. Therefore, 25 Gy in 10 fractions has become a standard dose for PCI.

Neurocognitive Toxicity

Whole brain RT, such as PCI, can result in cognitive decline, especially as a late effect in long-term survivors. However, there is little evidence that PCI at the recommended dose (≤25 Gy) results in neurocognitive changes. This may be due to use of less sensitive measurement tools in clinical trials, such as the Mini-Mental State Exam rather than more detailed neurocognitive testing (38). A French study randomized patients with SCLC and no CT evidence of brain metastases to either PCI (24 Gy in 12 fractions) or no PCI, and patients underwent baseline and follow-up neurocognitive testing by a neurologist (35). The cumulative 2-year rate of brain metastases was reduced in the PCI arm (67% vs. 40%), but there was no difference in the 2-year cumulative incidence of neuropsychological changes ($P = .19$–$.97$ for seven functional areas). The impact of this trial is limited by the lack of formal definitions of deficits or use of standardized scales to measure the parameters tested, including orientation, memory, judgment, language, and praxis.

Radiation dose likely affects neurocognitive function after PCI, with greater toxicity from higher doses. The RTOG 0212 trial formed part of the Intergroup trial discussed earlier (39). Neuropsychological testing was performed for patients in the low-dose and high-dose arms, and patients who received 25 Gy had less neurologic deterioration at 12 months than those who received

36 Gy, as defined by declines in memory, executive functioning, and other skills.

Novel strategies for reducing the neurocognitive toxicity of PCI are being explored. For instance, the NRG CC1432 phase II/III trial is testing hippocampal avoidance using intensity-modulated RT based on the promising results of a phase II trial in patients receiving therapeutic dose whole brain RT (30 Gy in 10 fractions) (40).

Patients with poor pretreatment neurocognitive function and those over 60 years old are at higher risk of neurotoxicity from PCI and this should be factored into decision making. In the RTOG 0212 trial, patients over 60 years old had an 83% rate of neurologic deterioration at 1 year compared to 59% for those 60 years old or younger (P = .02) (39). PCI should not be given concurrently with chemotherapy due to the increased risk of toxicity.

In summary, PCI to 25 Gy in 10 fractions over 2 weeks should be offered to patients who have had a partial or complete response to initial chemoradiotherapy and who have good performance status and neurocognitive function.

FOLLOW-UP AFTER TREATMENT

After completion of therapy, patients with LS-SCLC have a high risk of disease recurrence, both distant and local (19). Most recurrences occur in the first year after treatment completion (41). Patients should be followed with clinic visits and imaging such as contrast-enhanced chest CT. A reasonable schedule would be every 3 months for the first year, every 4 months for the second year, and less frequently after that. However, there is no high-quality evidence that detecting recurrences on surveillance imaging improves clinical outcomes. For patients who did not receive PCI, surveillance brain MRI can be considered since these patients are at high risk of developing brain metastases.

SUPPORTIVE CARE

Most patients with LS-SCLC will not be cured of their disease. Therefore, symptom management and efforts to minimize treatment-related decreases in quality of life are important. The NCCN has published guidelines on palliative care including best practices for the management of symptoms common in SCLC patients, such as pain, dyspnea, anorexia, and nausea (42). Early referral to a palliative care team may improve both quality-of-life and overall survival (43). There is strong evidence that continuing to smoke after a diagnosis of lung cancer reduces treatment effectiveness, increases side effects, and worsens overall survival (relative risk of death 2.36) (44). Therefore, current smokers should be encouraged to quit smoking and offered resources to assist with smoking cessation.

KEY POINTS

- LS-SCLC is potentially curable with definitive RT and chemotherapy.
- Standard treatment for limited-stage SCLC involves four to six cycles of chemotherapy, with thoracic RT given early during chemotherapy.
- Standard chemotherapy is four to six cycles of cisplatin or carboplatin plus etoposide.
- The optimal RT regimen has not been determined. In a randomized trial, accelerated hyperfractionated RT was found to be superior to the same dose of conventionally fractionated RT. Currently, standard RT regimens range from 45 Gy in 3 weeks using twice-daily treatment to 60 to 70 Gy in 6 to 7 weeks using once-daily treatment.
- Surgery may be appropriate for the rare patients with very limited burden of disease (T1-2 N0 M0).
- PCI should be considered for appropriate patients who respond well to initial therapy, though neurocognitive toxicity is a concern.
- Supportive care is important and early palliative care is likely beneficial. Smoking cessation interventions should be initiated for active smokers.

REFERENCES

1. Shepherd FA, Crowley J, Van Houtte P, et al. The International Association for the Study of Lung Cancer lung cancer staging project: proposals regarding the clinical staging of small cell lung cancer in the forthcoming (seventh) edition of the tumor, node, metastasis classification for lung cancer. *J Thorac Oncol*. 2007;2(12):1067-1077.
2. Jett JR, Schild SE, Kesler KA, Kalemkerian GP. Treatment of small cell lung cancer: Diagnosis and management of lung cancer, 3rd ed.: American College of Chest Physicians evidence-based clinical practice guidelines. *Chest*. 2013;143(5 suppl): e400S-419S.
3. Zelen M. Keynote address on biostatistics and data retrieval. *Cancer Chemother Rep 3*. 1973;4:31-42.
4. Sundstrom S, Bremnes RM, Kaasa S, et al. Cisplatin and etoposide regimen is superior to cyclophosphamide, epirubicin, and vincristine regimen in small-cell lung cancer: results from a randomized phase III trial with 5 years' follow-up. *J Clin Oncol*. 2002;20(24):4665-4672.
5. Bovelli D, Plataniotis G, Roila F; ESMO Guidelines Working Group. Cardiotoxicity of chemotherapeutic agents and radiotherapy-related heart disease: ESMO Clinical Practice Guidelines. *Ann Oncol*. 2010; 21(suppl 5):v277-v282.

6. Sklaros DV, Samantas E, Kosmidis P, et al. Randomized comparison of etoposide-cisplatin vs. etoposide-carboplatin and irradiation in small-cell lung cancer: a Hellenic Cooperative Oncology Group study. *Ann Oncol*. 1994;5:601-607.
7. Rossi A, DiMaio M, Chiodini P, et al. Carboplatin- or cisplatin-based chemotherapy in first-line treatment of small-cell lung cancer: the COCIS meta-analysis of individual patient data. *J Clin Oncol*. 2012;30:1692-1698.
8. National Comprehensive Cancer Network. NCCN Clinical Practice Guidelines in Oncology: Small Cell Lung Cancer, version 1.2016. Available at: http://www.nccn.org/professionals/physician_gls/pdf/sclc.pdf. Accessed March 13, 2016.
9. Kubota K, Hida T, Ishikura S, et al. Etoposide and cisplatin versus irinotecan and cisplatin in patients with limited-stage small-cell lung cancer treated with etoposide and cisplatin plus concurrent accelerated hyperfractionated thoracic radiotherapy (JCOG0202): a randomized phase 3 study. *Lancet Oncol*. 2013;15:106-113.
10. Antonia SJ, Bendell JC, Taylor MH, et al. Phase I/II study of nivolumab with or without ipilimumab for treatment of recurrent small cell lung cancer (SCLC): CA209-032. *J Clin Oncol*. 2015;33(suppl; abstr 7503).
11. Earl H, Rudd R, Spiro S, et al. A randomised trial of planned versus as required chemotherapy in small cell lung cancer: a Cancer Research Campaign trial. *Br J Cancer*. 1991;64(3):566-572.
12. Souhami RL, Spiro SG, Rudd RM, et al. Five-day oral etoposide treatment for advanced small-cell lung cancer: randomized comparison with intravenous chemotherapy. *J Natl Cancer Inst*. 1997;89(8):577-580.
13. Pignon J, Arriagada R, Ihde D, et al. A meta-analysis of thoracic radiotherapy for small-cell lung cancer. *N Engl J Med*. 1992;327:1618-1624.
14. Warde P, Payne D. Does thoracic irradiation improve survival and local control in limited-stage small-cell carcinoma of the lung? A meta-analysis. *J Clin Oncol*. 1992;10:890-895.
15. Murray N, Coy P, Pater J. Importance of timing for thoracic irradiation in the combined modality treatment of limited-stage small-cell lung cancer. *J Clin Oncol*. 1993;11:334-336.
16. Fried D, Morris D, Poole C, et al. Systematic review evaluating the timing of thoracic radiation therapy in combined modality therapy for limited-stage small-cell lung cancer. *J Clin Oncol*. 2004;22:4837-4845.
17. De Ruysscher D, Pijls-Johannesma M, Bentzen SM, et al. Time between the first day of chemotherapy and the last day of chest radiation is the most important predictor of survival in limited-disease small-cell lung cancer. *J Clin Oncol*. 2006;24(7):1057-1063.
18. Hu X, Bao Y, Zhang L, et al. Omitting elective nodal irradiation and irradiating postinduction versus preinduction chemotherapy tumor extent for limited-stage small cell lung cancer: interim analysis of a prospective randomized noninferiority trial. *Cancer*. 2012;118(1):278-287.
19. Turrisi A, Kyungmann K, Blum R, et al. Twice-daily compared with once-daily thoracic radiotherapy in limited small-cell lung cancer

treated concurrently with cisplatin and etoposide. *N Engl J Med.* 1999;340:265-271.

20. Movsas B, Moughan J, Komaki R, et al. Radiotherapy patterns of care study in lung carcinoma. *J Clin Oncol.* 2003;21(24):4553-4559.
21. McCracken J, Janaki L, Crowley J, et al. Concurrent chemotherapy/radiotherapy for limited small-cell lung carcinoma: a Southwestern Oncology Group study. *J Clin Oncol.* 1990;8:892-898.
22. Bonner JA, Sloan JA, Shanahan TG, et al. Phase III comparison of twice-daily split-course irradiation versus once-daily irradiation for patients with limited stage small-cell lung carcinoma. *J Clin Oncol.* 1999;17(9):2681-2691.
23. Choi NC, Herndon JE, Rosenman J, et al. Phase I study to determine the maximum-tolerated dose of radiation in standard daily and hyperfractionated-accelerated twice-daily radiation schedules with concurrent chemotherapy for limited-stage small-cell lung cancer. *J Clin Oncol.* 1998;16(11):3528-3536.
24. van Loon J, De Ruysscher D, Wanders R, et al. Selective nodal irradiation on basis of (18)FDG-PET scans in limited-disease small-cell lung cancer: a prospective study. *Int J Radiat Oncol Biol Phys.* 2010;77(2):329-336.
25. Shirvani SM, Komaki R, Heymach JV, et al. Positron emission tomography/computed tomography-guided intensity-modulated radiotherapy for limited-stage small-cell lung cancer. *Int J Radiat Oncol Biol Phys.* 2012;82(1):e91-97.
26. Lad T, Piantadosi S, Thomas P, et al. A prospective randomized trial to determine the benefit of surgical resection of residual disease following response of small cell lung cancer to combination chemotherapy. *Chest.* 1994;106(6 suppl):320S-323S.
27. Shepherd FA, Ginsberg RJ, Feld R, et al. Surgical treatment for limited small-cell lung cancer. The University of Toronto Lung Oncology Group experience. *J Thorac Cardiovasc Surg.* 1991;101(3):385-393.
28. Inoue M, Miyoshi S, Yasumitsu T, et al. Surgical results for small cell lung cancer based on the new TNM staging system. Thoracic Surgery Study Group of Osaka University, Osaka, Japan. *Ann Thorac Surg.* 2000;70(5):1615-1619.
29. Schreiber D, Rineer J, Weedon J, et al. Survival outcomes with the use of surgery in limited-stage small cell lung cancer: should its role be re-evaluated? *Cancer.* 2010;116(5):1350-1357.
30. Shioyama Y, Nagata Y, Komiyama T, Takay K. Multi-institutional retrospective study of stereotactic body radiation therapy for stage I small cell lung cancer: Japan Radiation Oncology Study Group (JROSG). *Int J Radiat Oncol Biol Phys.* 2015;93(3):S101.
31. Verma V, Simone CB, Zhen W. Stereotactic radiotherapy for stage I small cell lung cancer. *Oncologist.* 2016;21(2):131-133.
32. Slotman B, Faivre-Finn C, Kramer G, et al. Prophylactic cranial irradiation in extensive small-cell lung cancer. *N Engl J Med.* 2007;357(7):664-672.

33. Gregor A, Cull A, Stephens RJ, et al. Prophylactic cranial irradiation is indicated following complete response to induction therapy in small cell lung cancer: results of a multicentre randomised trial. United Kingdom Coordinating Committee for Cancer Research (UKCCCR) and the European Organization for Research and Treatment of Cancer (EORTC). *Eur J Cancer*. 1997;33(11):1752-1758.
34. Auperin A, Arriagada R, Pignon JP, et al. Prophylactic cranial irradiation for patients with small-cell lung cancer in complete remission. Prophylactic Cranial Irradiation Overview Collaborative Group. *N Engl J Med*. 1999;341(7):476-484.
35. Arriagada R, Le Chevalier T, Borie F, et al. Prophylactic cranial irradiation for patients with small-cell lung cancer in complete remission. *J Natl Cancer Inst*. 1995;87(3):183-190.
36. Fruh M, De Ruysscher D, Popat S, et al. Small-cell lung cancer (SCLC): ESMO Clinical Practice Guidelines for diagnosis, treatment and follow-up. *Ann Oncol*. 2013;24(suppl 6):vi99-105.
37. Le Pechoux C, Dunant A, Senan S, et al. Standard-dose versus higher-dose prophylactic cranial irradiation (PCI) in patients with limited-stage small-cell lung cancer in complete remission after chemotherapy and thoracic radiotherapy (PCI 99-01, EORTC 22003-08004, RTOG 0212, and IFCT 99-01): a randomised clinical trial. *Lancet Oncol*. 2009;10(5):467-474.
38. Meyers CA, Wefel JS. The use of the mini-mental state examination to assess cognitive functioning in cancer trials: no ifs, ands, buts, or sensitivity. *J Clin Oncol*. 2003;21(19):3557-3558.
39. Wolfson AH, Bae K, Komaki R, et al. Primary analysis of a phase II randomized trial Radiation Therapy Oncology Group (RTOG) 0212: impact of different total doses and schedules of prophylactic cranial irradiation on chronic neurotoxicity and quality of life for patients with limited-disease small-cell lung cancer. *Int J Radiat Oncol Biol Phys*. 2011;81(1):77-84.
40. Gondi V, Pugh SL, Tome WA, et al. Preservation of memory with conformal avoidance of the hippocampal neural stem-cell compartment during whole-brain radiotherapy for brain metastases (RTOG 0933): a phase II multi-institutional trial. *J Clin Oncol*. 2014;32(34):3810-3816.
41. Manapov F, Klöcking S, Niyazi M, et al. Timing of failure in limited disease (stage I-III) small-cell lung cancer patients treated with chemoradiotherapy: a retrospective analysis. *Tumori*. 2013;99(6):656-660.
42. National Comprehensive Cancer Network. NCCN Clinical Practice Guidelines in Oncology: Palliative Care, version 1.2016. https://www.nccn.org/professionals/physician_gls/f_guidelines.asp
43. Temel JS, Greer JA, Muzikansky A, et al. Early palliative care for patients with metastatic non-small-cell lung cancer. *N Engl J Med*. 2010;363(8):733-742.
44. Tao L, Wang R, Gao YT, Yuan JM. Impact of postdiagnosis smoking on long-term survival of cancer patients: the Shanghai cohort study. *Cancer Epidemiol Biomarkers Prev*. 2013;22(12):2404-2411.

Management of Extensive-Stage Small Cell Lung Cancer 11

Gregory P. Kalemkerian and James A. Hayman

INTRODUCTION

Small cell lung cancer (SCLC) is an aggressive, poorly differentiated neuroendocrine carcinoma with clinical, pathological, and molecular characteristics that are distinct from those of non–small-cell lung cancer (NSCLC). Clinically, SCLC is characterized by rapid growth, early lymphatic and hematogenous metastatic spread, initial responsiveness to chemotherapy and radiation, relapse with relatively chemoresistant disease, and poor overall prognosis.

STAGE CLASSIFICATION

The Veterans' Administration Lung Group classification is routinely used to stage SCLC. Limited-stage (LS) is defined as tumor confined to one hemithorax, with or without regional lymph node involvement, which can be safely encompassed in a tolerable radiation therapy (RT) port. Extensive-stage (ES) is defined as disease that has spread beyond this point, including malignant pleural or pericardial effusion, tumor nodules in different ipsilateral lung lobes, contralateral lung nodules, and other hematogenous metastases. Involvement of contralateral mediastinal and ipsilateral supraclavicular lymph nodes is usually considered LS, while involvement of contralateral supraclavicular and hilar lymph nodes is frequently deemed ES due to the toxicity associated with an extended radiation field. However, the decision on how to treat such patients needs to be individualized based on the potential risks and benefits as assessed by the managing care team. At least two-thirds of patients are found to have ES-SCLC at initial diagnosis.

The TNM staging system that is used for NSCLC could also be applied to SCLC since these T and N descriptors and the overall stage I to IV groupings, also predict prognosis in patients with SCLC (1) (Appendix A.1). In the TNM system, ES-SCLC can be defined as T1-4 N0-3 M1a/b or T3-4 due to multiple lung nodules that are too extensive or dispersed to be encompassed in a tolerable radiation port.

OVERVIEW OF CLINICAL MANAGEMENT

The management of ES-SCLC is frequently complicated by both the aggressiveness of the disease and the underlying health status of the patient. Many patients present with rapidly progressive, debilitating symptoms due to bulky intrathoracic disease, widespread metastases, and/or paraneoplastic syndromes. Due to long-term tobacco use, many patients also have comorbidities that contribute to their impaired performance status and limit the delivery of optimal therapy. These factors also complicate the enrollment of patients with SCLC onto clinical trials.

ES-SCLC is an incurable disease in which the goals of care are to palliate symptoms, optimize quality of life, and prolong survival. The mainstay of treatment is platinum-based, two-drug chemotherapy which yields an objective response rate of 60% to 70% and a complete response rate of up to 10%. Patients who attain a good response and maintain a good performance status are candidates for prophylactic cranial irradiation (PCI) and consolidative thoracic RT, based on clinical trials demonstrating improved survival. Although chemotherapy improves quality of life and prolongs survival in patients with ES-SCLC, nearly all relapse with relatively chemoresistant disease.

Single-agent chemotherapy is the standard treatment for patients with relapsed SCLC based on the demonstration of improvement in survival versus supportive care alone. Palliative RT is usually very useful for control of localizable symptoms, such as shortness of breath due to bronchial obstruction, superior vena cava syndrome, bone pain, or neurologic dysfunction due to brain metastases. The prognosis of patients with ES-SCLC has changed little since the 1970s, with 2-year overall survival improving only from 3.4% to 5.6% (2).

FIRST-LINE CHEMOTHERAPY

Historical Development

Historically, patients with ES-SCLC who did not receive therapy had a very poor prognosis, with a median survival of less than 2 months. Clinical trials with single-agent therapy revealed surprisingly high-response rates, resulting in an extensive list of active agents (Table 11.1). However, single-agent therapy yields few complete responses and a relatively short duration of response. In the 1970s, alkylator-based combination chemotherapy regimens, such as cyclophosphamide, doxorubicin, and vincristine (CAV), resulted in significant improvements in overall survival when compared to single-agent therapy (3). In patients with ES-SCLC, these regimens resulted in response rates of 60% to 80%, complete response rates of 15% to 25%, and median survival times of 7 to 10 months.

Table 11.1 Clinically active agents in small cell lung cancer

DNA intercalating agents	Cisplatin
	Carboplatin
Alkylating agents	Cyclophosphamide
	Ifosfamide
	Temozolomide
	Bendamustine
Topoisomerase 2 inhibitors	Etoposide
	Teniposide
Anthracyclines	Doxorubicin
	Epirubicin
	Amrubicin
Topoisomerase 1 inhibitors	Irinotecan
	Topotecan
Microtubule inhibitors	Vincristine
	Vinblastine
	Vinorelbine
Microtubule stabilizers	Paclitaxel
	Docetaxel
Antimetabolites	Methotrexate
	Gemcitabine
Immune checkpoint inhibitors	Pembrolizumab
	Nivolumab

Cisplatin Plus Etoposide

In the 1980s, the combination of etoposide and cisplatin (EP) was found to have response and survival rates similar to those of older alkylator-based regimens with a relatively favorable toxicity profile (4). Subsequently, randomized trials directly comparing CAV to EP failed to demonstrate the superiority of either regimen (5). Recently, a phase III study comparing EP to cyclophosphamide, epirubicin, and vincristine (CEV) in patients with both LS- and ES-SCLC reported that overall survival was significantly better with EP (10.2 vs. 7.8 months, P = .0004), although there was little difference noted in those with ES-SCLC (6). Meta-analyses have also demonstrated a modest survival advantage for cisplatin-based therapy (7). Therefore, EP has become the standard regimen for SCLC based on efficacy that is at least as good as other regimens, a reasonable toxicity profile, and the ease with which it can be combined with thoracic RT in patients with LS-SCLC.

Cisplatin Versus Carboplatin

Cisplatin is a relatively difficult drug, particularly in the palliative setting, due to its cumbersome administration and unpleasant side effects, including nausea/vomiting, ototoxicity, nephrotoxicity, and peripheral neuropathy. Due to these limitations, many oncologists freely substitute carboplatin in light of its ease of administration and more favorable nonhematologic toxicity profile. Thus far, only one trial has directly compared EP to etoposide plus carboplatin (EC). Sklaros et al. randomized 147 patients with LS- or ES-SCLC to six cycles of EP or EC, adding concurrent thoracic RT in those with LS (8). There was no difference in response rate (57% vs. 58%), time to progression (TTP; median, 8.4 vs. 8.6 months), or overall survival (median, 12.5 vs. 11.8 months) between EP and EC, respectively.

Recently, the COCIS meta-analysis of 663 patients from four trials compared cisplatin-based to carboplatin-based therapy for first-line treatment of both LS- and ES-SCLC (9). Two-thirds of patients had ES disease. This meta-analysis found no significant difference between cisplatin and carboplatin in any efficacy endpoint, including response rate (67% vs. 66%, P = .83), progression-free survival (PFS; median, 5.5 vs. 5.3 months, P = .25), and overall survival (median, 9.6 vs. 9.4 months, P = .37) (9). Carboplatin-based regimens were associated with more grade 3 to 4 cytopenia, while cisplatin predictably caused more nausea/vomiting, neurotoxicity, and nephrotoxicity. Based on these data demonstrating equivalent efficacy, it is most reasonable to use carboplatin-based regimens in patients with ES-SCLC given the palliative nature of therapy and the focus on maintenance of good quality of life.

Alternative First-Line Regimens

Topoisomerase I Inhibitors + Platinum

Irinotecan and topotecan are topoisomerase I inhibitors with single-agent activity against SCLC. Several regimens combining these agents with platinum analogs have been compared to platinum plus etoposide in patients with ES-SCLC (Table 11.2). In the first phase III trial of irinotecan plus cisplatin (IP), Noda et al. from the Japanese Cooperative Oncology Group (JCOG)

Table 11.2 Phase III randomized trials of cisplatin or carboplatin plus irinotecan or topotecan in ES-SCLC

			Response rate		Overall survival			
Trial	Arm	*N*	%	*P*	Median	1-y	2-y	*P*
Noda et al. (10)	IP	77	84	.02	12.8 mo	58.4%	19.5%	.002
	EP	77	68		9.4 mo	37.7%	5.2%	
Hanna et al. (11)	IP	221	48	NS	9.3 mo	35%	8%	.74
	EP	110	44		10.2 mo	35%	8%	
Lara et al. (12)	IP	324	60	.56	9.9 mo	41%	NR	.71
	EP	327	57		9.1 mo	34%	NR	
Zatloukal et al. (13)	IP	202	39	NS	10.2 mo	42%	16%	.06
	EP	203	47		9.7 mo	39%	8%	
Hermes et al. (14)	IC	105	17*	.02	8.5 mo	NR	NR	.02
	EC	104	7*		7.1 mo	NR	NR	
Eckardt et al. (15)	TP	389	63	NS	9.0 mo	31%	NR	.48
	EP	395	69		9.2 mo	31%	NR	
Fink et al. (16)	TP	358	56	.01	45 wk	40%	NR	.30
	EP	345	46		41 wk	36%	NR	

EC, etoposide + carboplatin; EP, etoposide + cisplatin; IC, irinotecan + carboplatin; IP, irinotecan + cisplatin; NS, not significant; NR, not reported; TP, topotecan + cisplatin.
*Complete response rate.

randomized 154 patients with previously untreated ES-SCLC to either EP or IP and reported that IP resulted in a significantly better response rate, PFS, and overall survival (Table 11.2) (10). IP resulted in significantly more diarrhea, while EP caused greater hematologic toxicity. Subsequent randomized trials in Western patients have failed to confirm the superiority of IP over EP. Hanna et al. compared a modified IP regimen to EP in 331 patients with previously untreated ES-SCLC and reported no difference in overall efficacy (Table 11.2) (11). As in the JCOG trial, EP resulted in more myelosuppression and febrile neutropenia, while IP caused more diarrhea. In a Southwest Oncology Group (SWOG) study from the United States, Lara et al. randomized 651 patients with previously untreated ES-SCLC to receive IP or EP using the same regimens and schedules as the initial JCOG trial (12). Again, there was no significant difference in response rate or survival between the two arms (Table 11.2). A European study by Zatloukal et al. randomized 405 patients with previously untreated ES-SCLC to receive IP or EP and reported noninferiority of IP, with the response rate and TTP favoring EP, but overall survival favoring IP (Table 11.2) (13).

The combination of irinotecan plus carboplatin (IC) has also been studied in patients with ES-SCLC. In a phase III trial, Hermes et al. randomized 209 patients with untreated ES-SCLC to receive IC or EC and reported a significant improvement in overall survival with IC, with similar quality of life outcomes in both arms (Table 11.2) (14).

Topotecan is generally considered to be more tolerable than irinotecan. Eckardt et al. randomized 784 patients with previously untreated ES-SCLC to receive either oral topotecan plus cisplatin (TP) or EP. Once again, efficacy was similar in both arms (Table 11.2) (15). As in the prior trials of IP versus EP, there was more neutropenia and febrile neutropenia in patients receiving EP and more diarrhea in those treated with TP. Quality of life analysis slightly favored EP ($P = .049$). A similar study by Fink et al. compared TP to EP in 703 patients with untreated ES-SCLC and reported a significant improvement in response rate and TTP with TP, but no difference in overall survival (Table 11.2) (16).

Meta-analyses of studies comparing platinum analogs plus either topoisomerase 1 inhibitors or etoposide have reported modest improvements in overall survival with platinum plus irinotecan or topotecan combinations (17). However, when balancing toxicity profiles and efficacy endpoints, it is clear that these regimens are not a significant advance, and EP or EC remain the standard-of-care for patients with ES-SCLC.

Other Chemotherapy Regimens

Phase II trials utilizing a variety of regimens, including carboplatin plus paclitaxel and paclitaxel plus topotecan, in patients with ES-SCLC have reported response and survival outcomes that appear similar to those achieved with standard regimens (18,19). Although these empiric combinations have not been evaluated in randomized trials, it is unlikely that they would result in significant improvements in survival.

Recent studies have demonstrated that amrubicin, a novel anthracycline, has clinically relevant activity in patients with SCLC. Early phase studies in previously untreated patients with ES-SCLC showed high response rates for both single-agent amrubicin and the combination of amrubicin plus cisplatin (AP). However, a phase III trial comparing AP to IP in 284 previously untreated patients with ES-SCLC was stopped early due to futility with similar response rates for AP and IP (78% vs. 72%, $P = .33$), but with PFS (median, 5.6 vs. 5.1 months; HR1.42, 95% CI 1.16–1.73) and overall survival (median, 17.7 vs. 15.0 months; HR 1.43, 95% CI 1.10–1.85) significantly favoring IP (20).

Other Chemotherapy-Based Strategies

Numerous chemotherapy-based strategies, including dose-intensification, dose-dense regimens, weekly administration, triplet therapy, high-dose consolidation, alternating or sequential non–cross-resistant regimens, maintenance therapy, and consolidation therapy, have failed to demonstrate consistent improvements in survival, and many of these more aggressive approaches have resulted in unacceptable toxicity.

As an example of three-drug therapy, CALGB 9732 randomized 587 patients with untreated ES-SCLC to receive six cycles of EP or EP plus paclitaxel (PET) (21). The response rates were 68% and 75% for EP and PET, respectively, with overlapping 95% confidence intervals. Similarly, there were no significant differences in failure-free survival (median, 5.9 vs. 6.4 months, $P = .18$) or overall survival (median, 9.9 vs. 10.6 months, $P = .17$) between EP and PET, respectively. However, PET was associated with an unacceptable increase in treatment-related deaths, primarily due to neutropenic sepsis (2.4% vs. 6.5%) despite the planned use of G-CSF.

In regard to consolidation therapy, ECOG 7593 evaluated EP for four cycles versus EP for four cycles followed by four cycles of topotecan in 402 patients with ES-SCLC (22). Although PFS was modestly but statistically significantly improved with the addition of topotecan (median, 3.6 vs. 2.3 months, $P < .001$), there was no difference in overall survival (median, 9.3 vs. 8.9 months, $P = .43$). As expected, consolidation topotecan did increase toxicity, but there was no significant difference in reported quality of life between the two arms. In addition to refuting the notion of consolidation topotecan (or early second-line therapy), this study indirectly supports the use of four, rather than six or more, cycles of initial chemotherapy.

Recommendations for First-Line Chemotherapy

Based on the available data and the palliative goals of care, four to six cycles of carboplatin AUC 5 on day 1 plus etoposide 100 mg/m^2 days 1 to 3 every 21 days should be considered the preferred first-line chemotherapy regimen for patients with ES-SCLC. Cisplatin 75 mg/m^2 plus etoposide 100 mg/m^2 days 1 to 3 every 21 days for four to six cycles is an option for younger patients with good performance status and normal organ function.

RADIATION THERAPY

General Principles

Since ES-SCLC is an incurable, systemic disease, RT has traditionally been used only to prevent or palliate symptoms. However, building on improvements in outcomes for patients with LS-SCLC with the addition of RT, several studies have been published over the past decade that have demonstrated improvement in survival with the addition of RT in patients with ES-SCLC, thereby expanding the role of RT in this setting.

Prophylactic Cranial Irradiation

SCLC has an extraordinarily high propensity to metastasize to the brain. PCI has been shown in a meta-analysis to improve survival in patients with SCLC who have had a complete response to initial treatment (23). Of note, approximately 85% of the patients included in this meta-analysis had LS disease and 75% received thoracic RT, raising questions as to the applicability of these findings to patients with ES-SCLC. To address the question of PCI in ES-SCLC, the European Organization for Research and Treatment of Cancer (EORTC) undertook a trial in which 286 patients with ES-SCLC and any response to chemotherapy were randomized to PCI or no further therapy (24). This study allowed four to six cycles of any type of chemotherapy and used a variety of different PCI schedules (e.g., 20 Gy in 5 or 8 fractions, 24 Gy in 12 fractions, 25 Gy in 10 fractions, 30 Gy in 10 or 12 fractions). In addition, repeat negative brain imaging after chemotherapy was not required for study entry. PCI decreased the incidence of symptomatic brain metastases from 40% to 15% at 1 year ($P < .001$) and increased the 1-year survival rate from 13% to 27% ($P = .003$) without a large decrement in quality of life (25). However, a more recent study from Japan, which has only been reported as an abstract, has questioned the use of PCI in ES-SCLC (26). This study required a negative brain MRI prior to enrollment and randomized patients with any response to platinum-based doublet chemotherapy to PCI of 25 Gy in 10 fractions or no further therapy. After enrolling 163 of a planned 330 patients, an interim analysis led to early termination of the study due to futility with patients in the PCI arm demonstrating a lower median overall survival than those on observation without PCI (10 vs. 15 months, $P = .09$).

Recommendations for PCI

At this time, PCI is still recommended for patients with ES-SCLC with a response to chemotherapy, good performance status, and no evidence of brain metastases on repeat brain imaging. Considering the poor prognosis and comorbidities of patients with ES-SCLC, the potential benefits and risks of PCI need to be carefully weighed for every patient. It is generally agreed that if PCI is planned it should be started soon after restaging. Most patients in the EORTC study received 20 Gy in 5 fractions or 30 Gy in 10 fractions. However, due to concerns about neurocognitive toxicity and data from a PCI trial in LS-SCLC that demonstrated better outcomes with 25 Gy than with 36 Gy, the use of 25 Gy in 10 fractions is favored (27). Data in patients with LS-SCLC also demonstrated that age is the most significant predictor of chronic neurotoxicity following PCI (28). Although long-term toxicity may be less relevant in patients with ES-SCLC due to their relatively poor prognosis, it is reasonable to withhold PCI in elderly patients and those with impaired baseline neurocognitive function.

Thoracic Radiation Therapy

Based on data demonstrating an improvement in survival with the addition of thoracic RT in patients with LS-SCLC and the fact that most patients with ES-SCLC will have symptomatic progression of thoracic disease after response to initial therapy, there has been increasing interest in adding thoracic RT in patients with ES disease. In a single institution study, Jeremic et al. reported on a subgroup of 109 patients with ES-SCLC who had at least a partial response in the chest and a complete response at distant sites following three cycles of EP who were randomized to accelerated hyperfractionated RT of 54 Gy in twice daily 1.5 Gy fractions with concurrent low-dose daily EP versus two more cycles of EP without RT (29). Patients in both arms then received PCI and two more cycles of EP. Patients on the RT arm had significantly better overall survival (median, 17 vs. 11 months; 5-year, 9.1% vs. 3.7%; $P = .041$). However, because these data came from a single institution study with a small sample size, required a complete response in all distant sites, and employed aggressive thoracic RT with concurrent chemotherapy, these results were generally viewed as hypothesis generating rather than practice changing.

Encouraging data from this trial and other smaller studies served as justification for the phase III European CREST trial in which 495 patients with ES-SCLC who had responded to initial chemotherapy were randomized to receive either thoracic RT (30 Gy in 10 fractions) or no thoracic RT (30). All patients received PCI and 88% of those on the thoracic RT arm underwent concurrent RT to both sites. While the addition of thoracic RT did not achieve a statistically significant improvement in the primary endpoint of 1-year overall survival (33% vs. 28%, $P = .066$), a secondary analysis did find significant improvement in 2-year overall survival (13% vs. 3%, $P = .004$).

Recommendation for Thoracic RT

Results from the CREST trial have led to the use of thoracic RT in patients with ES-SCLC who have had a response to chemotherapy and good performance status. As with PCI, the potential benefits and risks of thoracic RT must be carefully evaluated for each individual patient. Based on the design of this pivotal trial, thoracic RT and PCI are typically initiated concurrently within 2 to 7 weeks after chemotherapy. The standard dose of thoracic RT is 30 Gy in 10 fractions although some data support the use of doses up to 45 Gy in 15 fractions.

Radiation Therapy to Oligometastatic Sites

Approximately 60% of patients with ES-SCLC treated with chemotherapy, PCI, and thoracic RT progress at sites other than the chest and brain (30). This finding raises the question of whether there is a role for using RT to treat limited metastatic sites. In a randomized phase II Radiation Therapy Oncology Group (RTOG)/NRG trial, patients with one to four metastatic lesions with a response to four to six cycles of platinum-based chemotherapy and no brain metastases received PCI or PCI plus RT of 45 Gy in 15 fractions to the chest and to sites of metastatic disease. After enrolling 86 eligible patients, a preplanned interim analysis led to early termination of the study due to futility with no statistical difference in 1-year overall survival between the PCI only arm and the PCI plus thoracic and metastatic site RT arm (60% vs. 51%; $P = .21$) (31).

Recommendation for RT to Oligometastatic Sites

Given the lack of benefit in the RTOG/NRG trial, treating even a limited number of asymptomatic metastatic sites with RT in patients with ES-SCLC is not recommended.

Palliative Radiation Therapy

In patients with symptomatic metastatic lesions, RT can be highly effective in achieving symptom relief. For example, RT can relieve neurologic symptoms due to brain metastases or vertebral metastases causing spinal cord, cauda equina, or nerve root compression, pain from bone metastases, and respiratory symptoms due to bronchial obstruction from lung tumors or lymph node metastases. In addition, due to the fact that SCLC is generally very responsive to RT, patients with SCLC typically experience more rapid palliation of their symptoms with RT than patients with NSCLC.

In light of the high degree of responsiveness of SCLC to first-line chemotherapy, many focal symptoms in newly diagnosed patients, such as superior vena cava syndrome, airway obstruction, or bone pain, can be managed with prompt initiation of systemic chemotherapy, with RT held in reserve. However, in patients with spinal cord compression RT should be initiated urgently. For patients with asymptomatic brain metastases identified on initial staging evaluation, brain RT can be delayed in favor of early initiation of systemic first-line chemotherapy, which is frequently needed to control rapidly progressive systemic symptoms and declining performance status. In such situations, brain metastases usually respond to systemic therapy and brain scans should be repeated every two cycles with initiation of brain RT for any evidence of progressive CNS disease.

Recommendations for Palliative RT

The approach used for treating patients with symptomatic SCLC metastases is similar to that for treating patients with other primary cancers. For example, 30 Gy in 10 fractions is commonly used for symptomatic brain, bone, and thoracic metastases. However, there are several caveats. Because SCLC is so radiation-responsive, lower doses of RT are frequently employed (e.g., 20 Gy in 5 fractions). In addition, even in patients with a limited number of small brain metastases that may be amenable to stereotactic radiosurgery, its use is not recommended due to the responsiveness of the disease and the high likelihood of subclinical disease elsewhere in the brain. Instead, whole brain RT is recommended as initial treatment with radiosurgery reserved for salvage therapy in patients with progression in a limited number of lesions after whole brain RT.

CHEMOTHERAPY FOR RECURRENT DISEASE

Virtually all patients with ES-SCLC will relapse with relatively chemoresistant disease. Recurrent SCLC has traditionally been divided into two categories based on responsiveness to further therapy: (a) refractory/resistant disease is defined as primary progression or recurrence within 3 months of initial therapy, and (b) relapsed/sensitive disease is defined as recurrence more than 3 months after initial therapy. Response rates for subsequent therapy are substantially lower in patients with a shorter duration of response to initial treatment (i.e., refractory/resistant).

Topotecan

Topotecan is the only drug currently approved by the U.S. Food and Drug Administration (FDA) for use in patients with relapsed SCLC. The benefit of second-line therapy in patients with recurrent SCLC was demonstrated by O'Brien et al. in a randomized trial comparing oral topotecan to best supportive care in 141 patients with both sensitive and resistant relapse (32). Despite a response rate of only 7%, overall survival was significantly better in patients receiving oral topotecan (median, 26 vs. 14 weeks; 6-month, 49% vs. 26%; $P = .01$) (Table 11.3).

Phase II trials evaluating single-agents and combination regimens in patients with relapsed SCLC have generally demonstrated higher response rates with combination therapy, but no apparent improvement in overall survival. In addition, the toxicity of combination regimens is difficult for many patients with recurrent SCLC due to impaired performance status and significant comorbidities. A randomized phase III trial compared single-agent topotecan 1.5 mg/m^2 IV on days one to five every 21 days to CAV in 211 patients with SCLC who had relapsed more than 60 days after initial therapy (33). This trial reported no significant difference in response rate (24% vs. 18%, $P = .29$), TTP (median, 13 vs. 12 weeks, $P = .55$), or overall survival (median, 25 weeks both arms, $P = .79$) between topotecan and CAV, respectively (Table 11.3). However, hematologic toxicity was significantly greater with the combination regimen. In addition, patients receiving topotecan noted greater improvement in symptoms, such as dyspnea, anorexia, and fatigue, and a delay in eventual symptom progression. Based on these findings, single-agent chemotherapy became the standard treatment approach for patients with relapsed SCLC who have a good performance status.

A phase III randomized study compared oral versus intravenous (IV) topotecan in patients with recurrent SCLC and reported no statistically significant or clinically meaningful differences in response rate, PFS, or overall survival (Table 11.3) (34).

Table 11.3 Selected phase III randomized trials in relapsed small cell lung cancer

Trial/year	Arm	*N*		Time from initial therapy	Response rate	PFS or TTP (median)	Overall survival	
		Total	Sensitive/resistant				Median	1-y
O'Brien/2006 (32)	BSC	70	35/35	≥45 d	–	NR	13.9 wk	26%†
	Topotecan PO 2.3 mg/m²/d × 5d	71	30/41		7% (S 3%/R 10%)	NR	25.9 wk*	49%†*
von Pawel/1999 (33)	CAV	104	83/21	≥60 d	18% (S 22%/R 5%)	12.3 wk	24.7 wk	14.4%
	Topotecan IV 1.5 mg/m²/d × 5d	107	85/22		24% (S 27%/R 14%)	13.3 wk	25.0 wk	14.2%
Goto/2014 (47)	PEI	90	90/0	>90 d	84%*	5.7 mo*	18.2 mo*	NR
	Topotecan IV 1.0 mg/m²/d × 5d	90	90/0		27%	3.6 mo	12.5 mo	NR
Eckardt/2007 (34)	Topotecan IV 1.5 mg/m²/d × 5d	151	137/13	≥90 d	22%	14.6 wk	35 wk	29%
	Topotecan PO 2.3 mg/m²/d × 5d	153	134/15		18%	11.9 wk	33 wk	33%

(*continued*)

Table 11.3 Selected phase III randomized trials in relapsed small cell lung cancer (*continued*)

Trial/year	Arm	*N*		Time from initial therapy	Response rate	PFS or TTP (median)	Overall survival	
		Total	Sensitive/resistant				Median	1-y
Von Pawel/2014 (46)	Topotecan IV 1.5 mg/m²/d × 5d	213	117/96		17% (S 23%/R 9%)	3.5 mo	7.8 mo (S 9.9/ R 5.7)	NR
	Amrubicin 40 mg/m²/d × 3d	424	225/199		31%* (S 41%/R 20%)	4.1 mo*	7.5 mo (S 9.2/ R 6.2)	NR

BSC, best supportive care; CAV, cyclophosphamide + doxorubicin + vincristine; d, day(s); IV, intravenous; mo, months; NR, not reported; PEI, cisplatin + etoposide + irinotecan; PFS/TTP, progression-free survival or time-to-progression; PO, oral; R, resistant (relapse less than 90 days from completion of first-line therapy); S, sensitive (relapse ≥90 days from completion of first-line therapy); wk, weeks.

*Statistically significant ($P < .05$).

†6-month overall survival rate.

Quality of life measures were also similar, but oral topotecan did result in less severe neutropenia.

The standard regimen of topotecan 1.5 mg/m^2 IV on days one to five of a 21 day cycle induces severe myelotoxicity and fatigue. An attenuated dose regimen of topotecan 1.25 mg/m^2 IV on days one to five of a 21 day cycle adjusted for toxicity on subsequent cycles may be equally efficacious with lower toxicity (35). Weekly topotecan 4 mg/m^2 IV also appears to have lower toxicity than the standard regimen, but efficacy may be compromised (36). Pooled analyses have suggested that standard-dose topotecan is tolerable and effective in patients with relapsed SCLC and an ECOG performance status of two, but the high rate of treatment delays (46% for cycle 2), low dose-intensity (1.59 mg/m^2/week), and short overall survival (median, 16 weeks) raise serious questions about the utility of this regimen in this impaired patient population (37).

Other Chemotherapy Agents

Several other standard drugs have demonstrated modest activity in phase II studies in patients with relapsed SCLC, including irinotecan, oral etoposide, paclitaxel, docetaxel, vinorelbine, and gemcitabine (38). For example, oral etoposide has shown response rates of 23% to 45%, but little activity is noted in patients with resistant relapse (39). In contrast, paclitaxel had a response rate of 29% in patients who had received at least two prior lines of chemotherapy, suggesting that it is a reasonable option for patients with refractory/resistant disease (40).

The most recent additions to the list of active agents in relapsed SCLC are temozolomide and bendamustine. In a phase II trial, 64 patients who had one to two prior regimens received temozolomide 75 mg/m^2 for 21 days of a 28-day cycle. The overall response rate was around 20% in both the second- and third-line settings, and 38% in patients with brain metastases (41). A subsequent study with temozolomide 200 mg/m^2 on days 1–5 of a 28-day cycle reported a response rate of 12% with a more tolerable toxicity profile (42). Bendamustine, an alkylating agent used routinely in chronic lymphocytic leukemia, has demonstrated response rates of 26% and 29%, along with tolerable toxicity in two phase II trials in patients with relapsed SCLC (43,44).

A randomized phase II trial compared amrubicin to topotecan in 76 patients with recurrent SCLC and reported a significantly better response rate (44% vs. 15%, P = .02) with modest improvements in PFS and overall survival with amrubicin (45). However, a phase III trial in which 637 patients with recurrent SCLC were randomized to receive either amrubicin or topotecan reported a significant improvement in response rate (31% vs. 17%,

P = .0002) with amrubicin, but no difference in median PFS (4.1 vs. 4.0 months, P = .98) or overall survival (7.5 vs. 7.8 months, P = .17) (Table 11.3) (46). The disappointing survival outcomes in phase III trials with amrubicin in both the first-line and relapsed settings have dimmed enthusiasm for this agent.

Combination Chemotherapy

Recently, a phase III trial from Japan has challenged the standard of single-agent therapy for relapsed SCLC. In this study, 180 patients with SCLC that had relapsed more than 90 days after initial therapy were randomized to single-agent topotecan 1.0 mg/m^2 IV on days 1 to 5 every 21 days for four cycles or the combination of cisplatin 25 mg/m^2 in days 1 and 8, etoposide 60 mg/m^2 on days 1 to 3, and irinotecan 90 mg/m^2 on day 8 every 2 weeks for five cycles (PEI). (47). The PEI regimen significantly improved response rate (84% vs. 27%; P < .0001), PFS (median, 5.7 vs. 3.6 months; HR 0.50; P < .001), and overall survival (median, 18.2 vs. 12.5 months; HR 0.67; P = .008). However, 50% of patients receiving PEI required dose reductions and 31% developed febrile neutropenia despite routine use of G-CSF. Severe diarrhea and hematologic toxicity also occurred more frequently with PEI. While the efficacy of PEI is notable, the toxicity raises concerns as to the tolerability and generalizability of this regimen, and confirmatory trials with modified dosing are needed before adopting PEI as a standard treatment option.

Reinduction Chemotherapy

Reinitiation of the first-line chemotherapy regimen is recommended for patients with an initial response duration of greater than 6 months based on studies demonstrating response rates of 50% to 60% with this approach (48,49).

Recommendations for Subsequent Chemotherapy

Reinduction with the initial chemotherapy regimen is preferred for patients who relapse more than 6 months from first-line therapy. For patients relapsing within 6 months of initial treatment who have good performance status, single-agent chemotherapy is considered the standard-of-care, with topotecan or paclitaxel being the most commonly used agents. Close attention to toxicity is essential, with appropriate use of dose-modifications and treatment holds in order to maintain quality of life. Although the optimal duration of subsequent chemotherapy for SCLC has not been studied, cumulative toxicity is often limiting. Therefore, it is reasonable to continue subsequent chemotherapy until two cycles beyond best response, progression of disease, or development of unacceptable toxicity. Treatment beyond second-line chemotherapy remains an option for patients with a good performance status, but the low response rate associated with such treatment makes enrollment on a clinical trial a more attractive alternative.

MOLECULARLY TARGETED THERAPY

Future advances in the treatment of SCLC will rely on continued research into the biology of the disease and the identification of molecular targets that drive survival, proliferation, and metastasis. Although many rational, targeted therapies have already been evaluated in clinical trials in patients with SCLC, these approaches have demonstrated little clinical activity. Thus far, strategies demonstrating limited promise include antiangiogenic agents, metalloproteinase inhibitors, growth factor pathway inhibitors, retinoids, proapoptotic agents, therapeutic vaccines, and oncolytic tumor viruses (50). Despite these setbacks, an unprecedented number of novel molecular strategies are now being evaluated in preclinical and clinical studies in SCLC.

Identification of Molecular Targets

Several reports have recently been published on the application of advanced, next-generation molecular techniques for the identification of therapeutic targets and predictive biomarkers in SCLC. A consistent finding of these studies is the very high frequency of protein-altering mutations in SCLC, likely due to prolonged exposure to tobacco carcinogens (51–53). Another common finding is that the *TP53* and *RB1* tumor suppressor genes are mutated and inactivated in nearly all SCLCs. Many other candidates for targeted therapeutic strategies have been identified in genomic and proteomic studies in SCLC, including: *MYC*-family gene amplification; histone-modifiers (*CREBBP, MLL, EP300*); the *PI3K-PTEN* pathway; *FGFR1;* the neural cell migration mediator *SLIT2;* DNA repair mediators (*PARP1*); cell cycle checkpoint regulators (*EZH2*); and mediators of "stem-cell" characteristics (Notch, Hedgehog, *SOX2*) (51–54).

The most promising recent approach targets delta-like protein 3 (DLL3), a Notch ligand that is overexpressed in SCLC tumor-initiating cells. Rovalpituzumab tesirine (Rova-T) consists of a humanized monoclonal antibody targeting DLL3 linked to a DNA damaging toxin. A phase I study of Rova-T in patients with relapsed SCLC reported a response rate of 23% in all patients and 44% in those with high DLL3 tumor expression treated at the recommended phase II dose (55).

The technology now exists for rapid and broad characterization of molecular drivers in cancer cells. In SCLC and other cancers with high mutational burdens, the clinical validation of relevant therapeutic targets remains challenging. In such tumors, it is likely that tumor cell heterogeneity and the dysregulation of numerous pathways will limit the activity of any single molecularly targeted intervention and more complex approaches with combinations of agents will be needed to attain adequate tumor control or eradication.

Immunotherapy

Immune checkpoint inhibitors have shown promise in many tumor types, including SCLC. Ipilimumab is a human monoclonal antibody that binds to CTLA-4 and enhances T-cell activation in tumors. A randomized phase II trial enrolled 164 patients with ES-SCLC who received carboplatin and paclitaxel plus either concurrent or phased ipilumumab or placebo (56). Phased ipilumumab given after two cycles of chemotherapy resulted in a higher response rate and better overall survival than placebo (median, 13 vs. 10 months; HR, 0.75; $P = .13$), suggesting that chemotherapy may sensitize SCLC to immunotherapy.

Activated T-cells also express PD-1, another immune checkpoint receptor, and binding of PD-1 to its ligand PD-L1 inactivates T-cells. Many cancer cells produce PD-L1, resulting in localized immunosuppression that protects tumors from immune surveillance. A phase Ib trial of pembrolizumab, an anti-PD1 monoclonal antibody, yielded a response rate of 35% in 20 patients with PD-L1-positive SCLC (57). Another phase I/II study of patients with relapsed SCLC evaluated nivolumab, another anti-PD1 monoclonal antibody, and the combination of nivolumab plus ipilumumab (58). Response rates were 10% in 98 patients treated with single-agent nivolumab, and 21% in 115 patients treated with the combination. Further trials of immune checkpoint inhibitors in SCLC are currently under way.

CONCLUSION

ES-SCLC remains an incurable disease. Cytotoxic chemotherapy does improve survival and quality of life, but nearly all patients relapse within 1 to 2 years with relatively chemoresistant disease. Platinum-based chemotherapy has been the standard first-line therapy for the past 30 years, with cisplatin or carboplatin plus etoposide being favored worldwide. While many other chemotherapeutic strategies have been evaluated to improve outcomes, none have shown a clear benefit over standard platinum-based therapy. The use of PCI and sequential thoracic RT in patients with ES-SCLC is now part of routine care based on supportive data from randomized trials. However, the benefits of these interventions are modest. Given the disseminated nature of SCLC, more effective systemic therapy is clearly needed to have a greater impact on this disease. Advanced molecular analyses are now allowing the definition of many candidate driver mutations in SCLC. Future gains in treatment will depend on the development of strategies to successfully target the genetic and immunologic drivers of tumor growth and survival.

KEY POINTS

- Most patients with SCLC have ES disease with hematogenous metastases at initial presentation.
- The goals of care for patients with ES-SCLC are palliative and include shrinkage of tumor, relief of symptoms, maintenance of quality of life and prolongation of survival.
- The primary initial treatment for ES-SCLC is systemic chemotherapy. Given the palliative goals of care, the most reasonable regimen is carboplatin plus etoposide for a maximum of four to six cycles.
- PCI and consolidative thoracic radiation may improve survival for patients with good response to initial chemotherapy. The potential benefits and risks of these interventions must be thoroughly assessed in each patient before initiating therapy.
- Single-agent chemotherapy (e.g., topotecan or paclitaxel) remains the standard-of-care for patients with recurrent ES-SCLC.
- Palliative RT is effective for alleviating local symptoms and improving quality of life in patients with ES-SCLC.
- Molecularly targeted therapy has thus far failed to impact on overall survival. However, immune checkpoint inhibitors have shown promise in patients with ES-SCLC.
- ES-SCLC is incurable. The response rate to initial chemotherapy is about 60%. Median, 1-year, and 2-year overall survivals are 9 to 10 months, 30% to 40%, and less than 10%, respectively.
- It is essential to provide optimal palliative care and to maintain quality of life throughout the course of disease. If the side effects of treatment impair quality of life, then other options of care need to be explored.

REFERENCES

1. Shepherd FA, Crowley J, Van Houtte P, et al. The IASLC Lung Cancer Staging Project: proposals regarding the clinical staging of small cell lung cancer in the forthcoming (seventh) edition of the tumor, node, metastasis classification for lung cancer. *J Thorac Oncol*. 2007;2:1067-1077.
2. Navada S, Lai P, Schwartz AG, Kalemkerian GP. Temporal trends in small cell lung cancer: analysis of the national Surveillance, Epidemiology, and End-Results database. *J Clin Oncol*. 2006;24(18S):384s.
3. Lowenbraun S, Bartolucci A, Smalley RV, et al. The superiority of combination chemotherapy over single agent chemotherapy in small cell lung carcinoma. *Cancer*. 1979;44:406-413.
4. Evans WK, Shepherd FA, Feld R, et al. VP-16 and cisplatin as first-line therapy for small-cell lung cancer. *J Clin Oncol*. 1985;3:1471-1477.
5. Roth BJ, Johnson DH, Einhorn LH, et al. Randomized study of cyclophosphamide, doxorubicin, and vincristine versus etoposide and cisplatin versus alternation of these two regimens in extensive small-cell lung cancer: a phase III trial of the Southeastern Cancer Study Group. *J Clin Oncol*. 1992;10:282-291.
6. Sundstrøm S, Bremnes RM, Kaasa S, et al. Cisplatin and etoposide regimen is superior to cyclophosphamide, epirubicin, and vincristine regimen in small-cell lung cancer: results from a randomized phase III trial with 5 years' follow-up. *J Clin Oncol*. 2002;20:4665-4672.
7. Pujol JL, Carestia L, Duares JP. Is there a case for cisplatin in the treatment of small-cell lung cancer? A meta-analysis of randomized trials of a cisplatin-containing regimen versus a regimen without this alkylating agent. *Br J Cancer*. 2000;83:8-15.
8. Sklaros DV, Samantas E, Kosmidis P, et al. Randomized comparison of etoposide–cisplatin vs. etoposide–carboplatin and irradiation in small-cell lung cancer. *Ann Oncol*. 1994;5:601-607.
9. Rossi A, DiMaio M, Chiodini P, et al., Carboplatin- or cisplatin-based chemotherapy in first-line treatment of small-cell lung cancer: the COCIS meta-analysis of individual patient data. *J Clin Oncol*. 2012;30:1692-1698.
10. Noda K, Nishiwaki Y, Kawahara M, et al. Irinotecan plus cisplatin compared with etoposide plus cisplatin for extensive small-cell lung cancer. *N Engl J Med*. 2002;346:85-91.
11. Hanna N, Bunn PA, Langer C, et al. Randomized phase III trial comparing irinotecan/cisplatin with etoposide/cisplatin in patients with previously untreated extensive-stage small-cell lung cancer. *J Clin Oncol*. 2006;24:2038-2043.
12. Lara PN, Natale R, Crowley J, et al. Phase III trial of irinotecan/cisplatin compared with etoposide/cisplatin in extensive-stage small-cell lung cancer: clinical and pharmacogenomic results from SWOG S0124. *J Clin Oncol*. 2009;27:2530-2535.
13. Zatloukal P, Cardenal F, Szczesna A, et al. A multicenter international randomized phase III study comparing cisplatin in combination with irinotecan or etoposide in previously untreated small-cell

lung cancer patients with extensive disease. *Ann Oncol.* 2010;21: 1810-1816.

14. Hermes A, Bergman B, Bremmes R, et al. Irinotecan plus carboplatin versus oral etoposide plus carboplatin in extensive small-cell lung cancer: a randomized phase III trial. *J Clin Oncol.* 2008;26:4261-4267.
15. Eckardt JR, von Pawel J, Papai Z, et al. Open-label, multicenter, randomized, phase III study comparing oral topotecan/cisplatin versus etoposide/cisplatin as treatment for chemotherapy-naive patients with extensive-disease small-cell lung cancer. *J Clin Oncol.* 2006;24:2044-2051.
16. Fink TH, Huber RM, Heigener DF, et al. Topotecan/cisplatin compared with cisplatin/etoposide as first-line treatment for patients with extensive disease small-cell lung cancer. *J Thorac Oncol.* 2012;7:1432-1439.
17. Lima JP, dos Santos LV, Sasse EC, et al. Camptothecins compared with etoposide in combination with platinum analog in extensive stage small cell lung cancer: systematic review with meta-analysis. *J Thorac Oncol.* 2010;5:1986-1993.
18. Thomas P, Castelnau O, Paillotin, et al. Phase II trial of paclitaxel and carboplatin in metastatic small-cell lung cancer: a Groupe Francais de Pneumo-Cancerologie study. *J Clin Oncol.* 2001;19:1320-1325.
19. Lyss AP, Herndon JE, Lynch TJ, et al. Novel doublets in extensive-stage small-cell lung cancer: a randomized phase II study of topotecan plus cisplatin or paclitaxel. *Clin Lung Cancer.* 2002;3:205-210.
20. Satouchi M, Kotani Y, Shibata T, et al. Phase III study comparing amrubicin plus cisplatin with irinotecan plus cisplatin in the treatment of extensive-disease small-cell lung cancer: JCOG 0509. *J Clin Oncol.* 2014;32:1262-1268.
21. Niell HB, Herndon JE, Miller AA, et al. Randomized phase III Intergroup trial of etoposide and cisplatin with or without paclitaxel and granulocyte colony-stimulating factor in patients with extensive-stage small-cell lung cancer: Cancer and Leukemia Group B trial 9732. *J Clin Oncol.* 2005;23:3752-3759.
22. Schiller JH, Adak S, Cella D, et al. Topotecan versus observation after cisplatin plus etoposide in extensive-stage small-cell lung cancer: E7593—a phase III trial of the Eastern Cooperative Oncology Group. *J Clin Oncol.* 2001;19:2114-2122.
23. Auperin A, Arriagada R, Pignon JP, et al. Prophylactic cranial irradiation for patients with small-cell lung cancer in complete remission. Prophylactic Cranial Irradiation Overview Collaborative Group. *N Engl J Med.* 1999;341:476-484.
24. Slotman B, Faivre-Finn C, Kramer G, et al. Prophylactic cranial irradiation in extensive small-cell lung cancer. *N Engl J Med.* 2007;357:664-672.
25. Slotman BJ, Mauer ME, Bottomley A, et al. Prophylactic cranial irradiation in extensive disease small-cell lung cancer: short-term health-related quality of life and patient reported symptoms: results of an international phase III randomized controlled trial by the EORTC Radiation Oncology and Lung Cancer Groups. *J Clin Oncol.* 2009;27:78-84.

26. Seto T, Takahashi T, Yamanaka T, et al. Prophylactic cranial irradiation has a detrimental effect on the overall survival of patients with extensive disease small cell lung cancer: results of a Japanese randomized phase III trial. *J Clin Oncol.* 2014;32(15S):477s.
27. Le Pechoux C, Dunant A, Senan S, et al. Standard-dose versus higher-dose prophylactic cranial irradiation (PCI) in patients with limited-stage small-cell lung cancer in complete remission after chemotherapy and thoracic radiotherapy (PCI 99-01, EORTC 22003-08004, RTOG 0212, and IFCT 99-01): a randomised clinical trial. *Lancet Oncol.* 2009;10:467-474.
28. Wolfson AH, Bae K, Komaki R, et al. Primary analysis of a phase II randomized trial Radiation Therapy Oncology Group (RTOG) 0212: impact of different total doses and schedules of prophylactic cranial irradiation on chronic neurotoxicity and quality of life for patients with limited-disease small-cell lung cancer. *Int J Radiat Oncol Biol Phys.* 2011;81:77-84.
29. Jeremic B, Shibamoto Y, Nikolic N, et al. Role of radiation therapy in the combined-modality treatment of patients with extensive disease small-cell lung cancer: a randomized study. *J Clin Oncol.* 1999;17:2092-2099.
30. Slotman BJ, van Tinteren H, Praag JO, et al. Use of thoracic radiotherapy for extensive stage small-cell lung cancer: a phase 3 randomised controlled trial. *Lancet.* 2015;385:36-42.
31. Gore EM, Hu C, Sun A, et al. NRG Oncology/RTOG 0937: Randomized phase II study comparing prophylactic cranial irradiation (PCI) alone to PCI and consolidative extra-cranial irradiation for extensive disease small cell lung cancer. *Int J Radiat Oncol Biol Phys.* 2015;94:5.
32. O'Brien MER, Ciuleanu TE, Tsekov H, et al. Phase III trial comparing supportive care alone with supportive care with oral topotecan in patients with relapsed small-cell lung cancer. *J Clin Oncol.* 2006;24:5441-5447.
33. Von Pawel J, Schiller JH, Shepherd FA, et al. Topotecan versus cyclophosphamide, doxorubicin, and vincristine for the treatment of recurrent small-cell lung cancer. *J Clin Oncol.* 1999;17:658-667.
34. Eckardt JR, von Pawel J, Pujol JL, et al. Phase III study of oral compared with intravenous topotecan as second-line therapy in small-cell lung cancer. *J Clin Oncol.* 2007;25:2086-2092.
35. Huber RM, Reck M, Gosse H, et al. Efficacy of a toxicity-adjusted topotecan therapy in recurrent small cell lung cancer. *Eur Respir J.* 2006;27:1183-1189.
36. Shah C, Ready N, Perry M, et al. A multi-center phase II study of weekly topotecan as second-line therapy for small cell lung cancer. *Lung Cancer.* 2007;57:84-88.
37. Lilenbaum RC, Huber RM, Treat J, et al. Topotecan therapy in patients with relapsed small-cell lung cancer and poor performance status. *Clin Lung Cancer.* 2006;8:130-134.

38. Schneider BJ. Management of recurrent small cell lung cancer. *JNCCN*. 2008;6:323-331.
39. Johnson DH, Greco FA, Strupp J, et al. Prolonged administration of oral etoposide in patients with relapsed or refractory small-cell lung cancer: a phase II trial. *J Clin Oncol*. 1990;8:1613-1617.
40. Smit EF, Fokkema E, Biesma B, et al. A phase II study of paclitaxel in heavily pretreated patients with small-cell lung cancer. *Br J Cancer*. 1998;77:347-351.
41. Pietanza MC, Kadota K, Huberman K, et al. Phase II trial of temozolomide in patients with relapsed sensitive or refractory small cell lung cancer, with assessment of methylguanine-DNA methyltransferase as a potential biomarker. *Clin Cancer Res*. 2012;18:1138-1145.
42. Zauderer MG, Drilon A, Kadota K, et al. Trial of a 5-day dosing regimen of temozolomide in patients with relapsed small cell lung cancers with assessment of methylguanine-DNA methyltransferase. *Lung Cancer*. 2014;86:237-240.
43. Schmittel A, Knodler M, Hortig P, et al. Phase II trial of second-line bendamustine chemotherapy in relapsed small cell lung cancer patients. *Lung Cancer*. 2007;55:109-113.
44. Lammers PE, Shyr Y, Li CI, et al. Phase II study of bendamustine in relapsed chemotherapy sensitive or resistant small-cell lung cancer. *J Thorac Oncol*. 2014;9:559-562.
45. Jotte R, Conkling P, Reynolds C, et al. Randomized phase II trial of single-agent amrubicin or topotecan as second-line treatment in patients with small-cell lung cancer sensitive to first-line platinum-based chemotherapy. *J Clin Oncol*. 2011;29:287-293.
46. von Pawel J, Jotte R, Spigel DR, et al. Randomized phase III trial of amrubicin versus topotecan as second-line treatment for patients with small-cell lung cancer. *J Clin Oncol*. 2014;32:4012-4019.
47. Goto K, Ohe Y, Shibata T, et al. A randomized phase III study of cisplatin, etoposide and irinotecan versus topotecan as second-line chemotherapy in patients with sensitive relapsed small-cell lung cancer: Japan Clinical Oncology Group study JCOG0605. *J Clin Ocnol*. 2014;32(15S):478s.
48. Postmus PE, Berendsen HH, van Zandwijk N, et al. Retreatment with the induction regimen in small cell lung cancer relapsing after an initial response to short term chemotherapy. *Eur J Cancer Clin Oncol*. 1987;23:1409-1411.
49. Giaccone G, Ferrati P, Donadio M, et al. Reinduction chemotherapy in small cell lung cancer. *Eur J Cancer Clin Oncol*. 1987;23:1697-1699.
50. Schneider BJ, Kalemkerian GP. Personalized therapy of small cell lung cancer. In: Ahmad A, Gadgeel SM, eds. *Lung Cancer and Personalized Medicine: Novel Therapies and Clinical Management*. New York, NY: Springer; 2016:149-174.
51. Peifer M, Fernandez-Cuesta L, Sos ML, et al. Integrative genome analyses identify key somatic driver mutations of small-cell lung cancer. *Nat Genet*. 2012;44:1104-1110.

52. Rudin CM, Durnick S, Stawiski EW, et al. Comprehensive genomic analysis identifies SOX2 as a frequently amplified gene in small-cell lung cancer. *Nat Genet.* 2012;44:1111-1116.
53. George J, Lim JS, Jang SJ, et al. Comprehensive genomic profiles of small cell lung cancer. *Nature*. 2015;524:47-53.
54. Byers LA, Wang J, Nilsson MB, et al. Proteomic profiling identifies dysregulated pathways in small cell lung cancer and novel therapeutic targets including PARP1. *Cancer Discov*. 2012;2:798-811.
55. Pietanza MC, Spigel D, Bauer TM, et al. Safety, activity and response durability assessment of single-agent rovalpituzumab tesirine, a delta-like protein 3 (DLL3)-targeted antibody drug conjugate, in small cell lung cancer. *European Cancer Congress*. Vienna, Austria, September 25–29, 2015.
56. Reck M, Bondarenko I, Luft A, et al. Ipilimumab in combination with paclitaxel and carboplatin as first-line therapy in extensive-disease-small-cell lung cancer: results from a randomized, double-blind, multicenter phase 2 trial. *Ann Oncol*. 2013;24:75-83.
57. Ott PA, Fernandez MEE, Hiret S, et al. Pembrolizumab (MK-3475) in patients with extensive-stage small cell lung cancer: preliminary safety and efficacy results from KEYNOTE-028. *J Clin Oncol*. 2015;33(15S):400s.
58. Antonia SJ, Lopez-Martin JA, Bendell J, et al. Nivolumab alone and nivolumab plus ipilimumab in recurrent small-cell lung cancer (CheckMate 032): a multicentre, open-label, phase 1/2 trial. *Lancet Oncol*. 2016;17:883-895.

12 Management of Elderly and High-Risk Patients With Lung Cancer

Vinicius Ernani and Taofeek K. Owonikoko

INTRODUCTION

Lung cancer is the leading cause of cancer-associated mortality worldwide, causing an estimated 1.4 million deaths per year. In the United States, lung cancer occurs in a predominantly elderly population with a median age at diagnosis of 70 years (1). Indeed, two-thirds of newly diagnosed lung cancer patients are more than 65 years old and approximately 10% to 15% are 80 years old or older at diagnosis (2). An analysis of the Surveillance, Epidemiology, and End Results (SEER) database revealed that non–small-cell lung cancer (NSCLC) accounts for 84% of lung cancer cases in patients less than 70 years old, 85% among those aged 70 to 79 years, and 90% of those aged 80 years or older (2). The prevalence of the different histologic subtypes of lung cancer also varies with age. Squamous cell carcinoma accounts for approximately 20% of all cases in each of the three elderly age groups, while adenocarcinoma accounts for 33% of cases in the less than 70-year group, 27% in those 70 to 79 years, and 23% in those greater than 80 years old.

Although lung cancer is a disease of the elderly, there is no established consensus on the management of elderly patients due to the limited representation of this group in pivotal studies that established standard management algorithms. Indeed, only 25% of older patients receive cytotoxic chemotherapy for advanced disease (3). Moreover, due to age-related declines in physical capability and organ function (Figure 12.1), treatment approaches that are deemed safe in fit younger patients may require particular care and adjustment when applied to fit elderly patients and younger patients with significant comorbid conditions.

There are also no established consensus definitions for elderly or high-risk patients, but elderly is generally defined as ≥70 years of age, while significant impairment in neurologic, cardiopulmonary, hepatic, and renal function could place a patient at high risk for specific surgical, radiotherapeutic, or systemic interventions used to treat lung cancer. Significant heterogeneity exists within elderly and high-risk populations due to differences in the impact

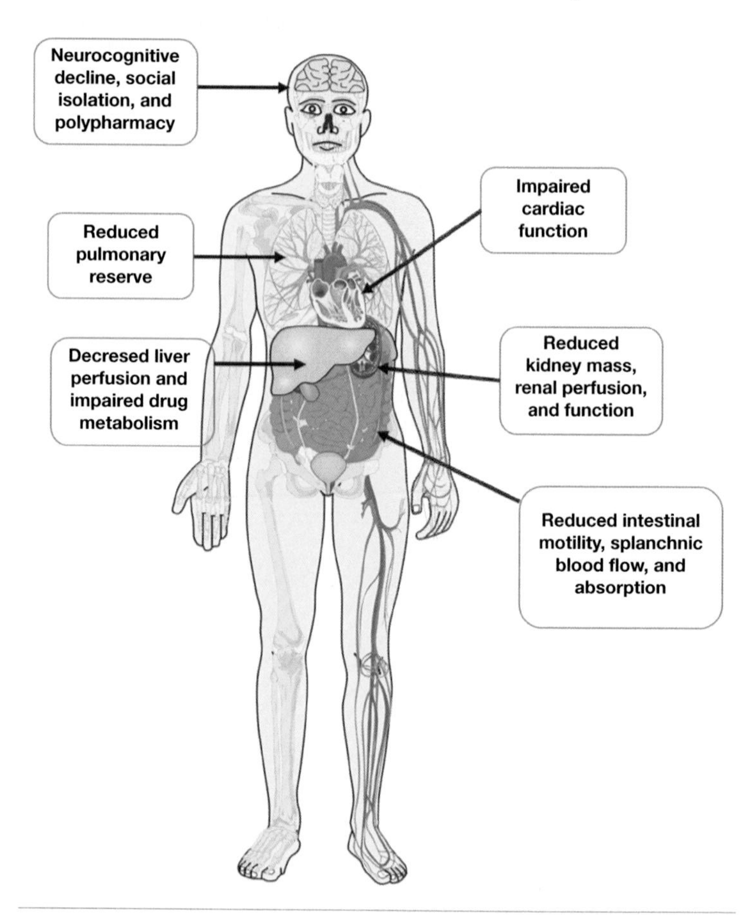

Figure 12.1 Age-Dependent Decline in Critical Organ Function Impacting Optimal Management of NSCLC in Elderly and High-Risk Patients

of specific organ dysfunction and comorbid illnesses. These differences may or may not correlate directly with functional status and capacity to tolerate the increasing array of therapies employed in the management of various stages of lung cancer. For the purpose of this review, elderly patients and "unfit" younger patients are considered the high-risk patient group requiring special attention when selecting optimal therapy.

GENERAL CONSIDERATIONS IN ELDERLY LUNG CANCER PATIENTS

The normal aging process involves a progressive deterioration in physiologic function, especially renal and hematopoietic function. In addition, older patients often have multiple comorbidities, including cardiac and pulmonary conditions, which put them at risk for surgical intervention. The elderly also have a greater likelihood of polypharmacy, which can interfere with efficient metabolism of anticancer agents (4,5). While chronological age is not the best parameter for determining fitness, existing validated tools may not be practical for routine patient care. However, a few of these tools, such as the Charlson comorbidity index and the more detailed Cumulative Illness Rating Scale-Geriatric, have been employed as research measures (6,7).

Performance status is a major prognostic factor in lung cancer patients and is generally employed to guide the selection of the most appropriate treatment. Performance status needs to be evaluated independently from comorbidities, because there is little correlation between comorbidity and functional status in elderly patients (8). The Comprehensive Geriatric Assessment (CGA; Table 12.1) encompasses multiple domains such as functional, emotional, and nutritional status, comorbid illnesses, polypharmacy, cognitive capacity, and the patient's social and environmental situations, and is more reliable than age alone in classifying patients as "fit," vulnerable, or frail and in aiding selection of patients for specific therapeutic interventions (9–11). In a prospective phase III trial, CGA outperformed the traditional tools of performance status and chronological age in assigning appropriate systemic therapy (12).

Table 12.1 Comprehensive Geriatric Assessment (CGA)

Parameters	Assessment methods
Functional status	Performance status, activities of daily living, instrumental activities of daily living, timed up-and-go
Comorbidities	Charlson comorbidity index, cumulative illness rating
Socioeconomic status	Income, transportation, living conditions, assistance
Cognitive status	Folstein mini-mental status score
Nutrition status	Body mass index, nutritional mini-questionnaire
Emotional status	Depression geriatric scale
Medications	Number, usefulness, interactions
Geriatric syndromes	Dementia, repeated falls, bone fractures, neglect, abuse

EARLY STAGE NSCLC

Surgical Considerations in Elderly and High-Risk Patients

Surgery is the primary treatment for patients with early stage lung cancer and should not be withheld from elderly patients based solely on their chronological age. Performance status and comorbid illnesses should be considered when deciding for or against surgery (13). Since elderly and high-risk patients are more likely to suffer from pulmonary complications following lung resection, preoperative cardiopulmonary evaluation is recommended for every patient undergoing surgery. In a study of patients of all ages, the Lung Cancer Study Group prospectively compared sublobar resection with lobectomy and demonstrated that limited resections were associated with higher rates of death and local recurrence. Thus, lobectomy is superior to sublobar resection in patients with early stage NSCLC (14). However, some retrospective studies support more limited operations, such as wedge resection or segmentectomy, in elderly patients with lung cancer (15,16). For standard-risk patients with operable disease, sublobar resections should be reserved for pure ground-glass lesions smaller than 2 cm located in the periphery of the lung. In patients at higher risk for surgical complications, sublobar resections can be performed more liberally.

Video-assisted thoracoscopic surgery (VATS) is a minimally invasive technique that enables an optimal oncologic resection with comparable cancer-specific outcomes to open surgical approaches. VATS is also associated with shortened hospital stay and lower rate of postoperative pulmonary complications (17). However, minimally invasive surgery does not obviate the need for proper selection of patients, especially those with impaired cardiac function or limited cardiopulmonary reserve, since frail patients are more likely than fit patients to have postoperative complications following minimally invasive surgery (18,19).

Radiation for Medically Inoperable Patients With Early Stage NSCLC

Stereotactic ablative radiotherapy (SABR) is now an established alternative to surgery in medically inoperable patients, including elderly and high-risk patients with significant comorbid illnesses that render surgery unsafe. Whether SABR is a legitimate alternative to surgery in fit elderly patients who may safely undergo surgery has not been clearly established because prospective studies that attempted to compare SABR to definitive surgery in operable patients have been unable to meet accrual targets. Nonetheless, pooled data from 58 patients with clinical stage I, operable NSCLC enrolled on two randomized, phase III trials stereotactic ablative radiotherapy (SABR) in stage I non–small-cell lung cancer patients who can undergo lobectomy (STARS) and trial of either surgery or stereotactic radiotherapy for early stage (IA) lung cancer (ROSEL) that were discontinued for poor accrual showed a 3-year overall survival rate of 95% versus 79% (HR 0.14, 95% confidence interval [CI] 0.02–1.19; $P = .037$) and a 3-year recurrence-free survival of 86% versus 80% (HR 0.69, 95% CI 0.21–2.29; $P = .54$) for SABR versus surgery, respectively. This limited dataset suggests that SABR could be considered in appropriately informed elderly patients with operable stage I NSCLC (20).

Adjuvant Chemotherapy in NSCLC

The Lung Adjuvant Cisplatin Evaluation (LACE) meta-analysis established that adjuvant cisplatin-based chemotherapy is associated with a 5.3% absolute increase in 5-year overall survival after complete surgical resection of NSCLC compared to no further treatment (21). Unfortunately, there are no elderly specific randomized trials in the adjuvant setting. Data supporting the use of adjuvant chemotherapy in the elderly come from two studies. The first was a pooled analysis that considered individual data from 4,584 patients enrolled in the five randomized trials registered in the LACE database. Outcome and toxicity data were compared between three age groups: less than 65 years old, 65 to 69 years old, and ≥70 years old. Elderly patients ≥70 years old received significantly fewer total doses of cisplatin and fewer cycles of chemotherapy. However, the survival benefit from cisplatin-based adjuvant chemotherapy was similar in patients in the three age groups, and there was no significant difference in treatment-related toxicity (22). Similarly, a retrospective analysis of the impact of age on survival, treatment delivery, and toxicity in 155 elderly patients (>65 years) enrolled on the JBR.10 study showed that adjuvant chemotherapy conferred a survival benefit in elderly patients that was comparable to that reported for the overall study population (23). Cisplatin-based regimens were used in the pivotal studies of adjuvant chemotherapy. However, carboplatin has a better safety profile, especially in the elderly. While there is no comparative data in this setting to establish the equivalence of carboplatin and cisplatin, extrapolation from a meta-analysis in patients with advanced-stage disease that showed no difference in efficacy between carboplatin and cisplatin (24) supports the use of carboplatin in elderly and high-risk patients with specific contraindication to cisplatin.

Postoperative Radiation Therapy in NSCLC

Patients who have undergone complete surgical resection for NSCLC and have a high risk of recurrence, especially those with mediastinal lymph node involvement, may benefit from postoperative radiation therapy (PORT) (25,26). While there is no robust prospective data regarding the impact of PORT in elderly patients, a retrospective analysis suggests a lack of benefit for PORT in the elderly (27).

LOCALLY ADVANCED NSCLC

Concurrent chemoradiotherapy (CCRT) is the standard of care for most patients with unresectable stage III NSCLC, but the majority of elderly patients with stage III disease do not receive combined modality therapy. At least three randomized phase III trials demonstrated improved survival with CCRT compared to a sequential approach in the general lung cancer population at the cost of higher toxicity (28–30). Post hoc analyses indicate that both elderly and younger patients achieve a comparable survival benefit from CCRT, but significant increases in both hematologic and nonhematologic toxicities in the elderly could potentially outweigh the benefits if patients are not carefully selected (31–33). In a phase III trial in Japanese patients, ≥70 years old with locally advanced NSCLC, CCRT using low-dose, single-agent carboplatin was superior to radiation alone (median overall survival, 22.4 vs. 16.9 months), at the expense of higher toxicity (34).

METASTATIC NSCLC

Cytotoxic Chemotherapy

Concerns regarding the risk of intolerable toxicity limited the use of cytotoxic chemotherapy in elderly patients until the European, phase III Elderly Lung Cancer Vinorelbine Italian Study Group (ELVIS) study compared single-agent vinorelbine versus best supportive care in patients ≥70 years of age and demonstrated that vinorelbine was both safe and beneficial (median overall survival, 28 vs. 21 weeks; $P = .03$) (35). A subsequent phase III trial comparing docetaxel to vinorelbine in 182 elderly Japanese patients ≥70 years old demonstrated a significant benefit with docetaxel in terms of progression-free survival (PFS), response rate, and disease-related symptoms (36). However, the phase III Multicenter Italian Lung Cancer in the Elderly Study (MILES) that compared single-agent vinorelbine or gemcitabine to the combination of vinorelbine plus gemcitabine in 698 patients ≥70 years old showed no survival advantage for the combination regimen (37). These trials established a role for single-agent chemotherapy as a safe and effective option for elderly patients with metastatic NSCLC.

Subsequently, a number of studies have examined the efficacy and tolerability of two-drug regimens in older and high-risk lung cancer patients. Retrospective subset analyses of randomized trials that enrolled fit patients of all ages with advanced NSCLC have generally shown similar outcomes with combination chemotherapy regardless of age (38–41). For example, a subset analysis of a study that compared cisplatin or carboplatin plus docetaxel to cisplatin plus vinorelbine showed no survival difference with age (39). Similarly, a retrospective analysis of a phase III study of gemcitabine plus carboplatin or paclitaxel versus carboplatin plus paclitaxel demonstrated no survival difference by age (40). Finally, a phase III trial that randomized 561 patients to paclitaxel alone versus carboplatin plus paclitaxel reported a nonsignificant improvement in survival with combination therapy with similar survival outcomes in elderly (≥70 years old) and younger patients (41). However, a combined analysis of data from two Southwest Oncology Group (SWOG) trials reported shorter overall survival in patients ≥70 years old who were treated with platinum-based, two-drug chemotherapy regimens (median, 7 vs. 9 months; $P = .04$) (42).

Recent prospective, elderly specific trials have also demonstrated a survival benefit with combination chemotherapy over single-agent therapy. (Table 12.2) Quoix et al. randomized 451 patients between 70 and 89 years of age to carboplatin plus paclitaxel × four cycles or single-agent vinorelbine or gemcitabine × five cycles, and reported improved overall survival with combination chemotherapy (10.3 vs. 6.2 months; $P < .0001$) (43). Another prospective study by Lilenbaum et al. in high-risk patients with advanced, untreated NSCLC and an ECOG performance status of two compared single-agent pemetrexed to the combination of carboplatin plus pemetrexed. A large proportion of the enrolled patients were elderly (median age, 65 years; range 40–91 years). All efficacy endpoints favored combination chemotherapy over single-agent therapy, including response rate (10% vs. 24%; $P = .032$), PFS (median, 2.8 vs. 5.8 months; HR 0.46, 95% CI 0.35–0.63; $P < .001$), and overall survival (median, 5.3 vs. 9.3 months; HR 0.62, 95% CI 0.46–0.83; $P = .001$) (44).

A recent comprehensive meta-analysis of 51 elderly focused studies evaluated the benefits of: (a) nonplatinum single-agents versus combination regimens and (b) nonplatinum combination regimens versus platinum-based combination regimens. Based on low-quality evidence from five randomized trials, nonplatinum single-agent therapy and combination regimens yielded similar overall survival (HR 0.92, 95% CI 0.72–1.17) and PFS (HR 0.94, 95% CI 0.83–1.07). In contrast, based on moderate-quality evidence, platinum-based combination therapy resulted in improved overall survival compared to nonplatinum combination regimens (HR 0.76, 95% CI 0.69–0.85), albeit at the cost of increased hematologic and nonhematologic toxicity (45).

Table 12.2 Selected prospective studies of cytotoxic chemotherapy in elderly or high-risk lung cancer patients

Study	*N*	Definition of elderly (years old)	Regimen	Overall survival (mo)	*P* value
Gridelli et al. (35)	191	≥70	Vinorelbine + BSC	7.0	.02
			BSC	5.0	
Kudoh et al. (36)	182	≥70	Vinorelbine	9.9	.138
			Docetaxel	14.3	
Gridelli et al. (37)	698	≥70	Vinorelbine + Gemcitabine vs. Gemcitabine	7.5 vs. 7.0	.69
			Vinorelbine + Gemcitabine vs. Vinorelbine	7.5 vs. 9.0	.93
Gridelli et al. (64)	159	>70	Cisplatin + Gemcitabine	10.9	NR
			Cisplatin + Vinorelbine	8.2	
Abe et al. (65)	221	≥70	Cisplatin + Docetaxel	13.3	NR
			Docetaxel	14.8	
Biesma et al. (66)	181	≥70	Carboplatin + Gemcitabine	8.6	NR
			Carboplatin + Paclitaxel	6.9	
Quoix et al. (43)	451	≥70	Gemcitabine or Vinorelbine	6.2	NR
			Carboplatin + Paclitaxel	10.3	
Zukin et al. (44)	205	NA	Pemetrexed	5.3	<.001
			Carboplatin + Pemetrexed	9.3	

BSC, best supportive care; NR, not reported.

Antiangiogenic Agents

The addition of bevacizumab, a monoclonal antibody targeting vascular endothelial growth factor (VEGF), to cytotoxic chemotherapy is a standard option for first-line treatment of advanced, non-squamous NSCLC. The benefit of bevacizumab was reported in ECOG 4599, which randomized 878 patients of all ages with advanced NSCLC to carboplatin plus paclitaxel alone versus carboplatin, paclitaxel plus bevacizumab followed by maintenance bevacizumab. Patients treated with chemotherapy plus bevacizumab demonstrated improved overall survival (median, 12.3 vs. 10.3 months; HR 0.79; *P* = .003) (46). Subsequently, the PointBreak trial failed to demonstrate the superiority of carboplatin, pemetrexed plus bevacizumab followed by maintenance pemetrexed plus bevacizumab over carboplatin, paclitaxel plus bevacizumab followed by maintenance bevacizumab. A combined retrospective analysis of outcome by age using individual data from patients treated with carboplatin, paclitaxel, plus bevacizumab on the E4599 and PointBreak studies showed a significant benefit with the addition of bevacizumab when compared to patients treated with carboplatin plus paclitaxel alone in E4599, but only in patients younger than 75 years of age. Elderly patients not only did not seem to benefit from bevacizumab, but also had increased toxicity when treated with it (47).

Epidermal Growth Factor Receptor-Tyrosine Kinase Inhibitors

EGFR gene mutations are more commonly observed in younger patients and never-smokers. However, these alterations are also found in elderly patients and smokers, albeit at a lower frequency. Thus, molecular testing for *EGFR* mutations and other targetable genetic alterations should not be restricted based on patient age or other clinical or demographic factors (48). Epidermal growth factor receptor-tyrosine kinase inhibitors (EGFR-TKIs) (erlotinib, gefitinib, and afatinib) are now established as the preferred front-line treatment for metastatic NSCLC harboring sensitizing *EGFR* mutations. There are no prospective data to suggest which EGFR-TKI might be preferred for the treatment of elderly patients. However, elderly specific studies and subgroup analyses of randomized trials comparing EGFR-TKIs to platinum-based chemotherapy have demonstrated the safety and efficacy of these agents in elderly patients (Table 12.3) (49,50). Moreover, these studies have reported no significant differences in clinical outcome between elderly and younger patients (51–53). Therefore, elderly patients with *EGFR*-mutated NSCLC should be treated with the same algorithms as used for younger patients.

Anaplastic Lymphoma Kinase Inhibitors

Anaplastic lymphoma kinase (*ALK*) rearrangement is the second most common targetable alteration, after *EGFR* mutations, in NSCLC. *ALK* rearrangement is frequently observed in younger, never-smokers, but its presence is not dependent solely on these clinical characteristics (48). Given the relatively small number of

Table 12.3 Elderly specific studies and subgroup analyses of trials evaluating EGFR-TKIs

Study	*N*	Definition of elderly (years old)	Median progression-free survival (mo, unless noted)	Median overall survival (mo, unless noted)
Yoshioka et al. (67)	9,907	>75	<75 y = 65 days 75–85 y = 74 days ≥85 y = 72 days	NR
Kurishima et al. (68)	304	>75	<75 y = 46 days ≥75 y = 62 days (*P* = .25)	<75 y =146 days ≥75 y = 170 days (*P* = .76)
Jackman et al. (69)	80	75	3.5	10.9
Wheatley-Price et al. (70)	488	NR	<70 y = 2.1 ≥70 y = 3.0	<70 y = 6.4 ≥70 y = 7.6
Platania et al. (71)	43	73	3.0	8.4
Chen et al. (72)	57	77	4.6	11.7
Morikawa et al. (73)	71	75	14.3	30.8
Takahashi et al. (74)	20	79.5	10.0	26.4
Maemondo et al. (75)	31	80	12.1	33.8
Inoue et al. (76)	22	72	6.5	17.8
Nakao et al. (50)	21	85	5.9	12.1

EGFR-TKIs, Epidermal growth factor receptor-tyrosine kinase inhibitors; NR, not reported.

patients with *ALK*-rearranged NSCLC, elderly specific studies are not feasible. Moreover, formal subset analyses based on age are also impractical since the overwhelming majority of patients are younger. Nonetheless, clinical trials that established the efficacy of crizotinib, ceritinib, and alectinib for the treatment of *ALK*-rearranged NSCLC did enroll some elderly patients and revealed no age-based differences in safety or efficacy (54,55).

Immunotherapy

Agents targeting the PD-1 signaling pathway are now approved for the treatment of squamous and non-squamous NSCLC that progressed after treatment with platinum-based therapy. While there is a progressive natural diminution in immunologic response with age, post hoc subset analyses of the pivotal studies leading to the approval of the PD-1 antagonists nivolumab and pembrolizumab did not suggest any differences in treatment efficacy based on age. A recent meta-analysis of nine randomized, controlled trials of immune checkpoint inhibitors enrolling 5,265 patients evaluated efficacy in both younger and older (≥65–70 years old) patients and found a consistent overall survival benefit favoring immunotherapy in both younger (HR 0.75, 95% CI 0.68–0.82) and older (HR 0.73, 95% CI 0.62–0.87) patient subgroups (56).

SMALL CELL LUNG CANCER

Small cell lung cancer (SCLC) commonly occurs in the elderly, with 43% of patients being diagnosed at 70 years of age or older (2). Patients with SCLC also frequently present with poor performance status due to preexisting comorbidities and the aggressiveness of the disease. However, few randomized trials have specifically focused on the treatment of SCLC in the elderly, and many have combined elderly and poor performance status patients without reporting outcomes separately for the two groups. Therefore, deriving appropriate treatment guidelines for the elderly and other high-risk patients is challenging.

A common theme in clinical trials for elderly patients with SCLC is to compare the efficacy and toxicity of lower intensity regimens to standard regimens (Table 12.4). In one randomized trial that enrolled only elderly patients, Ardizzoni et al. compared standard cisplatin plus etoposide (PE) to a reduced-dose PE regimen in 95 patients ≥70 years old with performance status of 0 to 2. Although reduced-dose PE was less toxic, it also yielded a lower response rate and overall survival (57). Two other randomized trials included both elderly and poor performance status patients. Okamoto et al. compared PE to carboplatin plus etoposide in 220 patients with extensive-stage SCLC. Ninety-two percent of patients were ≥70 years old with a performance status of 0 to 1 and 8% were less than 70 years old with a performance status of 3. There were no significant differences in response rate or survival between the two arms in the overall study population or in the subgroup of elderly patients (58). Souhami et al. compared single-agent etoposide to a regimen

Table 12.4 Randomized trials in elderly patients with small cell lung cancer

Trial/y	Eligibility	Arms	*N* (LS/ES)	Median age (range)	Response rate	Median PFS	Overall Survival Median	1 y
Ardizzoni et al. (57)	≥70 y old and PS 0–2	P 25 mg/m² d1–2 + E 60 mg/m² d1–3 × 4 cycles	28 (16/12)	74(70–80)	39%	NR	31 wk	18%
		P 40 mg/m² d1–2 + E 100 mg/m² d1–3 + G-CSF × 4 cycles	67 (36/31)	73 (70–79)	69%	NR	41 wk	39%
Okamoto et al. (58)	≥70 y old and PS 0–1 (92%); or <70 y old and PS 3 (8%)	C AUC 5 d1 + E 80 mg/m² d1–3 × 4 cycles	110 (0/110)	74 (56–86) [≥70 = 93%]	73%	5.2 mo	10.6 mo [≥70 = 11 mo]	41% [≥70 = 43%]
		P 25 mg/m² d1–3 + E 80 mg/m² d1–3 × 4 cycles	110 (0/110)	74 (55–85) [≥70 = 91%]	73%	4.7 mo (*P* = .20)	9.9 mo [≥70 = 10 mo]	35% [≥70 = 34%] (*P* = .54)
Souhami et al. (59)	≥75 y old and any PS; or <75 y old and PS 2–3	E 100 mg PO BID d1–5 × 6 cycles	75 (7/66)	67 (49–80)	33%	3.6 mo	4.8 mo	10%
		PE alternating with CAV × 6 cycles	80 (4/72)	66 (50–86)	46% (*P* < .01)	5.6 mo (*P* = .001)	5.9 mo	19% (*P* < .05)

AUC, area under curve; BID, twice-a-day; C, carboplatin; CAV, cyclophosphamide + doxorubicin + vincristine; d, day(s); E, etoposide; ES, extensive-stage; G-CSF, granulocyte-colony stimulating factor; LS, limited-stage; mo, months; NR, not reported; P, cisplatin; PE, cisplatin + etoposide; PFS, progression-free survival; PO, oral; S, performance status; wk, weeks; y, year.

that alternated PE with CAV (cyclophosphamide, doxorubicin, vincristine) in 155 patients who were either ≥75 years old with any performance status or less than 75 years old with performance status of 2 to 3. All efficacy endpoints, including response rate, PFS, overall survival, and quality of life, were significantly worse in the single-agent etoposide arm (59). However, this trial did not report outcomes separately for elderly or poor performance status patients.

Several large clinical trials have been retrospectively analyzed to evaluate the effect of age on outcome in SCLC. Yuen et al. reported a retrospective, age-specific analysis of INT-0096 in which 381 patients with limited-stage SCLC and performance status 0 to 2 were randomized to receive standard PE with either once-daily or twice-daily radiation therapy (RT). Only 13% of patients were ≥70 years old. Response rates (88% vs. 80%; $P = .11$) and PFS (5 years, 19% vs. 16%; $P = .18$) were similar in both younger and older patients, but toxicity was greater in the elderly. Overall survival was better in younger patients (median, 22 vs. 14 months; $P = .05$), mainly due to a higher treatment-related death rate in elderly patients (10% vs. 1%). Among elderly patients, twice-daily radiation did result in better overall survival compared to once-daily RT, but this difference did not reach statistical significance (60). Schild et al. performed a retrospective age-specific analysis on NCCTG 89-20-52, a similar trial that randomized 263 patients with limited-stage SCLC and performance status 0 to 2 to standard PE with either once-daily or twice-daily RT. In this study, 21% of patients were ≥70 years old. Overall survival was nonsignificantly lower in elderly patients compared to younger patients (5-year, 17% vs. 22%; $P = .14$). Again, the treatment-related death rate (5.6% vs. 0.5%, $P = .03$) was significantly greater in the elderly (61).

Two recent retrospective analyses also support the use of chemotherapy and RT in appropriate elderly patients, though treatment selection-bias may confound the results of such studies. A retrospective study of the National Lung Cancer Database evaluated 8,637 patients ≥70 years of age with limited-stage SCLC who were treated with either chemotherapy alone or chemoradiotherapy. The use of chemoradiotherapy declined with increasing age, higher TNM stage, and greater comorbidities, and was associated with better overall survival (median, 15.6 vs. 9.3 months; $P < .001$) (62). Similarly, an analysis of 10,428 patients ≥65 years old with SCLC who were enrolled in the SEER-Medicare database reported that the use of chemotherapy and RT were both associated with better survival, even in patients ≥85 years old, with chemotherapy improving overall survival by 6.9 months (63).

In general, elderly patients with limited-stage SCLC and good performance status should be considered for treatment with platinum-based chemotherapy plus thoracic RT with close attention to treatment-related toxicity. Elderly patients with extensive-stage SCLC and good performance status should be considered for treatment with carboplatin-based chemotherapy, while those with poor performance status may still benefit from palliative chemotherapy or RT, particularly if their debility is due to SCLC.

KEY POINTS

- Lobectomy with lymph node dissection is safe in elderly patients with good performance status and good pulmonary function, but lung-sparing, sublobar resections may be considered in high-risk patients.
- SABR is an alternative in medically inoperable elderly and high-risk patients with early stage lung cancer.
- Elderly patients derive a comparable survival benefit from adjuvant chemotherapy as younger patients, and carboplatin-based regimens may be used to improve tolerability.
- CCRT should be offered to elderly patients with unresectable, stage III NSCLC with good performance status. Sequential chemoradiotherapy is an option in elderly patients with borderline performance status and in high-risk patients with stage III NSCLC, but combined-modality therapy is not appropriate for frail or unfit patients regardless of age.
- Selected platinum-based, two-drug chemotherapy regimens are safe and beneficial for elderly patients with advanced NSCLC and good performance status, but single-agent chemotherapy remains a reasonable standard treatment.
- EGFR-TKIs, ALK inhibitors, and ROS1 inhibitors are the standard of care for patients with advanced *EGFR*-mutated, *ALK*-rearranged, and *ROS1*-rearranged NSCLC, respectively, regardless of age.
- Immune checkpoint inhibitors are safe and effective in fit elderly patients with relapsed NSCLC.
- Elderly patients with limited-stage SCLC and performance status 0 to 2 should be considered for treatment with platinum-based chemotherapy plus thoracic RT.
- Elderly patients with extensive-stage SCLC and performance status 0 to 2 should be considered for treatment with carboplatin-based chemotherapy.

REFERENCES

1. Siegel R, Ma J, Zou Z, Jemal A. Cancer statistics, 2014. *CA Cancer J Clin.* 2014;64(1):9-29. Epub 2014/01/09. doi:10.3322/caac.21208. PubMed PMID: 24399786.
2. Owonikoko TK, Ragin CC, Belani CP, et al. Lung cancer in elderly patients: an analysis of the surveillance, epidemiology, and end results database. *J Clin Oncol.* 2007;25(35):5570-5577. Epub 2007/12/11. doi:10.1200/JCO.2007.12.5435. PubMed PMID: 18065729.
3. Davidoff AJ, Tang M, Seal B, Edelman MJ. Chemotherapy and survival benefit in elderly patients with advanced non-small-cell lung cancer. *J Clin Oncol.* 2010;28(13):2191-2197. Epub 2010/03/31. doi:10.1200/JCO.2009.25.4052. PubMed PMID: 20351329.
4. Repetto L, Audisio RA. Elderly patients have become the leading drug consumers: it's high time to properly evaluate new drugs within the real targeted population. *J Clin Oncol.* 2006;24(35):e62-e63. Epub 2006/12/13. doi:10.1200/JCO.2006.09.3039. PubMed PMID: 17158531.
5. Shayne M, Culakova E, Poniewierski MS, et al. Dose intensity and hematologic toxicity in older cancer patients receiving systemic chemotherapy. *Cancer.* 2007;110(7):1611-1620. Epub 2007/08/21. doi:10.1002/cncr.22939. PubMed PMID: 17705197.
6. Charlson ME, Pompei P, Ales KL, MacKenzie CR. A new method of classifying prognostic comorbidity in longitudinal studies: development and validation. *J Chronic Dis.* 1987;40(5):373-383. Epub 1987/01/01. PubMed PMID: 3558716.
7. Harboun M, Ankri J. Comorbidity indexes: review of the literature and application to studies of elderly population. *Rev Epidemiol Sante Publique.* 2001;49(3):287-298. Epub 2001/06/28. PubMed PMID: 11427831.
8. Extermann M, Overcash J, Lyman GH, et al. Comorbidity and functional status are independent in older cancer patients. *J Clin Oncol.* 1998;16(4):1582-1587. Epub 1998/04/29. PubMed PMID: 9552069.
9. Quoix E, Westeel V, Zalcman G, Milleron B. Chemotherapy in elderly patients with advanced non-small cell lung cancer. *Lung Cancer.* 2011;74(3):364-368. Epub 2011/09/07. doi:10.1016/j.lungcan.2011.06.006. PubMed PMID: 21893363.
10. Repetto L, Fratino L, Audisio RA, et al. Comprehensive geriatric assessment adds information to Eastern Cooperative Oncology Group performance status in elderly cancer patients: an Italian Group for Geriatric Oncology Study. *J Clin Oncol.* 2002;20(2):494-502. Epub 2002/01/12. PubMed PMID: 11786579.
11. Presley C, Lilenbaum R. The treatment of advanced lung cancer in the elderly: the role of a comprehensive geriatric assessment and doublet chemotherapy. *Cancer J.* 2015;21(5):392-397. Epub 2015/09/22. doi:10.1097/PPO.0000000000000145. PubMed PMID: 26389764.
12. Corre R, Greillier L, Le Caer H, et al. Use of a comprehensive geriatric assessment for the management of elderly patients with advanced non-small-cell lung cancer: the phase III randomized

ESOGIA-GFPC-GECP 08-02 study. *J Clin Oncol*. 2016;34(13): 1476-1483. doi:10.1200/JCO.2015.63.5839. PubMed PMID: 26884557.

13. Pallis AG, Gridelli C, van Meerbeeck JP, et al. EORTC Elderly Task Force and Lung Cancer Group and International Society for Geriatric Oncology (SIOG) experts' opinion for the treatment of non-small-cell lung cancer in an elderly population. *Ann Oncol*. 2010;21(4): 692-706. Epub 2009/09/01. doi:10.1093/annonc/mdp360. PubMed PMID: 19717538.
14. Ginsberg RJ, Rubinstein LV. Randomized trial of lobectomy versus limited resection for T1 N0 non-small cell lung cancer. Lung Cancer Study Group. *Ann Thorac Surg*. 1995;60(3):615-622; discussion 22-23. Epub 1995/09/01. PubMed PMID: 7677489.
15. Mery CM, Pappas AN, Bueno R, et al. Similar long-term survival of elderly patients with non-small cell lung cancer treated with lobectomy or wedge resection within the surveillance, epidemiology, and end results database. *Chest*. 2005;128(1):237-245. Epub 2005/07/09. doi:10.1378/chest.128.1.237. PubMed PMID: 16002941.
16. Okami J, Ito Y, Higashiyama M, et al. Sublobar resection provides an equivalent survival after lobectomy in elderly patients with early lung cancer. *Ann Thorac Surg*. 2010;90(5):1651-1656. Epub 2010/10/26. doi:10.1016/j.athoracsur.2010.06.090. PubMed PMID: 20971281.
17. Schuchert MJ, Pettiford BL, Pennathur A, et al. Anatomic segmentectomy for stage I non-small-cell lung cancer: comparison of video-assisted thoracic surgery versus open approach. *J Thorac Cardiovasc Surg*. 2009;138(6):1318-1325 e1. Epub 2009/11/26. doi: 10.1016/j.jtcvs.2009.08.028. PubMed PMID: 19931665.
18. Revenig LM, Canter DJ, Master VA, et al. A prospective study examining the association between preoperative frailty and postoperative complications in patients undergoing minimally invasive surgery. *J Endourol*. 2014;28(4):476-480. doi:10.1089/end.2013.0496. PubMed PMID: 24308497.
19. Sepehri A, Beggs T, Hassan A, et al. The impact of frailty on outcomes after cardiac surgery: a systematic review. *J Thorac Cardiovasc Surg*. 2014;148(6):3110-3117. doi:10.1016/j.jtcvs.2014.07.087. PubMed PMID: 25199821.
20. Chang JY, Senan S, Paul MA, et al. Stereotactic ablative radiotherapy versus lobectomy for operable stage I non-small-cell lung cancer: a pooled analysis of two randomised trials. *Lancet Oncol*. 2015;16(6): 630-637. doi:10.1016/S1470-2045(15)70168-3. PubMed PMID: 25981812; PubMed Central PMCID: PMC4489408.
21. Pignon JP, Tribodet H, Scagliotti GV, et al. Lung adjuvant cisplatin evaluation: a pooled analysis by the LACE Collaborative Group. *J Clin Oncol*. 2008;26(21):3552-3559. Epub 2008/05/29. doi:10.1200/JCO.2007.13.9030. PubMed PMID: 18506026.
22. Fruh M, Rolland E, Pignon JP, et al. Pooled analysis of the effect of age on adjuvant cisplatin-based chemotherapy for completely resected non-small-cell lung cancer. *J Clin Oncol*. 2008;26(21):3573-3581. Epub 2008/07/22. doi:10.1200/JCO.2008.16.2727. PubMed PMID: 18640938.

23. Pepe C, Hasan B, Winton TL, et al. Adjuvant vinorelbine and cisplatin in elderly patients: National Cancer Institute of Canada and Intergroup Study JBR.10. *J Clin Oncol*. 2007;25(12):1553-1561. Epub 2007/04/20. doi:10.1200/JCO.2006.09.5570. PubMed PMID: 17442999.

24. de Castria TB, da Silva EM, Gois AF, Riera R. Cisplatin versus carboplatin in combination with third-generation drugs for advanced non-small cell lung cancer. *Cochrane Database Syst Rev*. 2013;8:CD009256. doi:10.1002/14651858.CD009256.pub2. PubMed PMID: 23949842.

25. Douillard JY, Rosell R, De Lena M, et al. Impact of postoperative radiation therapy on survival in patients with complete resection and stage I, II, or IIIA non-small-cell lung cancer treated with adjuvant chemotherapy: the adjuvant Navelbine International Trialist Association (ANITA) randomized trial. *Int J Radiat Oncol Biol Phys*. 2008;72(3):695-701. doi:10.1016/j.ijrobp.2008.01.044. PubMed PMID: 18439766.

26. Mikell JL, Gillespie TW, Hall WA, et al. Postoperative radiotherapy is associated with better survival in non-small cell lung cancer with involved N2 lymph nodes: results of an analysis of the National Cancer Data Base. *J Thorac Oncol*. 2015;10(3):462-471. doi: 10.1097/JTO.0000000000000411. PubMed PMID: 25384064; PubMed Central PMCID: PMC4336617.

27. Wisnivesky JP, Halm EA, Bonomi M, et al. Postoperative radiotherapy for elderly patients with stage III lung cancer. *Cancer*. 2012; 118(18):4478-4485. doi:10.1002/cncr.26585. PubMed PMID: 22331818; PubMed Central PMCID: PMC3355220.

28. Furuse K, Fukuoka M, Kawahara M, et al. Phase III study of concurrent versus sequential thoracic radiotherapy in combination with mitomycin, vindesine, and cisplatin in unresectable stage III non-small-cell lung cancer. *J Clin Oncol*. 1999;17(9):2692-2699. Epub 1999/11/24. PubMed PMID: 10561343.

29. Curran WJ Jr., Paulus R, Langer CJ, et al. Sequential vs. concurrent chemoradiation for stage III non-small cell lung cancer: randomized phase III trial RTOG 9410. Journal of the National Cancer Institute. 2011;103(19):1452-1460. Epub 2011/09/10. doi:10.1093/jnci/djr325. PubMed PMID: 21903745; PubMed Central PMCID: 3186782.

30. Zatloukal P, Petruzelka L, Zemanova M, et al. Concurrent versus sequential chemoradiotherapy with cisplatin and vinorelbine in locally advanced non-small cell lung cancer: a randomized study. *Lung Cancer*. 2004;46(1):87-98. Epub 2004/09/15. doi:10.1016/j.lungcan.2004.03.004. PubMed PMID: 15364136.

31. Schild SE, Stella PJ, Geyer SM, et al. The outcome of combined-modality therapy for stage III non-small-cell lung cancer in the elderly. *J Clin Oncol*. 2003;21(17):3201-3206. Epub 2003/07/23. doi:10.1200/JCO.2003.12.019. PubMed PMID: 12874270.

32. Rocha Lima CM, Herndon JE 2nd, Kosty M, et al. Therapy choices among older patients with lung carcinoma: an evaluation of two trials of the Cancer and Leukemia Group B. *Cancer*. 2002;94(1):181-187. Epub 2002/01/30. PubMed PMID: 11815975.

33. Pfister DG, Johnson DH, Azzoli CG, et al. American Society of Clinical Oncology treatment of unresectable non-small-cell lung cancer guideline: update 2003. *J Clin Oncol*. 2004;22(2):330-353. Epub 2003/12/24. doi:10.1200/JCO.2004.09.053. PubMed PMID: 14691125.
34. Atagi S, Kawahara M, Yokoyama A, et al. Thoracic radiotherapy with or without daily low-dose carboplatin in elderly patients with non-small-cell lung cancer: a randomised, controlled, phase 3 trial by the Japan Clinical Oncology Group (JCOG0301). *Lancet Oncol*. 2012;13(7):671-678. Epub 2012/05/25. doi:10.1016/S1470-2045(12)70139-0. PubMed PMID: 22622008.
35. The Elderly Lung Cancer Vinorelbine Italian Study Group. Effects of vinorelbine on quality of life and survival of elderly patients with advanced non-small-cell lung cancer. *J Natl Cancer Inst*. 1999;91(1):66-72. Epub 1999/01/16. PubMed PMID: 9890172.
36. Kudoh S, Takeda K, Nakagawa K, et al. Phase III study of docetaxel compared with vinorelbine in elderly patients with advanced non-small-cell lung cancer: results of the West Japan Thoracic Oncology Group Trial (WJTOG 9904). *J Clin Oncol*. 2006;24(22):3657-3663. Epub 2006/08/01. doi:10.1200/JCO.2006.06.1044. PubMed PMID: 16877734.
37. Gridelli C, Perrone F, Gallo C, et al. Chemotherapy for elderly patients with advanced non-small-cell lung cancer: the Multicenter Italian Lung Cancer in the Elderly Study (MILES) phase III randomized trial. *J Natl Cancer Inst*. 2003;95(5):362-372. Epub 2003/03/06. PubMed PMID: 12618501.
38. Langer CJ, Manola J, Bernardo P, et al. Cisplatin-based therapy for elderly patients with advanced non-small-cell lung cancer: implications of Eastern Cooperative Oncology Group 5592, a randomized trial. *J Natl Cancer Inst*. 2002;94(3):173-181. Epub 2002/02/07. PubMed PMID: 11830607.
39. Belani CP, Fossella F. Elderly subgroup analysis of a randomized phase III study of docetaxel plus platinum combinations versus vinorelbine plus cisplatin for first-line treatment of advanced nonsmall cell lung carcinoma (TAX 326). *Cancer*. 2005;104(12):2766-2774. Epub 2005/11/17. doi:10.1002/cncr.21495. PubMed PMID: 16288485.
40. Ansari RH, Socinski MA, Edelman MJ, et al. A retrospective analysis of outcomes by age in a three-arm phase III trial of gemcitabine in combination with carboplatin or paclitaxel vs. paclitaxel plus carboplatin for advanced non-small cell lung cancer. *Crit Rev Oncol Hematol*. 2011;78(2):162-171. Epub 2010/04/24. doi:10.1016/j.critrevonc.2010.03.003. PubMed PMID: 20413322.
41. Lilenbaum RC, Herndon JE 2nd, List MA, et al. Single-agent versus combination chemotherapy in advanced non-small-cell lung cancer: the cancer and leukemia group B (study 9730). *J Clin Oncol*. 2005;23(1):190-196. Epub 2004/12/31. doi:10.1200/JCO.2005.07.172. PubMed PMID: 15625373.
42. Blanchard EM, Moon J, Hesketh PJ, et al. Comparison of platinum-based chemotherapy in patients older and younger than 70 years: an analysis of Southwest Oncology Group Trials 9308 and 9509.

J Thorac Oncol. 2011;6(1):115-120. Epub 2010/11/26. doi:10.1097/JTO.0b013e3181fbebfd. PubMed PMID: 21107287; PubMed Central PMCID: 3075557.

43. Quoix E, Zalcman G, Oster JP, et al. Carboplatin and weekly paclitaxel doublet chemotherapy compared with monotherapy in elderly patients with advanced non-small-cell lung cancer: IFCT-0501 randomised, phase 3 trial. *Lancet*. 2011;378(9796):1079-1088. Epub 2011/08/13. doi:10.1016/S0140-6736(11)60780-0. PubMed PMID: 21831418.
44. Zukin M, Barrios CH, Pereira JR, et al. Randomized phase III trial of single-agent pemetrexed versus carboplatin and pemetrexed in patients with advanced non-small-cell lung cancer and Eastern Cooperative Oncology Group performance status of 2. *J Clin Oncol*. 2013;31(23):2849-2853. Epub 2013/06/19. doi:10.1200/JCO.2012.48.1911. PubMed PMID: 23775961.
45. Santos FN, de Castria TB, Cruz MR, Riera R. Chemotherapy for advanced non-small cell lung cancer in the elderly population. *Cochrane Database Syst Rev*. 2015;10:CD010463. doi:10.1002/14651858.CD010463.pub2. PubMed PMID: 26482542.
46. Sandler A, Gray R, Perry MC, et al. Paclitaxel–carboplatin alone or with bevacizumab for non-small-cell lung cancer. *N Engl J Med*. 2006;355(24):2542-2550. PubMed PMID: 17167137.
47. Langer CJ, Socinski MA, Patel JD, et al. Isolating the role of bevacizumab in elderly patients with previously untreated non-squamous non-small cell lung cancer: secondary analyses of the ECOG 4599 and PointBreak trials. *Am J Clin Oncol*. 2015. doi:10.1097/COC.0000000000000163. PubMed PMID: 25628268.
48. Rekhtman N, Leighl NB, Somerfield MR. Molecular testing for selection of patients with lung cancer for epidermal growth factor receptor and anaplastic lymphoma kinase tyrosine kinase inhibitors: American Society of Clinical Oncology endorsement of the College of American Pathologists/International Association for the study of lung cancer/association for molecular pathology guideline. *J Clin Oncol*. 2015;11(2):135-136. Epub 2014/12/18. doi:10.1200/JOP.2014.002303. PubMed PMID: 25515718.
49. Hohenforst-Schmidt W, Zarogoulidis P, Steinheimer M, et al. Tyrosine kinase inhibitors for the elderly. *J Cancer*. 2016;7(6):687-693. doi: 10.7150/jca.14819. PubMed PMID: 27076850; PubMed Central PMCID: PMC4829555.
50. Nakao M, Muramatsu H, Sone K, et al. Epidermal growth factor receptor-tyrosine kinase inhibitors for non-small-cell lung cancer patients aged 80 years or older: a retrospective analysis. *Mol Clin Oncol*. 2015;3(2):403-407. doi:10.3892/mco.2014.453. PubMed PMID: 25798276; PubMed Central PMCID: PMC4360513.
51. Wu YL, Zhou C, Hu CP, et al. Afatinib versus cisplatin plus gemcitabine for first-line treatment of Asian patients with advanced non-small-cell lung cancer harbouring EGFR mutations (LUX-Lung 6): an open-label, randomised phase 3 trial. *Lancet Oncol*. 2014;

15(2):213-222. Epub 2014/01/21. doi:10.1016/S1470-2045(13)70604-1. PubMed PMID: 24439929.

52. Zhou C, Wu YL, Chen G, et al. Erlotinib versus chemotherapy as first-line treatment for patients with advanced EGFR mutation-positive non-small-cell lung cancer (OPTIMAL, CTONG-0802): a multicentre, open-label, randomised, phase 3 study. *Lancet Oncol*. 2011;12(8):735-742. Epub 2011/07/26. doi:10.1016/S1470-2045(11)70184-X. PubMed PMID: 21783417.

53. Rosell R, Carcereny E, Gervais R, et al. Erlotinib versus standard chemotherapy as first-line treatment for European patients with advanced EGFR mutation-positive non-small-cell lung cancer (EURTAC): a multicentre, open-label, randomised phase 3 trial. *Lancet Oncol*. 2012;13(3):239-246. Epub 2012/01/31. doi:10.1016/S1470-2045(11)70393-X. PubMed PMID: 22285168.

54. Solomon BJ, Mok T, Kim DW, et al. First-line crizotinib versus chemotherapy in ALK-positive lung cancer. *N Engl J Med*. 2014;371(23):2167-2177. Epub 2014/12/04. doi:10.1056/NEJMoa1408440. PubMed PMID: 25470694.

55. Shaw AT, Kim DW, Mehra R, et al. Ceritinib in ALK-rearranged non-small-cell lung cancer. *N Engl J Med*. 2014;370(13):1189-1197. doi:10.1056/NEJMoa1311107. PubMed PMID: 24670165; PubMed Central PMCID: PMC4079055.

56. Nishijima TF, Muss HB, Shachar SS, Moschos SJ. Comparison of efficacy of immune checkpoint inhibitors (ICIs) between younger and older patients: a systematic review and meta-analysis. *Cancer Treat Rev*. 2016;45:30-37. doi:10.1016/j.ctrv.2016.02.006. PubMed PMID: 26946217.

57. Ardizzoni A, Favaretto A, Boni L, et al. Platinum–etoposide chemotherapy in elderly patients with small-cell lung cancer: results of a randomized multicenter phase II study assessing attenuated-dose or full-dose with lenograstim prophylaxis—a Forza Operativa Nazionale Italiana Carcinoma Polmonare and Gruppo Studio Tumori Polmonari Veneto (FONICAP-GSTPV) study. *J Clin Oncol*. 2005;23(3):569-575. Epub 2005/01/22. doi:0.1200/JCO.2005.11.140. PubMed PMID: 15659503.

58. Okamoto H, Watanabe K, Kunikane H, et al. Randomised phase III trial of carboplatin plus etoposide vs split doses of cisplatin plus etoposide in elderly or poor-risk patients with extensive disease small-cell lung cancer: JCOG 9702. *Br J Cancer*. 2007;97(2):162-169. Epub 2007/06/21. doi:10.1038/sj.bjc.6603810. PubMed PMID: 17579629; PubMed Central PMCID: 2360311.

59. Souhami RL, Spiro SG, Rudd RM, et al. Five-day oral etoposide treatment for advanced small-cell lung cancer: randomized comparison with intravenous chemotherapy. *J Natl Cancer Inst*. 1997;89(8):577-580. Epub 1997/04/16. PubMed PMID: 9106647.

60. Yuen AR, Zou G, Turrisi AT, et al. Similar outcome of elderly patients in intergroup trial 0096: cisplatin, etoposide, and thoracic radiotherapy administered once or twice daily in limited stage small cell lung

carcinoma. *Cancer*. 2000;89(9):1953-1960. Epub 2000/11/07. PubMed PMID: 11064352.

61. Schild SE, Stella PJ, Brooks BJ, et al. Results of combined-modality therapy for limited-stage small cell lung carcinoma in the elderly. *Cancer*. 2005;103(11):2349-2354. Epub 2005/04/27. doi:10.1002/cncr.21034. PubMed PMID: 15852407.
62. Corso CD, Rutter CE, Park HS, et al. Role of chemoradiotherapy in elderly patients with limited-stage small-cell lung cancer. *J Clin Oncol*. 2015;33(36):4240-4246. Epub 2015/10/21. doi:10.1200/JCO.2015.62.4270. PubMed PMID: 26481366; PubMed Central PMCID: 4678178.
63. Caprario LC, Kent DM, Strauss GM. Effects of chemotherapy on survival of elderly patients with small-cell lung cancer: analysis of the SEER-medicare database. *J Thorac Oncol*. 2013;8(10):1272-1281. Epub 2014/01/25. doi:10.1097/JTO.0b013e3182a007ba. PubMed PMID: 24457238; PMCID: 3901951.
64. Gridelli C, Maione P, Illiano A, et al. Cisplatin plus gemcitabine or vinorelbine for elderly patients with advanced non small-cell lung cancer: the MILES-2P studies. *J Clin Oncol*. 2007;25(29):4663-4669. Epub 2007/10/11. doi:10.1200/JCO.2007.12.5708. PubMed PMID: 17925563.
65. Abe T, Takeda K, Ohe Y, et al. Randomized phase III trial comparing weekly docetaxel plus cisplatin versus docetaxel monotherapy every 3 weeks in elderly patients with advanced non-small-cell lung cancer: the intergroup trial JCOG0803/WJOG4307L. *J Clin Oncol*. 2015;33(6):575-581. Epub 2015/01/15. doi:10.1200/JCO.2014.55.8627. PubMed PMID: 25584004.
66. Biesma B, Wymenga AN, Vincent A, et al. Quality of life, geriatric assessment and survival in elderly patients with non-small-cell lung cancer treated with carboplatin–gemcitabine or carboplatin–paclitaxel: NVALT-3 a phase III study. *Ann Oncol*. 2011;22(7):1520-1527. Epub 2011/01/22. doi:10.1093/annonc/mdq637. PubMed PMID: 21252061.
67. Yoshioka H, Komuta K, Imamura F, et al. Efficacy and safety of erlotinib in elderly patients in the phase IV POLARSTAR surveillance study of Japanese patients with non-small-cell lung cancer. *Lung Cancer*. 2014;86(2):201-206. Epub 2014/10/05. doi:10.1016/j.lungcan.2014.09.015. PubMed PMID: 25280386.
68. Kurishima K, Satoh H, Kaburagi T, et al. Erlotinib for elderly patients with non-small-cell lung cancer: subset analysis from a population-based observational study by the Ibaraki Thoracic Integrative (POSITIVE) Research Group. *Mol Clin Oncol*. 2013;1(5):828-832. Epub 2014/03/22. doi:10.3892/mco.2013.154. PubMed PMID: 24649255; PubMed Central PMCID: 3915644.
69. Jackman DM, Yeap BY, Lindeman NI, et al. Phase II clinical trial of chemotherapy-naive patients ≥70 years of age treated with erlotinib for advanced non-small-cell lung cancer. *J Clin Oncol*. 2007;25(7):760-766. Epub 2007/01/18. doi:10.1200/JCO.2006.07.5754. PubMed PMID: 17228019.

70. Wheatley-Price P, Ding K, Seymour L, et al. Erlotinib for advanced non-small-cell lung cancer in the elderly: an analysis of the National Cancer Institute of Canada Clinical Trials Group Study BR.21. *J Clin Oncol*. 2008;26(14):2350-2357. Epub 2008/05/10. doi:10.1200/JCO.2007.15.2280. PubMed PMID: 18467727.

71. Platania M, Agustoni F, Formisano B, et al. Clinical retrospective analysis of erlotinib in the treatment of elderly patients with advanced non-small cell lung cancer. *Target Oncol*. 2011;6(3):181-186. Epub 2011/06/15. doi:10.1007/s11523-011-0185-6. PubMed PMID: 21667119.

72. Chen YM, Tsai CM, Fan WC, et al. Phase II randomized trial of erlotinib or vinorelbine in chemonaive, advanced, non-small cell lung cancer patients aged 70 years or older. *J Thorac Oncol*. 2012; 7(2):412-418. Epub 2011/12/14. doi:10.1097/JTO.0b013e31823a39e8. PubMed PMID: 22157367.

73. Morikawa N, Minegishi Y, Inoue A, et al. First-line gefitinib for elderly patients with advanced NSCLC harboring EGFR mutations. A combined analysis of North-East Japan Study Group studies. *Expert Opin Pharmacother*. 2015;16(4):465-472. Epub 2015/01/20. doi:10.1517/14656566.2015.1002396. PubMed PMID: 25597331.

74. Takahashi K, Saito H, Hasegawa Y, et al. First-line gefitinib therapy for elderly patients with non-small cell lung cancer harboring EGFR mutation: Central Japan Lung Study Group 0901. *Cancer Chemother Pharmacol*. 2014;74(4):721-727. Epub 2014/08/05. doi:10.1007/s00280-014-2548-z. PubMed PMID: 25087097.

75. Maemondo M, Minegishi Y, Inoue A, et al. First-line gefitinib in patients aged 75 or older with advanced non-small cell lung cancer harboring epidermal growth factor receptor mutations: NEJ 003 study. *J Thorac Oncol*. 2012;7(9):1417-1422. Epub 2012/08/17. doi:10.1097/JTO.0b013e318260de8b. PubMed PMID: 22895139.

76. Inoue A, Kobayashi K, Usui K, et al. First-line gefitinib for patients with advanced non-small-cell lung cancer harboring epidermal growth factor receptor mutations without indication for chemotherapy. *J Clin Oncol*. 2009;27(9):1394-1400. Epub 2009/02/20. doi:10.1200/JCO.2008.18.7658. PubMed PMID: 19224850.

13 Management of Pulmonary Neuroendocrine Tumors

Ying Wang, Cheryl Ho, and Janessa Laskin

INTRODUCTION

Pulmonary neuroendocrine tumors (NETs) are a spectrum of lung malignancies that arise from the neuroendocrine (NE) cells of the bronchopulmonary epithelium (1). The term encompasses a wide range of clinicopathological traits and biologic behaviors; at one end of the spectrum are low-grade, slow-growing tumors, while at the other end are high-grade, aggressive tumors. Several classification schemes have been developed to describe these differing entities, all encompassed by the broad category of NET. In this chapter, we focus on the management of well-differentiated neuroendocrine tumors (WD-NET), a term that includes typical and atypical carcinoid (AC) tumors, and poorly differentiated large-cell neuroendocrine carcinoma (LCNEC). Small-cell lung cancer (SCLC), another high-grade, poorly differentiated NET, is covered in detail in Chapters 10 and 11.

CLASSIFICATION AND EPIDEMIOLOGY

Well-Differentiated Pulmonary NETs

WD-NETs, also called bronchopulmonary carcinoids (BPC), are rare tumours originating from the lung. WD-NETs can be further subclassified into low-grade typical carcinoids (TC), accounting for 90% of BPCs, and intermediate-grade AC, accounting for 10% of BPCs (Table 13.1) (2). Pulmonary WD-NETs are estimated to account for 1% to 2% of all adult lung malignancies and the incidence has increased over the last 30 years by approximately 6% per year (3). Potential explanations for this increasing incidence include higher sensitivity of detection by improved imaging techniques and a more specific diagnostic classification. Overall, the incidence rate ranges between 0.2 and 2 per 100,000 people per year (4). Approximately, 5% of pulmonary WD-NETs are associated with multiple endocrine neoplasm type 1 (MEN1) (5). WD-NETs more commonly arise in the gastrointestinal (GI) tract, with GI NETs accounting for two-thirds of all WD-NETs. It is not uncommon for both GI and pulmonary NETs to be included within

Table 13.1 Comparison of pulmonary neuroendocrine tumors

	Grade	Morphology	Mitoses per 10 HPFs	Necrosis
Typical carcinoid	Low	Well differentiated	<2	None
Atypical carcinoid	Intermediate	Well differentiated	2–10	Yes (focal)
Large cell neuroen-docrine carcinoma	High	Poorly differentiated	>10	Yes (extensive)
Small-cell lung carcinoma	High	Poorly differentiated	>10	Yes (extensive)

HPFs, high-power fields.

the same clinical trial, a practice that confounds the development of appropriate treatment algorithms since WD-NETs occurring in different locations do not always exhibit the same biological behavior or response to specific therapy.

Large-Cell Neuroendocrine Carcinoma

LCNEC is a high grade, poorly differentiated NET that has only been recognized as a distinct NET over the past 25 years (6,7). LCNEC is distinguished from other large cell carcinomas by NE cellular differentiation and histologic architecture, and from WD-NETs by its higher mitotic rates, worse prognosis, and more aggressive behavior (Table 13.1). Histologically, LCNEC shares the qualities of poor differentiation and higher grade with SCLC, but is distinguished from SCLC by larger cell size. LCNEC accounts for approximately 3% of lung malignancies, but many aspects of this entity remain unclear given its low incidence and relatively recent classification (4).

CLINICAL PRESENTATION

Tumor Location

The majority of pulmonary NETs arise within the central airways of the lung, and because of this location approximately 60% of patients present with dyspnea, hemoptysis, cough, pneumonia, chest discomfort, and/or unilateral wheezing. Peripheral pulmonary NETs are usually asymptomatic and are commonly discovered incidentally (5).

Secretory Tumors

Hormonally active pulmonary NETs are much less common than their GI counterparts, and are rarely diagnosed at an early stage. Only 1% to 2% of patients with pulmonary NETs present with symptoms associated with classic carcinoid syndrome, such as flushing, diarrhea, wheezing, and right-sided valvular heart disease (2,5,8). Patients should be monitored for carcinoid crisis following radiotherapy or procedural manipulation, but the risk is low enough that routine prophylaxis with a somatostatin analogue (SSA) is not recommended. Another 1% to 6% of patients with pulmonary NETs present with Cushing syndrome caused by ectopic adenocorticotrophic hormone (ACTH) production, with symptoms such as new onset glucose intolerance, proximal myopathy, hirsutism, facial plethora, and/or centripetal obesity. Though hormonal production is uncommon, all patients with pulmonary NETs should be clinically screened for paraneoplastic syndromes, with further laboratory and radiographic evaluation based on clinical suspicion (8,9).

DIAGNOSIS AND EVALUATION

Imaging

The European Neuroendocrine Tumor Society (ENETS) recommends the use of contrast CT as the gold standard for detecting pulmonary NETs (9). Complete staging should include a preoperative CT of the chest, abdomen, and pelvis for patients with potentially resectable disease. For those with metastatic disease, directed imaging with multiphasic CT or MRI is recommended for further elucidation of possible metastases, particularly to the liver (9).

Based on small retrospective studies, fluorodeoxyglucose-positron emission tomography (FDG-PET) has limited use in the detection of primary or metastatic WD-NETs due to their low metabolic activity (10). In contrast, LCNECs have much higher uptake of FDG with a usual mean standardized uptake value (SUV) of 9 to 12, which is comparable to that of SCLC. Therefore, FDG-PET can be useful in staging patients with LCNEC (5).

Indium-111 pentetreotide scintigraphy (octreotide scan) can be used to detect somatostatin subtype receptors (SSTR) on WD-NETs, although its routine use is not universally recommended (5).

Other Diagnostic Modalities

Patients with pulmonary NETs who are potentially eligible for curative resection must undergo a thorough preoperative clinical assessment to fully define tumor histology, location, and stage, as well as perioperative risk (8). For tumors in the central portion of the lung, a full workup includes bronchoscopy, potentially with endobronchial ultrasound-guided evaluation of mediastinal lymph nodes. Patients presenting with carcinoid syndrome or potential cardiovascular compromise should be considered for echocardiography. Pulmonary function tests should also be obtained prior to surgery, especially in high-risk patients such as those with preexisting lung disease (9).

Laboratory Investigations

Baseline biochemical investigations should be performed on all patients diagnosed with a pulmonary NET. This includes assessment of renal function, liver enzymes, calcium, glucose, and a plasma chromogranin A level. Paraneoplastic syndromes should be investigated if clinical assessment is suspicious for a hormonally secretory tumor. Potentially useful tests include a 24-hour urine for 5-hydroxy-indole-acetic acid (5-HIAA) to evaluate for carcinoid syndrome, and a serum ACTH level for suspected Cushing syndrome. Genetic assessment for *MEN1* mutation should only be undertaken if there is a strong suspicion based on family history, or if the patient presents with other features of the MEN1 syndrome (9).

PROGNOSIS

In general, the prognosis of TC is better than AC, and both are considerably better than LCNEC. There are wide variations in survival outcomes within each category of tumor in different reports since patient numbers are generally small. Lewis and Yao analyzed the survival of 187,991 patients with WD-NETs or LCNEC from the Surveillance Epidemiology and End Results (SEER) database and reported that median overall survival duration was 201 months for TC, 101 months for AC, and 6 months for LCNEC. For patients with metastatic disease the 5-year overall survival rates are 40% to 50% for TC, 20% for AC, and <5% for LCNEC (11).

MANAGEMENT OF EARLY STAGE WD-NET

Localized Therapy

For localized TC, due to the more indolent nature of disease, lung-preserving resection using sleeve, wedge, or segmental resection is generally preferred over either more extensive resections or watchful waiting without surgery (8,12). In contrast, a more extensive resection, such as lobectomy or pneumonectomy, is usually required for AC based on its higher incidence of lymph node involvement (30%–70% in AC vs. 5%–20% in TC) (13,14). Full mediastinal lymph node dissection is recommended if initial sampling is positive for lymph node involvement (9,13,14).

Bronchoscopic resection of intraluminal tumor has been studied in small series and has demonstrated good long-term survival for patients with central, endobronchial TC. In one study, of 28 patients who underwent bronchoscopic resection, the 10-year survival rate was 84% (15). However, careful patient selection is crucial, as endobronchial procedures result in a higher rate of recurrence compared to standard lung resections (13).

Stereotactic ablation radiotherapy (SABR) may also be considered for localized stage I pulmonary NETs, particularly in patients who are not good candidates for surgical resection. However, there is minimal data available on the long-term outcomes associated with the use of SABR for pulmonary NETs.

Surveillance Without Treatment

One retrospective series of patients with biopsy-proven, lymph node-negative TC who did not undergo resection reported 5-year disease-specific survival (DFS) rates of 87% for patients with T2 tumors and 92% for those with T1 tumors (12). Thus, careful clinical monitoring without intervention may be a viable option for a small subset of patients with asymptomatic, clinical stage I TC who prefer to avoid therapeutic intervention.

Adjuvant Therapy

Currently, there is a paucity of high-quality evidence addressing the role of adjuvant chemotherapy or radiotherapy in patients with resected WD-NETs. Existing data are primarily from small, retrospective series with many of these reports providing conflicting results.

In TC, the most recent and largest retrospective analysis suggested a trend toward worse 5-year survival rates in patients who underwent adjuvant chemotherapy. In this study, Nussbaum, et al. evaluated data from 629 patients with lymph node-positive TC, of whom 37 underwent adjuvant chemotherapy. Baseline characteristics were similar between those who received chemotherapy and those who did not. The 5-year overall survival rates for the chemotherapy versus no chemotherapy groups were 70% and 82%, respectively ($P = .042$), although this difference was not statistically significant after propensity matching ($P = .096$) (16).

Even published guidelines provide no consensus on the utility of adjuvant therapy. For example, ENETS states that only patients with AC and nodal involvement should be considered for adjuvant therapy (9). Similarly, the NCCN supports the use of chemotherapy with or without radiation for resected stage I to III AC and for stage IIIB TC (17). However, the North American Neuroendocrine Tumor Society (NA-NET) does not recommend adjuvant radiotherapy, chemotherapy, or chemoradiation, given the lack of evidence for prolongation of disease-free or overall survival (8).

Recommendations for Early Stage WD-NET

The standard of care in early stage pulmonary NET is complete surgical resection with the goal of R0 resection while maximizing the preservation of lung function. Alternative treatment modalities and surveillance should only be employed in patients who are not surgical candidates or who decide against surgical intervention. Given the lack of evidence of benefit, the routine use of adjuvant chemotherapy cannot be recommended for WD-NETs. However, adjuvant platinum-based chemotherapy could be considered in high-risk individuals on a case-by-case basis, particularly for those with node-positive AC.

Follow-Up After Resection

Disease recurrence occurs mostly within the first 5 years for AC, and first 10 years for TC. Although there is limited evidence that early detection of recurrence changes patient outcomes, given the indolent nature of most WD-NETs, the goal of active surveillance should be to detect recurrences that are amenable to further curative intervention.

Long-term surveillance after local resection is recommended at regular intervals by multiple guideline organizations, though there is no consensus on the timing of investigations (8,9,18). More frequent follow-up is generally recommended in the first year following surgery with chest radiographs and/or CT scans every 3 to 6 months. Subsequently, CT imaging every 1 to 2 years is suggested. If octreotide scan was positive preoperatively, the follow-up scans may be considered at a similar interval. If any biomarkers, such as serum chromogranin A or urinary 5-HIAA were elevated preoperatively, then these should also be followed at regular intervals. The use of other investigations should be guided by clinical findings. In general, AC requires a more intensive follow-up strategy since the recurrence risk is higher. Since WD-NETs are usually indolent in nature, follow-up evaluation is recommended for at least 10 years and could be considered indefinitely.

MANAGEMENT OF METASTATIC WD-NET

Currently, there is no standard international consensus on a step-wise treatment of pulmonary WD-NETs, mainly due to the lack of high-quality clinical evidence to guide treatment decision making. The goals of treatment, however, are clear, to control tumor growth, minimize cancer-related symptoms, improve quality-of-life, and prolong survival. Generally, treatment decisions are made according to prognosis and symptoms (5,9). Good prognostic indicators are TC histology, lack of symptoms, and disease stability over the preceding 6 months. Treatment choices in this group of patients include active surveillance without anticancer therapy, local-regional therapy, and SSAs. Poor prognostic indicators include AC histology, symptomatic disease, and documentation of growth within the last 6 months. Multiple agents have been explored in this group of patients, including targeted therapies, peptide-receptor radiotherapy (PRRT), and palliative chemotherapy.

Traditional Chemotherapy

Few clinical trials have evaluated the use of chemotherapy in pulmonary WD-NETs. As a result, treatment recommendations have been extrapolated from studies in patients with GI NETs and SCLC. Retrospective studies highlight the diversity of treatments that have been used in WD-NETs, including 5-fluoruracil (5FU) plus streptozocin or doxorubicin, cisplatin plus etoposide, and capecitabine plus temozolomide, oxaliplatin, or liposomal doxorubicin (19–21). These studies demonstrate mixed results, with objective responses ranging from 7% to 56%, and median duration of response ranging from 4 to 102 months (Table 13.2). Cisplatin (usually combined with etoposide, as in SCLC) is probably the most commonly used cytotoxic chemotherapy regimen, though responses appear to be substantially higher for patients with AC than with TC. Temozolamide has shown promise as a single-agent with partial responses seen in up to 31% of patients with pulmonary WD-NET (21).

In general, cytotoxic chemotherapy may be considered for symptomatic, bulky, or progressive disease, particularly for patients with AC. Given the small size and mixed results of existing studies, there is no specific chemotherapy regimen that can be recommended, and patient participation in a clinical trial is strongly encouraged.

Targeted Therapy

NETs, including the well-differentiated subtypes, are vascular tumors that often express targetable factors within pathways related to cellular proliferation and angiogenesis (e.g., VEGF/VEGFR, PDGF/PDGFR, IGF1/IGFR) (27). Thus, many targeted antiproliferative agents have been studied, mainly in small clinical trials that included patients with tumors of various subtypes and primary sites (Table 13.2).

Table 13.2 Selected studies of systemic therapy for advanced pulmonary carcinoid

Study	Number (pulmonary)	Treatment	RR	DCR	Results Median PFS (months)	Median overall survival (months)
Chong et al. Retrospective (20)	13	Etoposide + platinum	23%	69%	7	NR
	14	Temozolamide-based	14%	57%	10	
	11	Other cytoxic therapy	20%	70%	4	
	20	Octreotide-based	10%	70%	15	
Sun et al. Phase 2/3 (19)	22	5FU + streptozocin	16%	5.3	NR	24.3*
		5FU + doxorubicin	16%	4.5		15.7
Crona et al. Retrospective (21)	31	Temozolomide	14%	45%	5.3	23.2
Radiant-4 Phase 3 (22)	63	Everolimus	NR	NR	11*	NR
	27	Placebo			3.9	
RAMSETE Phase 2 (23)	19	Everolimus	63% (SD)	NR	6.2	NR

(*continued*)

Table 13.2 Selected studies of systemic therapy for advanced pulmonary carcinoid (*continued*)

Study	Number (pulmonary)	Treatment	RR	DCR	Results: Median PFS (months)	Results: Median overall survival (months)
Radiant-2 Phase 3 (24)	33	Octerotide LAR + Everolimus	67%†	NR	13.6	NR
	11	Octreotide LAR	27%†		5.6	
ITMO Group Phase 2 (25)	11	Octerotide LAR + Everolimus	18%*	NR	NR	NR
Kulke et al. Phase 2 (26)	14 (foregut)	Sunitinib	2.4%	82.9%*	10.2 (TTP)*	NR

DCR, disease control rate; 5FU, 5-fluorouracil; LAR, long-acting repeatable; NR, not reported; PFS, progression-free survival; RR, response rate; SD, stable disease rate; TTP, time to progression.

*These figures reflect the outcomes for all NETs and may not be representative for the pulmonary NET subgroup.

†Minor tumor response, not objective response by RECIST criteria.

MTOR Inhibition

The mammalian target of rapamycin (mTOR) is a kinase that is implicated in cell growth, metabolism, and angiogenesis in NETs. Everolimus is an mTOR inhibitor that has shown the most promising activity in recent trials. RADIANT-4 was a multicenter, randomized, controlled, phase III clinical trial comparing everolimus versus placebo as first- or second-line treatment of nonfunctional NETs of lung or GI origin (22). The study included 90 patients with pulmonary WD-NET, 63 of whom received everolimus. Progression-free survival (PFS) by central review for the entire cohort of NET patients was significantly better in patients treated with everolimus (11 vs. 3.9 months; HR 0.48, 95% confidence interval [CI] 0.35–0.67; $P < .00001$). For the lung NET cohort, the PFS hazard ratio was 0.50 (95% CI 0.28–0.88) suggesting a significant benefit in disease control. For the whole group, overall survival at the first interim analysis favored the everolimus arm, with a 36% reduction in estimated risk of death compared to placebo. This is the first prospective, randomized trial demonstrating significant PFS benefit in pulmonary WD-NETs. Adverse events were similar to those noted in prior everolimus studies, with stomatitis (63%), diarrhea (31%), and fatigue (13%) being the predominant toxicities. The RADIANT-4 results are consistent with the results of the phase II RAMSETE trial of everolimus in patients with advanced and metastatic, asymptomatic NETs (23). Nineteen patients with bronchial, thymic, or mediastinal NETs were included and everolimus was associated with a median PFS of 6.2 months and stable disease rate of 63%.

Based on this accumulating evidence, we suggest that everolimus be considered for the treatment of incurable pulmonary WD-NETs. In some cases, everolimus is appropriate as a first-line therapy option, particularly for patients whose tumors are somatostatin receptor-negative. In February 2016, the U.S. Food and Drug Administration (FDA) has approved everolimus for the treatment of pulmonary WD-NETs in patients who have advanced or unresectable disease.

Combinations of MTOR Inhibitors Plus Hormonal Therapy

The RADIANT-2, phase III trial randomized 429 patients with hormonally active NETs and carcinoid syndrome to octreotide-LAR with or without everolimus as first- or subsequent-line treatment (28). A subset analysis of the 44 patients with pulmonary WD-NETs demonstrated a median PFS of 13.6 months in the combination arm versus 5.6 months in the octreotide-LAR alone arm, and a "tumour shrinkage" rate (not by RECIST criteria) of 67% for combination therapy versus 27% for octreotide-LAR alone (24).

In a similar trial, 50 patients with advanced NETs (11 with lung primary) were evaluated in the Italian Trials in Medical Oncology (ITMO) Group phase II study to assess octreotide-LAR plus everolimus as first-line therapy. The response rate was 18% (2% with complete response) and the stable disease rate was 74% (25). This suggests a possible role for this combination as first-line treatment in patients with NET. The ongoing LUNA trial is a 3-arm randomized study evaluating everolimus versus pasireotide-LAR versus the combination of both agents as any line of therapy.

Other Targeted Agents

Due to the highly vascular nature of NETs antiangiogenic pathways are an obvious target, but the data from studies of antiangiogenic agents is still preliminary and most responses have been seen in pancreatic NETs as opposed to pulmonary tumors. For example, the oral multikinase inhibitor, sunitinib, which is active against multiple angiogenic pathways was tested in 107 patients with advanced NETs (26). Of these, 37 had carcinoids cancers, 14 of which were from the "foregut" which includes the lungs and stomach. In the carcinoid group, 44% of patients had tumor shrinkage, though most represented stable disease, with more activity noted in those with pancreatic NETs. The authors concluded that without further study it is difficult to clearly determine the efficacy of sunitinib in carcinoid tumors. Currently, there is no evidence to support the use of antiangiogenic agents in pulmonary NETs outside of a clinical trial.

Somatostatin Analogues

Somatostatin is a naturally occurring peptide that inhibits the release of growth hormone and multiple GI hormones. SSAs, such as octreotide, lanreotide, and pasireotide, are most commonly used to treat the symptoms associated with carcinoid syndrome. Cushing syndrome, which occurs in 1% to 6% of pulmonary WD-NETs does not respond to SSAs, but can be treated with ketoconazole, aminoglutethimide, metyrapone, or mifeprisonte (9). Acromegaly secondary to paraneoplastic growth hormone releasing hormone secretion is rare in NETs, but usually responds to SSAs or surgical tumor debulking (9). SSAs typically have a tolerable side-effect profile, though they can cause GI symptoms, and a small risk of hyperglycemia or cholelithiasis. Long acting formulations of SSAs should be considered as first-line treatment in functional WD-NETs as these agents can be extremely helpful for symptom control.

In GI NETs, SSAs have also been shown to inhibit tumor growth and can therefore be utilized as active anticancer treatment.

The most frequently studied long-acting SSAs are octreotide-LAR and lanreotide, which are available as once-a-month injections in intramuscular or subcutaneous formulations. The U.S. FDA has approved two SSAs, octreotide and lanreotide, based on the results of randomized phase III trials that demonstrated improved antitumor activity versus placebo in nonpulmonary NETs (29,30). For example, in one study, median PFS was 14.3 for octreotide versus 6 months for placebo ($P < .001$), although overall survival was similar in both groups. Unfortunately, these trials explicitly excluded pulmonary NETs, so the potential antiproliferative effect in this setting remains unclear. A randomized phase II study is currently underway to assess lanreotide versus placebo in selected pulmonary and thymic NETs with positive receptor uptake on octreotide scan.

Radiotherapy and Radionuclides

Pulmonary NETs are relatively radiotherapy-resistant, and radiotherapy should typically only be considered when surgery is not feasible, after an incomplete resection, or for palliation of focal tumor-associated symptoms, such as painful bone metastases (5).

Radiolabeled SSAs have demonstrated effectiveness in small studies, but are not widely available. For example, PRRT technology links the radionuclides yttrium-90 or lutetium-177 to an SSA in order to target somatostatin-receptor-expressing tumor cells. The largest study of such therapy was a phase II trial of ^{90}Y-DOTA-Tyr-octreotide in 1,109 patients with 25 different NET subtypes, including 84 who had pulmonary NETs with a positive octreotide scan (31). A "morphologic response" was reported in 34% of patients in the overall study population, though the majority of these patients were not evaluable by RECIST criteria. While intriguing, this treatment has considerable toxicity with 9% of patients experiencing permanent, grade 4 to 5 renal toxicity. The use of radiopeptides remains investigational and is unavailable in North America for pulmonary WD-NETs, although it is widely accepted as a treatment for GI NETs.

Directed Therapy for Metastatic Sites

The liver is the primary metastatic site for WD-NETs, and liver dysfunction due to metastatic involvement is the most frequent cause of death for patients with BPCs (5,8). Both the NCCN and IASLC guidelines suggest that surgical intervention may be attempted for curative intent in patients with indolent behaving pulmonary WD-NETs and limited hepatic metastases. However, this strategy is an extrapolation from the experience with GI NETs and it is not clear that it would be curative or even beneficial in patients with a pulmonary WD-NET since liver metastases in lung malignancies indicate systemic (rather than portal) hematogenous spread (17). In symptomatic patients with functional cancers, consideration of noncurative surgical debulking can be considered (17). Local tumour control via radiofrequency ablation (RFA), stereotactic radiotherapy, hepatic arterial chemoembolization, or radioisotope yttrium-90 eluting beads may also be considered on an individual basis, primarily for management of symptomatic metastases.

In summary, surgery can palliate symptoms and may provide a survival benefit for patients with GI NETs, but no evidence exists to support the use of surgical debulking or targeted ablation of metastases in pulmonary WD-NETs.

MANAGEMENT OF LCNEC

LCNEC was first identified as a distinct entity in 1991 and remains a relatively rare diagnosis (32). Currently, there is no standard treatment for pulmonary LCNEC, and there is an ongoing debate as to whether LCNEC should be managed using SCLC or NSCLC regimens. From a practical perspective, the general algorithm for treating LCNEC, particularly early stage disease, is the same as that for NSCLC, but the preferred chemotherapy regimens are the same as those used for SCLC.

Early Stage LCNEC

Surgery

Similar to NSCLC, stage I to II LCNEC is best treated with surgical resection with curative intent (33). Unfortunately, many patients are not surgical candidates since approximately 40% have distant metastatic disease and 60% to 80% have mediastinal lymph node involvement at time of diagnosis (34). Although there have been no randomized trials assessing methods of surgical resection for LCNEC, lobectomy with mediastinal lymph node sampling or dissection is the most frequently performed procedure, achieving an R0 resection in 84% to 100% (35–40). In summary, early stage (stage I–II) LCNEC should be treated like NSCLC and considered for complete surgical resection after appropriate preoperative evaluation as noted previously.

Adjuvant Therapy

There is little evidence of benefit from adjuvant chemotherapy or radiotherapy after complete resection of LCNEC. The majority of the data comes from retrospective studies in which approximately one-third of patients underwent adjuvant chemotherapy (Table 13.3) (35–40). In 2006, Iyoda et al. conducted a small prospective, single-armed, phase II trial of 15 patients with surgically

Table 13.3 Selected studies of adjuvant chemotherapy for resected large cell neuroendocrine carcinoma

Study	Number	Regimen	5-Year overall survival rate
Iyoda et al. Phase II & retrospective (35)	15 23	Cisplatin + etoposide Observation	88% 47.2%
Kenmotsu et al. Phase II (37)	40 (23 LCNEC; 17 SCLC)	Cisplatin + irinotecan	86%*
Sarkaria et al. Retrospective (39)	93	Platinum + other agent	51%
Tanaka et al. Retrospective (40)	23 40	Platinum + other agent Observation	74.4% 32.3%

LCNEC, large-cell neuroendocrine carcinoma; SCLC, small cell lung cancer.
*3-year overall survival rate.

resected LCNEC (35). Eleven patients had stage I disease. Patients were given two cycles of adjuvant cisplatin plus etoposide within 60 days of surgery. The outcomes of these patients were compared to 23 retrospectively identified patients with comparable characteristics who did not undergo adjuvant chemotherapy. There was a significant difference in survival between the two groups, with a better 5-year overall survival rate in adjuvantly treated patients (88% vs. 47%). Although this survival rate with adjuvant chemotherapy is quite high compared to that of other studies (28%–89%), this was the first demonstration of a potential survival benefit with the use of adjuvant chemotherapy in LCNEC. The same investigators later published their retrospective observations of a larger cohort of 72 patients with stage IA to IV LCNEC, 30 who received platinum-based adjuvant chemotherapy and 42 who did not (36). Most patients had recurrence within 3 years of surgery (91.7%) and the incidence of brain metastases was high. In a multivariate analysis, disease stage and the use of adjuvant chemotherapy emerged as independent prognostic variables with patients who received adjuvant therapy having a lower rate of tumor recurrence and a longer DFS (59% vs. 33%).

Sarkaria et al. retrospectively examined the survival of 93 patients with LCNEC, mostly with stage I to II disease; 22 received neoadjuvant platinum-based therapy and 71 received adjuvant treatment (39). Survival was similar with both treatment approaches, suggesting that in some cases neoadjuvant therapy may be a reasonable consideration. A prospective, randomized, double blind, phase III clinical trial is ongoing in Japan comparing adjuvant cisplatin plus irinotecan to cisplatin plus etoposide for patients with resected stage I to IIIA LCNEC. The choice of chemotherapy in this study reflects the standards for SCLC, particularly in Japan (41).

In summary, retrospective studies and extrapolation from prospective trials in NSCLC suggest that adjuvant chemotherapy could be beneficial for patients with completely resected stage II to III LCNEC. It is difficult to recommend adjuvant therapy for stage I LCNEC since this is not the standard of care for NSCLC and LCNEC does not typically respond to chemotherapy as well as SCLC does. Although the optimal regimen has not been defined, cisplatin plus etoposide has been the most commonly used combination because of the histological similarity to SCLC. Beyond the choice of chemotherapy, LCNEC is not generally treated like SCLC. For example, prophylactic cranial irradiation is not used in the adjuvant setting. The role of adjuvant radiation for resected N2 disease remains undefined and will likely follow whatever emerges as standard for NSCLC once more definitive trials have been completed. We do recommend that patients be referred to medical oncology for consideration of adjuvant therapy and that treatment decisions be made on a case-by-case basis with multidisciplinary input given the poor prognosis and high risk of recurrence (40%–60%) associated with LCNEC.

Locally Advanced LCNEC

Patients with locally advanced, unresectable stage III LCNEC are treated in a similar fashion as those with stage III NSCLC or limited-stage SCLC with four cycles of platinum-based chemotherapy plus concurrent definitive radiotherapy given with curative intent.

Metastatic LCNEC

Chemotherapy

Advanced LCNEC has a poor prognosis, and treatment is based primarily on small or retrospective studies. However, there is general agreement that platinum-based regimens do convey some advantage (Table 13.4). Three retrospective studies of systemic therapy have been conducted in patients with advanced LCNEC. Rossi et al. conducted a retrospective analysis of 83 patients with LCNEC across a broad range of stages. Regardless of stage, patients who received a "SCLC-like regimen" (primarily platinum plus etoposide) fared better than those who received a variety of typical "NSCLC regimens." In the small group of patients with metastatic disease, 12 received a SCLC regimen and 15 a NSCLC regimen,

Table 13.4 Selected studies of chemotherapy for advanced large cell neuroendocrine carcinoma

Study	Number	Regimen	Response rate	Results	
				Median PFS (months)	Median overall survival (months)
Rossi et al. Retrospective (38)	12	Platinum + etoposide	29% (combined)	NR	51
	15	"NSCLC regimens"			21
Sun et al. Retrospective (42)	11	Platinum + etoposide	73%	NR	16.5
	34	"NSCLC regimens"	50%		9.2
Le treut et al. Phase 2 (43)	29	Cisplatin + etoposide	31%	5	8
Niho et al. Phase 2 (44)	30	Cisplatin + irinotecan	44.7%	5.8	12.6

NR, not reported; NSCLC, non–small-cell lung cancer; PFS, progression-free survival.

with a higher response rate and a survival advantage noted for the SCLC treatment group (51 vs. 21 months; $P < .001$) (38).

In slight contrast, Sun et al. conducted a retrospective review of 45 consecutive patients with advanced LCNEC comparing the SCLC regimen of cisplatin plus etoposide ($n = 11$) against a variety of NSCLC regimens, including two patients treated with EGFR-directed therapy (42). Overall response rates were similar in both groups (SCLC regimen = 73% vs. NSCLC regiment = 50%; $P = .19$). Interestingly, there was an overall survival trend favoring the SCLC-treatment group (median, 16.5 vs. 9.2 months; $P = .10$).

Two small, single-arm, prospective phase II studies have been conducted in patients with advanced LCNEC examining cisplatin plus either etoposide or irinotecan. Le Treut et al. enrolled 42 patients with a centrally confirmed diagnosis of stage III or IV LCNEC on a phase II study of cisplatin plus etoposide for six cycles (43). Central pathology review reclassified 11 patients as having SCLC or another diagnosis other than LCNEC, highlighting one of the major challenges of drawing conclusions from studies in this disease entity. In the subgroup of 29 evaluable patients with confirmed LCNEC, 31% had a partial response and 34% had stable disease, with a median PFS of 5 months and median overall survival of 8 months. Another prospective phase II trial of 44 patients with advanced LCNEC assessed cisplatin plus irinotecan for four cycles (44). Again, 25% of patients were reclassified as SCLC. The response rate in patients with confirmed LCNEC was 47% with a median PFS of 5.8 months and a median overall survival of 12.6 months. Although the results of these prospective trials are not as encouraging as those from retrospective studies, they are likely more reflective of the reality of LCNEC, a disease that is nearly as aggressive as SCLC, but is as poorly responsive to therapy as NSCLC.

In summary, we recommend that metastatic LCNEC should be treated with one of the platinum-based chemotherapy regimens typically used to treat SCLC. Close attention should be paid to the potential side effects of therapy, since stage IV LCNEC is an incurable disease and maintenance of quality-of-life is a primary goal of care.

Molecularly Targeted Therapy

Despite the recent advances in targeted therapy and genomic profiling in NSCLC, there are little data to support the use of any specific targeted treatment in patients with LCNEC. Case reports suggest that EGFR activating mutations can occur in LCNEC and that these patients may respond to EGFR tyrosine kinase inhibitors, but such events appear to be rare (45).

Since LCNEC is a NET, Filosso et al. evaluated the use of adjuvant octreotide alone or in combination with radiotherapy in 10 patients with completely resected stage IB to IIIA LCNEC who had a positive preoperative octreotide scan (46). While there were some suggestions of a survival advantage with octreotide, the limitations of this study preclude any conclusion as to the activity of octreotide in this setting. Given the dearth of evidence supporting any specific targeted agent for patients with LCNEC, we strongly encourage participation in clinical trials.

KEY POINTS

- Pulmonary NETs account for one-third of all NETs and encompass a range of tumors with distinct biology, clinical presentation, treatment pathways, and prognoses.
- Pulmonary WD-NETs include TC, which have indolent behavior and rarely metastasize, and AC, which are intermediate-grade tumors with an increased propensity to metastasize to both regional lymph nodes and distant sites.
- LCNEC is a distinct, poorly differentiated pulmonary NET that exhibits aggressive behavior similar to that of SCLC.
- Hormone over-production syndromes, such as carcinoid syndrome and Cushing syndrome, are rare in pulmonary WD-NETs, but when they occur, they should be treated with SSAs.
- For patients with early stage TC, AC, and LCNEC, surgery is the recommended primary treatment. The role of adjuvant therapy is poorly defined.
- For patients with stage IV pulmonary WD-NET, particularly TC, everolimus is a reasonable first-line therapy.
- For patients with stage IV AC or LCNEC, platinum-based chemotherapy with regimens that are typically used to treat SCLC is the primary first-line treatment.
- Pulmonary NETs are an uncommon and diverse group of cancers. Therefore, treatment decisions should be individualized in consultation with a multidisciplinary team. Enrollment into clinical trials should be strongly encouraged.

REFERENCES

1. Klimstra DS, Modlin IR, Coppola D, et al. The pathologic classification of neuroendocrine tumors: a review of nomenclature, grading, and staging systems. *Pancreas*. 2010;39(6):707-712.
2. Gustafsson BI, Kidd M, Chan A, et al. Bronchopulmonary neuroendocrine tumors. *Cancer*. 2008;113(1):5-21.
3. Boyar Cetinkaya R, Aagnes B, Thiis-Evensen E, et al. Trends in incidence of neuroendocrine neoplasms in Norway: a report of 16,075 cases from 1993 through 2010. *Neuroendocrinology*. Published online on November 13, 2015. doi: 10.1159/000442207 [Epub ahead of print].
4. Yao JC, Hassan M, Phan A, et al. One hundred years after "carcinoid": epidemiology of and prognostic factors for neuroendocrine tumors in 35,825 cases in the United States. *J Clin Oncol*. 2008;26(18):3063-3072.
5. Noonan K, Derks J, Laskin J, Dingemans A. Neuroendocrine tumors of the lung other than small cell lung cancer. In: Pass H, Scagliotti GV, Ball D, eds. *The IASLC Multidisciplinary Approach to Thoracic Oncology*. International Association for the Study of Lung Cancer; 2013: 765-786.
6. Travis WD, Linnoila RI, Tsokos MG, et al. Neuroendocrine tumors of the lung with proposed criteria for large-cell neuroendocrine carcinoma. An ultrastructural, immunohistochemical, and flow cytometric study of 35 cases. *Am J Surg Pathol*. 1991;15(6):529-553.
7. Travis WD. Pathology of lung cancer. *Clin Chest Med*. 2002;23(1): 65-81, viii.
8. Phan AT, Oberg K, Choi J, et al. NANETS consensus guideline for the diagnosis and management of neuroendocrine tumors: well-differentiated neuroendocrine tumors of the thorax (includes lung and thymus). *Pancreas*. 2010;39(6):784-798.
9. Caplin ME, Baudin E, Ferolla P, et al. Pulmonary neuroendocrine (carcinoid) tumors: European Neuroendocrine Tumor Society expert consensus and recommendations for best practice for typical and atypical pulmonary carcinoids. *Ann Oncol*. 2015;26(8):1604-1620.
10. Tatci E, Ozmen O, Gokcek A, et al. 18F-FDG PET/CT rarely provides additional information other than primary tumor detection in patients with pulmonary carcinoid tumors. *Ann Thorac Med*. 2014;9(4):227-231.
11. Lewis M, Yao J. Bronchial neuroendocrine neoplasms: Surveillance Epidemiology and End Results (SEER) database review of demographics and survival in 187,911 cases. *J Clin Oncol*. 2015;33(15S):233s.
12. Raz DJ, Nelson RA, Grannis FW, et al. Natural history of typical pulmonary carcinoid tumors: a comparison of nonsurgical and surgical treatment. *Chest*. 2015;147(4):1111-1117.
13. Detterbeck FC. Management of carcinoid tumors. *Ann Thorac Surg*. 2010;89(3):998-1005.
14. Filosso PL, Rena O, Guerrera F, et al. Clinical management of atypical carcinoid and large-cell neuroendocrine carcinoma: a multicentre study on behalf of the European Association of Thoracic Surgeons

(ESTS) Neuroendocrine Tumours of the Lung Working Group dagger. *Eur J Cardiothorac Surg*. 2015;48(1):55-64.

15. Luckraz H, Amer K, Thomas L, et al. Long-term outcome of bronchoscopically resected endobronchial typical carcinoid tumors. *J Thorac Cardiovasc Surg*. 2006;132(1):113-115.
16. Nussbaum DP, Speicher PJ, Gulack BC, et al. Defining the role of adjuvant chemotherapy after lobectomy for typical bronchopulmonary carcinoid tumors. *Ann Thorac Surg*. 2015;99(2):428-434.
17. Kulke MH, Shah MH, Benson AB, 3rd, et al. Neuroendocrine tumors, version 1.2015. *J Natl Compr Canc Netw*. 2015;13(1):78-108.
18. Oberg K, Hellman P, Ferolla P, et al. Neuroendocrine bronchial and thymic tumors: ESMO Clinical Practice Guidelines for diagnosis, treatment and follow-up. *Ann Oncol*. 2012;23(suppl 7):vii120-vii123.
19. Sun W, Lipsitz S, Catalano P, et al. Phase II/III study of doxorubicin with fluorouracil compared with streptozocin with fluorouracil or dacarbazine in the treatment of advanced carcinoid tumors: Eastern Cooperative Oncology Group Study E1281. *J Clin Oncol*. 2005;23(22):4897-4904.
20. Chong CR, Wirth LJ, Nishino M, et al. Chemotherapy for locally advanced and metastatic pulmonary carcinoid tumors. *Lung Cancer*. 2014;86(2):241-246.
21. Crona J, Fanola I, Lindholm DP, et al. Effect of temozolomide in patients with metastatic bronchial carcinoids. *Neuroendocrinology*. 2013;98(2):151-155.
22. Yao JC, Fazio N, Singh S, et al. Everolimus for the treatment of advanced, non-functional neuroendocrine tumours of the lung or gastrointestinal tract (RADIANT-4): a randomised, placebo-controlled, phase 3 study. *Lancet*. 2015;387(10022):968-977.
23. Pavel ME, Wiedenmann B, Capdevila J, et al. RAMSETE: a single-arm, multicenter, single-stage phase II trial of RAD001 (everolimus) in advanced and metastatic silent neuro-endocrine tumours in Europe. *J Clin Oncol*. 2012;30(15s):268s.
24. Fazio N, Granberg D, Grossman A, et al. Everolimus plus octreotide long-acting repeatable in patients with advanced lung neuroendocrine tumors: analysis of the phase 3, randomized, placebo-controlled RADIANT-2 study. *Chest*. 2013;143(4):955-962.
25. Bajetta E, Catena L, Fazio N, et al. Everolimus in combination with octreotide long-acting repeatable in a first-line setting for patients with neuroendocrine tumors: an ITMO group study. *Cancer*. 2014;120(16):2457-2463.
26. Kulke MH, Lenz HJ, Meropol NJ, et al. Activity of sunitinib in patients with advanced neuroendocrine tumors. *J Clin Oncol*. 2008;26:3403-3410.
27. Marquez-Medina D, Popat S. Systemic therapy for pulmonary carcinoids. *Lung Cancer*. 2015;90(2):139-147.
28. Pavel ME, Hainsworth JD, Baudin E, et al. Everolimus plus octreotide long-acting repeatable for the treatment of advanced neuroendocrine

tumours associated with carcinoid syndrome (RADIANT-2): a randomised, placebo-controlled, phase 3 study. *Lancet*. 2011;378(9808): 2005-2012.

29. Rinke A, Wittenberg M, Schade-Brittinger C, et al. Placebo controlled, double-blind, prospective, randomized study on the effect of octreotide LAR in the control of tumor growth in patients with metastatic neuroendocrine midgut tumors (PROMID): results on long-term survival. *Neuroendocrinology*. Published online on January 6, 2016. doi:10.1159/000443612 [Epub ahead of print].
30. Caplin ME, Pavel M, Cwikla JB, et al. Lanreotide in metastatic enteropancreatic neuroendocrine tumors. *N Engl J Med*. 2014;371(3): 224-233.
31. Imhof A, Brunner P, Marincek N, et al. Response, survival, and long-term toxicity after therapy with the radiolabeled somatostatin analogue [90Y-DOTA]-TOC in metastasized neuroendocrine cancers. *J Clin Oncol*. 2011;29(17):2416-2423.
32. Lewis M, Yao J. Bronchial neuroendocrine neoplasms: Surveillance Epidemiology and End Results (SEER) database review of demographics and survival in 187911 cases. *J Clin Oncol*. 2015; 33(15S):233s.
33. Darling GE, Allen MS, Decker PA, et al. Randomized trial of mediastinal lymph node sampling versus complete lymphadenectomy during pulmonary resection in the patient with N0 or N1 (less than hilar) non-small cell carcinoma: results of the American College of Surgery Oncology Group Z0030 Trial. *J Thorac Cardiovasc Surg*. 2011;141(3):662-670.
34. Fasano M, Della Corte CM, Papaccio F, et al. Pulmonary large-cell neuroendocrine carcinoma: from epidemiology to therapy. *J Thorac Oncol*. 2015;10(8):1133-1141.
35. Iyoda A, Hiroshima K, Moriya Y, et al. Prospective study of adjuvant chemotherapy for pulmonary large cell neuroendocrine carcinoma. *Ann Thorac Surg*. 2006;82(5):1802-1807.
36. Iyoda A, Hiroshima K, Moriya Y, et al. Postoperative recurrence and the role of adjuvant chemotherapy in patients with pulmonary large-cell neuroendocrine carcinoma. *J Thorac Cardiovasc Surg*. 2009;138(2):446-453.
37. Kenmotsu H, Niho S, Ito T, et al. A pilot study of adjuvant chemotherapy with irinotecan and cisplatin for completely resected high-grade pulmonary neuroendocrine carcinoma (large cell neuroendocrine carcinoma and small cell lung cancer). *Lung Cancer*. 2014;84(3):254-258.
38. Rossi G, Cavazza A, Marchioni A, et al. Role of chemotherapy and the receptor tyrosine kinases KIT, PDGFRalpha, PDGFRbeta, and Met in large-cell neuroendocrine carcinoma of the lung. *J Clin Oncol*. 2005;23(34):8774-8785.
39. Sarkaria IS, Iyoda A, Roh MS, et al. Neoadjuvant and adjuvant chemotherapy in resected pulmonary large cell neuroendocrine

carcinomas: a single institution experience. *Ann Thorac Surg*. 2011; 92(4):1180-1186.

40. Tanaka Y, Ogawa H, Uchino K, et al. Immunohistochemical studies of pulmonary large cell neuroendocrine carcinoma: a possible association between staining patterns with neuroendocrine markers and tumor response to chemotherapy. *J Thorac Cardiovasc Surg*. 2013;145(3):839-846.
41. Eba J, Kenmotsu H, Tsuboi M, et al. A Phase III trial comparing irinotecan and cisplatin with etoposide and cisplatin in adjuvant chemotherapy for completely resected pulmonary high-grade neuroendocrine carcinoma (JCOG1205/1206). *Jpn J Clin Oncol*. 2014;44(4):379-382.
42. Sun JM, Ahn MJ, Ahn JS, et al. Chemotherapy for pulmonary large cell neuroendocrine carcinoma: similar to that for small cell lung cancer or non-small cell lung cancer? *Lung Cancer*. 2012;77(2):365-370.
43. Le Treut J, Sault MC, Lena H, et al. Multicentre phase II study of cisplatin-etoposide chemotherapy for advanced large-cell neuroendocrine lung carcinoma: the GFPC 0302 study. *Ann Oncol*. 2013;24(6):1548-1552.
44. Niho S, Kenmotsu H, Sekine I, et al. Combination chemotherapy with irinotecan and cisplatin for large-cell neuroendocrine carcinoma of the lung: a multicenter phase II study. *J Thorac Oncol*. 2013;8(7):980-984.
45. Iyoda A, Makino T, Koezuka S, et al. Treatment options for patients with large cell neuroendocrine carcinoma of the lung. *Gen Thorac Cardiovasc Surg*. 2014;62(6):351-356.
46. Filosso PL, Ruffini E, Oliaro A, et al. Large-cell neuroendocrine carcinoma of the lung: a clinicopathologic study of eighteen cases and the efficacy of adjuvant treatment with octreotide. *J Thorac Cardiovasc Surg*. 2005;129(4):819-824.

14 Management of Pleural Mesothelioma

Anish Thomas and Raffit Hassan

INTRODUCTION

Malignant mesothelioma is an aggressive tumor that arises from the serosal surfaces of pleura, pericardium, peritoneum, or the tunica vaginalis. Up to 3,000 patients are affected annually in the United States. The pleura is the most common primary site, accounting for 80% to 90% of cases, and the majority of patients are older adults with a median age at presentation of 74 years (1). Although most cases are attributed to asbestos exposure, roughly 20% of patients have no significant exposure to asbestos. Nonasbestos-related risk factors are not fully understood, but include prior radiation exposure, exposure to nonasbestos mineral fibers, such as erionite, and genetic predisposition. The latter includes germline mutations in the gene encoding BRCA1-associated protein-1 (*BAP1*) that are linked to susceptibility to mesothelioma, uveal and cutaneous melanoma, renal cell cancer, and possibly other cancers (2,3).

CLINICAL PRESENTATION AND DIAGNOSIS

Mesothelioma is a locally invasive tumor, which usually presents with unilateral involvement of the pleural cavity (Figures 14.1 and 14.2). Early symptoms reflect the pleural origin of the tumor and include dyspnea on exertion and chest discomfort. Invasion of adjacent structures, including the lungs, mediastinum, and chest wall, frequently manifests as pleuritic chest pain, dry, nonproductive cough, chest wall masses, and dysphagia. Constitutional symptoms, such as anorexia, weight loss, fever, and night sweats, are common. Distant metastases are uncommon in the early stages of disease, but do occur in patients with advanced disease. Common findings on physical exam include those indicative of a unilateral pleural effusion.

Diagnostic work-up commonly starts with imaging studies, usually chest CT, and thoracentesis with cytological analysis of pleural fluid in cases with pleural effusion. However, pleural fluid analysis and closed pleural biopsy are inconclusive in the majority of cases. Video-assisted thoracoscopic surgery (VATS) is the

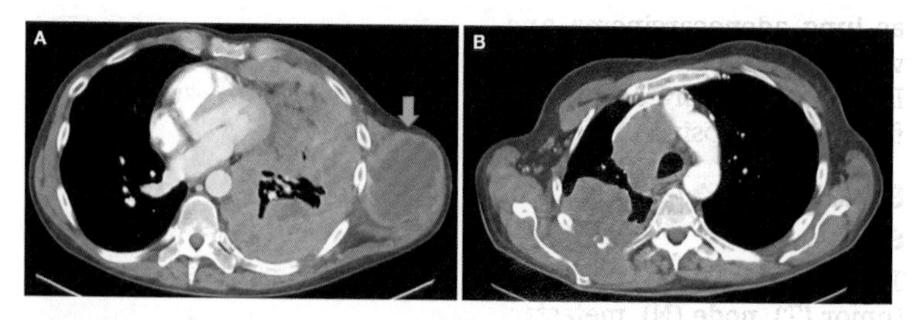

Figure 14.1 **CT Showing Pleural Mesothelioma: (A) Involving the Left Hemithorax and Chest Wall (Indicated by the Bold Arrow); (B) Right Hemithorax, Chest Wall, and Mediastinum**

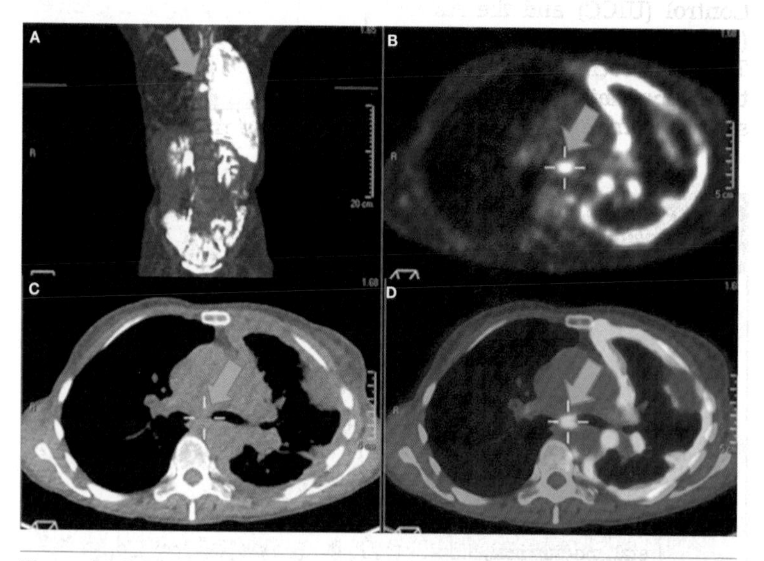

Figure 14.2 **Positron-Emission Tomography (PET; A and B), CT (C), and PET-CT Fusion (D) Showing Pleural Mesothelioma Involving the Left Hemithorax in a Characteristic Rind-Like Pattern With an Enlarged, Metabolically Active Subcarinal Lymph Node (Indicated by the Bold Arrow)**

preferred method for surgical diagnosis of mesothelioma. This procedure yields sufficient tissue to establish the diagnosis of mesothelioma, characterize the histological subtype, and distinguish mesothelioma from other tumors.

Three major histologic subtypes have been recognized: epithelioid, sarcomatoid, and a mixture of both, referred to as the biphasic subtype (4). Of the three subtypes, epithelioid tumors are the most common and have a better prognosis than biphasic or sarcomatoid tumors. A panel of immunohistochemical stains can usually differentiate mesothelioma from other malignancies, such as lung adenocarcinoma and sarcoma. Typically, mesothelioma will stain positively for calretinin, WT-1, cytokeratin 5/6, and D2-40, while lung adenocarcinoma will usually stain positively for TTF-1, Napsin A, CEA, BerEP4, and LeuM1.

STAGING AND PROGNOSIS

Staging

The most widely used staging system for mesothelioma is the tumor (T), node (N), metastasis (M) classification that was developed by the International Association for the Study of Lung Cancer (IASLC) and the International Mesothelioma Interest Group (IMIG), and accepted by the Union for International Cancer Control (UICC) and the American Joint Committee on Cancer (AJCC) (Tables 14.1 and 14.2) (5). It is challenging to obtain the T and N descriptors using current imaging modalities alone due to the anatomical location and pattern of spread along the pleural surface. Hence, TNM staging is most applicable for patients who

Table 14.1 TNM classification for pleural mesothelioma

Primary tumor (T)	
TX	Primary tumor cannot be assessed
T0	No evidence of primary tumor
T1	Tumor limited to the ipsilateral parietal pleura with or without mediastinal pleura and with or without diaphragmatic pleural involvement
T1a	No involvement of the visceral pleura
T1b	Tumor also involving the visceral pleura
T2	Tumor involving each of the ipsilateral pleural surfaces (parietal, mediastinal, diaphragmatic, and visceral pleura) with at least one of the following: Involvement of the diaphragmatic muscle Extension of tumor from the visceral pleura into the underlying pulmonary parenchyma
T3	Locally advanced but potentially resectable tumor; tumor involving all of the ipsilateral pleural surfaces (parietal, mediastinal, diaphragmatic, and visceral pleura) with at least one of the following: Involvement of the endothoracic fascia Extension into the mediastinal fat Solitary, completely resectable focus of tumor extending into the soft tissue of the chest wall Nontransmural involvement of the pericardium

(continued)

Table 14.1 TNM classification for pleural mesothelioma (*continued*)

T4	Locally advanced, technically unresectable tumor; tumor involving all of the ipsilateral pleural surfaces (parietal, mediastinal, diaphragmatic, and visceral pleura) with at least one of the following: Diffuse extension or multifocal masses of tumor in the chest wall, with or without associated rib destruction Direct diaphragmatic extension of the tumor to the peritoneum Direct extension of the tumor to the contralateral pleura Direct extension of the tumor to a mediastinal organ Direct extension of the tumor into the spine Tumor extending through to the internal surface of the pericardium with or without a pericardial effusion or tumor involving the myocardium
Regional lymph nodes (N)	
NX	Regional lymph node(s) cannot be assessed
N0	No regional lymph node metastases
N1	Metastases in the ipsilateral bronchopulmonary or hilar lymph node
N2	Metastases in the subcarinal or in the ipsilateral mediastinal lymph node, including the ipsilateral internal mammary and peridiaphragmatic nodes
N3	Metastases in the contralateral mediastinal, contralateral internal mammary, ipsilateral, or contralateral supraclavicular lymph nodes
Distant metastases (M)	
M0	No distant metastasis
M1	Distant metastasis

Table 14.2 Anatomic stage/prognostic groups for mesothelioma

Stage	T	N	M
I	T1	N0	M0
IA	T1a	N0	M0
IB	T1b	N0	M0
II	T2	N0	M0
III	T1, T2	N1	M0
	T1, T2	N2	M0
	T3	N0-2	M0
IV	T4	Any N	M0
	Any T	N3	M0
	Any T	Any N	M1

have undergone exploratory or cytoreductive surgery. Clinical staging is performed using CT and positron-emission tomography (PET) in patients with potentially resectable disease. However, these techniques have major limitations in assessing the extent of disease and have proven unreliable for staging in some studies (6).

Stage I disease is limited to the ipsilateral parietal pleura with or without mediastinal or diaphragmatic pleural involvement. Stage II involves each of the ipsilateral pleural surfaces (parietal, mediastinal, diaphragmatic, and visceral) with involvement of the diaphragmatic muscle or extension into the underlying pulmonary parenchyma. Stage III involves subcarinal or ipsilateral mediastinal lymph nodes with or without local extension of tumor into the chest wall or mediastinum. Stage IV includes contralateral mediastinal lymph node involvement, direct extension into the peritoneum through the diaphragm, diffuse involvement of the chest wall, and/or distant metastatic disease.

Prognostic Factors

In the absence of a reliable staging system, scoring systems that take into account factors beyond the extent of disease may prove to be useful to determine prognosis. Two major prognostic scoring systems have been developed: the Cancer and Leukemia Group B (CALGB) prognostic index (7) and the European Organization for Research and Treatment of Cancer (EORTC) prognostic system (8). The CALGB prognostic index was derived by examining the effect of various pretreatment clinical characteristics on the survival of patients with pleural and peritoneal mesothelioma who were accrued to various phase II clinical trials conducted by the CALGB. By univariate analyses, poor prognostic factors were poor Eastern Cooperative Oncology Group (ECOG) performance status (PS), chest pain, dyspnea, platelet count greater than 400,000/mcL, weight loss, serum lactate dehydrogenase (LDH) level greater than 500 IU/L, pleural involvement, low hemoglobin level, high white blood cell (WBC) count, and age greater than 75 years. In a multivariate analysis, pleural involvement, serum LDH greater than 500 IU/L, poor ECOG PS, chest pain, platelet count greater than 400,000/mcL, nonepithelioid histologic subtype, and age greater than 75 years predicted poor survival. Median survival ranged from 13.9 months for the best prognostic subgroup (PS 0 and age <49 years; or PS 0, age ≥49 years and hemoglobin ≥14.6) to 1.4 months for the worst subgroup (PS 1–2 and WBC ≥15.6/mcL).

The EORTC prognostic system was derived from previously untreated patients with pleural mesothelioma who were enrolled in EORTC clinical trials. In this system, the following variables predicted a poor outcome: poor PS, a high WBC count, a probable/possible histologic diagnosis of mesothelioma, male gender, and sarcomatoid histologic subtype. The median survival ranged from 10.8 months for the low-risk group (0–2 poor prognostic factors) to 5.5 months for the high-risk group (3–5 poor prognostic factors).

MANAGEMENT OF PLEURAL MESOTHELIOMA

Pleural mesothelioma remains localized to the hemithorax for most of the disease course. Regardless of the stage at diagnosis, drainage of malignant pleural effusions can effectively palliate effusion-related symptoms, such as dyspnea and pain. Periodic thoracentesis can be used to manage pleural effusions that reaccumulate slowly. Various approaches including pleurodesis and indwelling pleural catheters (which can be drained periodically) may be used to address rapidly reaccumulating pleural effusions. Pleurodesis involves complete drainage of the effusion via a chest tube or thoracoscopy followed by obliteration of the pleural space by forming adhesions between the visceral and parietal pleura. This is achieved by introducing agents, such as talc, which induce an inflammatory response in the pleural space. Video-assisted thoracoscopic partial pleurectomy (VAT-PP) involves thoracoscopic debulking of tumor along the parietal pleura and visceral pleural decortication to release trapped lung. VAT-PP may provide good symptom control in patients with malignant pleural effusions. However, the MesoVATS trial found no improvement in overall survival for patients who underwent VAT-PP compared with talc pleurodesis (1 year, 52% vs. 57%, respectively) (9). Additionally, the surgical complication rate and duration of hospital stay were significantly longer after VAT-PP.

Local control of disease with surgery is an important aspect of the care of patients who present with early stage disease, generally defined as stage I and II and selected patients with stage III, where the goal is macroscopic complete resection. The first step is to determine if the tumor is surgically resectable or not. This determination is based on a number of factors including the extent of disease (denoted by stage), extent of comorbid illnesses, cardiopulmonary status, and PS. Approximately 20% of newly diagnosed patients present with a good PS and stage I to III disease. These patients have potentially resectable disease and are treated with multimodality therapy consisting of surgery, chemotherapy, and radiation therapy (RT), since surgery alone is rarely curative. The majority of patients, however, present with advanced disease and/or comorbidities that preclude surgical resection, and are therefore unresectable or inoperable. These patients are generally treated with systemic chemotherapy or palliative care.

Surgically Resectable Disease

Surgery

There are two main surgical procedures used to achieve macroscopic complete resection in mesothelioma, pleurectomy/decortication (P/D), and extrapleural pneumonectomy (EPP). EPP involves en bloc removal of the ipsilateral parietal and visceral pleura, lung, pericardium, and hemidiaphragm. P/D is a less-invasive procedure involving removal of the parietal pleura from the chest wall, mediastinum, and diaphragm, as well as removal of the visceral pleura from the ipsilateral lung. The key difference between the procedures is that the lung is removed in EPP allowing administration of definitive doses of RT postoperatively with the goal of reducing the risk of local recurrence. However, EPP is associated with substantial postoperative morbidity and mortality, which in most large volume centers is below 8% (10,11). P/D preserves the lung parenchyma and provides good control of malignant pleural effusions with a lower rate of perioperative mortality, typically in the 0% to 5% range.

In a large retrospective series of over 600 patients who underwent resection from 1990 to 2006, Flores et al. reported an operative mortality of 7% for EPP (27/385 patients) and 4% for P/D (13/278 patients) (11). Multivariate analysis demonstrated better overall survival with P/D (HR = 1.4 for EPP; $P < .001$) when controlling for stage, histology, gender, and multimodality therapy. In another retrospective series of 1,365 patients who underwent resection from 1982 to 2012, the 30-day mortality was similar between patients who underwent EPP and P/D (4.1% vs. 2.6%, respectively; $P = .4$) (12). Patients with good prognostic factors (age <70 years, epithelioid subtype, received chemotherapy) had a similar overall survival with P/D or EPP.

Although there have been no randomized comparisons of efficacy between EPP and P/D, the Mesothelioma and Radical Surgery (MARS) study did assess the feasibility of a trimodality approach in the context of EPP (13). In this study, 112 patients underwent induction platinum-based chemotherapy and 50 were then randomly assigned to EPP followed by postoperative hemithorax RT or to no EPP. Median survival was 14.4 months (95% CI 5.3–18.7) for the EPP group and 19.5 months (95% CI 13.4—not reached) for the no EPP group. It is difficult to draw definitive conclusions from this trial since it was not adequately powered to detect a survival difference between the groups, but it does reinforce concerns regarding the utility of EPP. Decisions regarding surgery for patients with mesothelioma should be made on a case-by-case basis within a multidisciplinary team consisting of experienced thoracic surgeons, radiation oncologists, medical oncologists, pulmonologists, pathologists, and radiologists.

Adjuvant RT

RT to the ipsilateral chest cavity and chest wall after EPP improves local control (14). While intensity-modulated techniques can minimize the risk of RT-induced toxicity to adjacent organs, the possibility of lethal pulmonary injury exists for patients undergoing extensive pleural RT without having undergone EPP. Therefore, RT to the lung and chest wall is not standard practice after P/D (15). The role of hemithoracic RT after neoadjuvant chemotherapy and EPP was evaluated in the randomized SAKK 17/04 trial, which enrolled patients 18 to 70 years old with resectable stage I to III (T1–3 N0–2 M0) disease and good PS (16). Patients received three cycles of neoadjuvant cisplatin plus pemetrexed followed by EPP, and those with R0-R1 resection were randomly assigned to receive high-dose RT or observation. Overall, 151 patients received neoadjuvant chemotherapy, 113 went on to EPP, and 54 were randomized to RT or observation. Median local-regional relapse-free survival was similar in both arms (9.4 months for RT vs. 7.6 months for no RT).

Adjuvant and Neoadjuvant Chemotherapy

In patients with potentially resectable mesothelioma, chemotherapy can be given preoperatively (17, 18) or postoperatively (19). In the SAKK 17/04 trial, 34% of patients who received neoadjuvant chemotherapy achieved an objective response and 75% underwent EPP, with 64% achieving an R0/R1 resection (16). Chemotherapy agents used in this setting are essentially the same as those used in patients with unresectable disease and are described in more detail in the following.

Unresectable Disease

Role of Chemotherapy

Patients with surgically unresectable disease should be considered for palliative systemic chemotherapy. Although definitive comparisons are lacking, a large body of evidence suggests that chemotherapy offers improvements in symptom control, quality of life, and survival over best supportive care alone. One trial that randomized patients to active symptom control (ASC) with or without vinorelbine or mitomycin C, vinblastine, and cisplatin (MVP) closed prematurely due to poor accrual (20). In this study, the ASC alone arm ($n = 136$) and the ASC plus chemotherapy arms (vinorelbine, $n = 136$; MVP, $n = 137$) had a similar median survival of approximately 8 months when the chemotherapy arms were combined. However, when the chemotherapy arms were analyzed independently versus ASC alone, the vinorelbine arm demonstrated a 2-month survival benefit that approached statistical significance (HR 0.80, $P = .08$). There was no evidence of a survival benefit with MVP versus ASC alone (HR 0.99, $P = .95$). Only 140 patients in the chemotherapy arms underwent formal tumor assessment after treatment, with response rates of only 10% for MVP and 16% for vinorelbine. Notably, the chemotherapy agents used in this trial are not as active as the agents currently in use.

First-Line Chemotherapy

In patients with previously untreated, advanced mesothelioma, the pivotal EMPHACIS trial demonstrated that the combination of cisplatin plus pemetrexed provided an overall survival benefit over cisplatin alone (median, 12.1 vs. 9.3 months; HR 0.77, $P = .02$) (21) (Table 14.3). This trial randomized 456 patients who were not eligible for curative surgery to pemetrexed 500 mg/m^2 plus cisplatin 75 mg/m^2 or cisplatin 75 mg/m^2 alone every 21 days. In addition to improved survival, response rates were also higher with the combination regimen (41.3% vs. 16.7%, $P < .0001$). Based on this data, the U.S. Food and Drug Administration (FDA) approved pemetrexed plus cisplatin for the treatment of patients with malignant pleural mesothelioma whose disease is either unresectable or who are not otherwise candidates for curative surgery. A similar survival benefit has been seen with the combination of raltitrexed plus cisplatin versus cisplatin alone, with survival improving from 8.8 to 11.4 months (22).

Table 14.3 First-line chemotherapy regimens for pleural mesothelioma

Chemotherapy regimen	Schedule	Reference
Cisplatin 75 mg/m^2 Pemetrexed 500 mg/m^2 Bevacizumab 15 mg/kg*	Every 3 wk	23
Cisplatin 75 mg/m^2 Pemetrexed 500 mg/m^2	Every 3 wk	21
Carboplatin AUC 5 Pemetrexed 500 mg/m^2	Every 3 wk	27
Cisplatin 75 mg/m^2 Gemcitabine 1,000–1,250 mg/m^2	Every 3–4 wk	31

*Six cycles of the three-drug combination followed by maintenance bevacizumab 15 mg/kg until disease progression or excessive toxicity.

Role of Bevacizumab

Since its approval in 2003, pemetrexed plus cisplatin was the standard first-line therapy for patients with unresectable mesothelioma. In 2016, a randomized phase III trial (IFCT-GFPC-0701) reported that the addition of bevacizumab 15 mg/kg to pemetrexed plus cisplatin significantly improved overall survival from 16.1 months to 18.8 months (HR 0.77, *P* =·.167) (23). Patients enrolled in this study were 18 to 75 years old with PS 0 to 2 and no substantial cardiovascular comorbidity. Patients on therapeutic doses of anticoagulants or antiplatelet agents and those with uncontrolled hypertension, hemoptysis, or recent major surgery were excluded. Treatment-related drug discontinuation (24.3% vs. 6%) and bevacizumab-related adverse events, such as hypertension, hemorrhage, arterial and venous thromboembolic events, and proteinuria, were higher in patients receiving bevacizumab. Of note, median overall survival of 16.1 months in the control arm in this trial was much longer than that reported with cisplatin plus pemetrexed in the EMPHACIS trial. Based on these results, the combination of bevacizumab, pemetrexed, and cisplatin may be considered a standard regimen for selected patients with unresectable malignant pleural mesothelioma who are not amenable to curative surgery and have no contraindications to bevacizumab.

Supportive Care

The addition of folic acid and vitamin B_{12} resulted in a significant reduction in toxicity, particularly grade 3/4 neutropenia and leukopenia, in the pemetrexed plus cisplatin arm of the pivotal EMPHACIS trial. Folic acid 400 to 1,000 mcg daily should be administered orally beginning 7 days prior to treatment with pemetrexed and continued during treatment and for 21 days after the last pemetrexed dose. Vitamin B_{12} 1,000 mcg should be administered intramuscularly prior to treatment initiation and repeated every three cycles. Dexamethasone 4 mg orally is administered twice a day for 3 days beginning the day before treatment to minimize cutaneous reactions from pemetrexed. Cisplatin is highly emetogenic and nephrotoxic, so the routine use of pretreatment antiemetics and hydration is recommended.

Response Assessment

Response to chemotherapy is assessed using CT scans performed at baseline and then every two to three cycles during treatment. PET scans, although not recommended for routine follow-up, may supplement CT in selected cases by providing an indication of response or progression at an earlier time point. Serum biomarkers such as mesothelin may have a role in noninvasive tumor load assessment, but have not been prospectively validated in the clinical setting (24).

Duration of First-Line Therapy

Although combination chemotherapy improves survival and has a palliative effect on symptom control and quality-of-life, it is not curative. Based on pivotal trials discussed previously (23, 25), four to six cycles is considered the optimal duration of chemotherapy. Continuation of the first-line, combination regimen beyond this point is not thought to offer any benefit in terms of response, symptom relief, quality-of-life, or survival. In addition, cumulative toxicity occurs more frequently in patients who received longer durations of treatment.

Maintenance Therapy

The role of maintenance chemotherapy after four to six cycles of first-line chemotherapy is not known. In the IFCT-GFPC-0701 trial, the group that was randomized to receive bevacizumab, pemetrexed, and cisplatin was allowed maintenance bevacizumab after six cycles of combination chemotherapy until disease progression. A randomized phase II study is addressing the role of maintenance pemetrexed (NCT01085630). In this study, patients with pleural mesothelioma who have a response or stable disease after four cycles of pemetrexed plus cisplatin or carboplatin will be randomized to continue treatment with pemetrexed alone or to observation.

Alternative First-Line Regimens

The combination of pemetrexed plus carboplatin is a reasonable alternative for patients who cannot tolerate or have contraindications to cisplatin, based on results from large phase II trials and the expanded access experience showing comparable response rates and survival times (26–28). In an Italian phase II trial with 76 patients, pemetrexed plus carboplatin resulted in an overall response rate of 25% and median survival of 14 months (27).

Second-Line Chemotherapy

The vast majority of patients who receive first-line chemotherapy for mesothelioma will eventually experience disease progression. A number of agents have shown activity in the second-line setting and beyond, but none have been evaluated in randomized clinical trials. The most studied agent is pemetrexed, although this data was primarily derived when pemetrexed was not widely used as first-line therapy (29). A phase III trial randomized patients who had relapsed after first-line chemotherapy that did not include pemetrexed to receive pemetrexed plus best supportive care or best supportive care alone. Although patients who received pemetrexed had a higher response rate (18.7% vs. 1.7%; $P < .0001$) and better progression-free survival (median, 3.6 vs. 1.5 months; $P = .148$), overall survival was not significantly different between the arms (median, 9 months). Data on the utility of retreatment with pemetrexed are not available in patients who have received pemetrexed as part of their first-line regimens. Nevertheless, re-treatment with pemetrexed is considered a reasonable second-line option in patients who had disease control on prior pemetrexed-based therapy. Other second-line chemotherapy options include vinorelbine and gemcitabine. Single-agent vinorelbine resulted in a response rate of 16% and median overall survival of 9.6 months in patients with relapsed disease (30). The reported activity with single-agent gemcitabine monotherapy has been variable, but response rates of approximately 20% have been reported in combination with platinum (31).

Immunotherapy

Immune checkpoint inhibitors remain investigational in mesothelioma, although preliminary results are encouraging. In an open-label, single arm, phase II trial, the anti-CTLA4 monoclonal antibody tremelimumab showed a disease control rate of 31% and a 1-year survival of 48% in 21 patients with progression of disease on first-line platinum plus pemetrexed (32). An updated analysis continued to show clinical benefit with a median overall survival of 11.3 months (33). However, a phase III randomized, placebo-controlled trial failed to show superiority in overall survival for tremelimumab as second- or third-line therapy in 571 patients with pleural or peritoneal mesothelioma who were randomized to tremelimumab versus placebo (median, 7.7 vs. 7.3 months; HR = 0.92, $P = .408$) (34). In another trial, 25 patients with malignant pleural mesothelioma that was positive for PD-L1 expression received pembrolizumab, an anti-PD-1 antibody, and seven experienced a partial response with 12 having stable disease (35). Avelumab, an anti-PD-L1 antibody, resulted in unconfirmed responses in 9% (5 of 53) of patients in a trial which included patients with both PD-L1-positive and PD-L1-negative pleural or peritoneal mesothelioma (36).

Palliative RT

A short course of RT can effectively control pain in some patients with mesothelioma involving the chest wall. In a single-arm phase II trial of palliative RT (20 Gy in 5 fractions), 14 of 40 (35%) patients had a clinically meaningful improvement in pain 5 weeks after treatment (37). A wide variety of doses and fractionation schemes have been used for palliative RT.

KEY POINTS

- Pleural mesothelioma is a locally invasive tumor which usually presents with unilateral involvement.
- VATS is the preferred method for surgical diagnosis of pleural mesothelioma; pleural fluid analyses and closed pleural biopsies are usually inconclusive and do not provide histological subtyping.
- For patients with recurrent pleural effusions, pleurodesis or pleural catheters may provide palliation from dyspnea and pain.
- For patients with stage I to II and selected patients with stage III mesothelioma, surgery can provide good local control where the goal is macroscopic complete resection. Since surgery alone is rarely curative, surgery is usually followed by chemotherapy and/or RT.
- There are two main surgical procedures used to achieve macroscopic complete resection, P/D, and EPP; decisions regarding the utility of surgery for a patient should be individualized through discussion with a multidisciplinary team.
- Patients with surgically unresectable disease are considered for palliative systemic chemotherapy. Cisplatin or carboplatin plus pemetrexed for four to six cycles is the standard first-line regimen. Selected patients may benefit from the addition of bevacizumab to first-line chemotherapy.
- Gemcitabine or vinorelbine can be used as second-line or third-line therapy, though activity is limited. Clinical trials should be strongly encouraged in this setting.

REFERENCES

1. National Institute for Occupational Safety and Health (NIOSH). Malignant mesothelioma. Number of deaths by sex, race, age, median age at death, and anatomical site, U.S. residents age 15 and over, 1999–2007. Mortality multiple cause-of-death data from National Center for Health Statistics, National Vital Statistics System. https://wwwn.cdc.gov/eworld/Data/Malignant_mesothelioma_Number_of_deaths_by_sex_race_age_group_and_median_age_at_death_US_residents_age_15_and_over_20012010/434
2. Testa JR, Cheung M, Pei J, et al. Germline BAP1 mutations predispose to malignant mesothelioma. *Nat Genet*. 2011;43(10):1022-1025.
3. Carbone M, Yang H, Pass HI, et al. BAP1 and cancer. *Nat Rev Cancer*. 2013;13(3):153-159.
4. Travis WD, Brambilla E, Muller-Hermelink H, Harris CC. *Pathology and Genetics of Tumours of the Lung, Pleura, Thymus, and Heart*. World Health Organization Classification of Tumours. Lyon, France: IARC Press; 2004.
5. American Joint Committee on Cancer. Pleural mesothelioma. In: Edge SB, Byrd DR, Compton CC, Fritz AG, Greene FL, Trotti A, et al. *Pleural Mesothelioma. AJCC Cancer Staging Manual*. 7th ed. New York, NY: Springer; 2010:chap 26.
6. Steele JP. Prognostic factors in mesothelioma. *Semin Oncol*. 2002; 29(1):36-40.
7. Herndon JE, Green MR, Chahinian AP, et al. Factors predictive of survival among 337 patients with mesothelioma treated between 1984 and 1994 by the Cancer and Leukemia Group B. *Chest*. 1998;113(3):723-731.
8. Curran D, Sahmoud T, Therasse P, et al. Prognostic factors in patients with pleural mesothelioma: the European Organization for Research and Treatment of Cancer experience. *J Clin Oncol*. 1998;16(1):145-152.
9. Rintoul RC, Ritchie AJ, Edwards JG, et al. Efficacy and cost of video-assisted thoracoscopic partial pleurectomy versus talc pleurodesis in patients with malignant pleural mesothelioma (MesoVATS): an open-label, randomised, controlled trial. *Lancet*. 2014;384(9948):1118-1127.
10. Rusch VW, Piantadosi S, Holmes EC. The role of extrapleural pneumonectomy in malignant pleural mesothelioma. A Lung-Cancer Study-Group trial. *J Thorac Cardiovasc Surg*. 1991;102(1):1-9.
11. Flores RM, Pass HI, Seshan VE, et al. Extrapleural pneumonectomy versus pleurectomy/decortication in the surgical management of malignant pleural mesothelioma: results in 663 patients. *J Thorac Cardiovasc Surg*. 2008;135(3):620-626.
12. Bovolato P, Casadio C, Bille A, et al. Does surgery improve survival of patients with malignant pleural mesothelioma?: a multicenter retrospective analysis of 1365 consecutive patients. *J Thorac Oncol*. 2014;9(3):390-396.
13. Treasure T, Lang-Lazdunski L, Waller D, et al. Extra-pleural pneumonectomy versus no extra-pleural pneumonectomy for patients

with malignant pleural mesothelioma: clinical outcomes of the Mesothelioma and Radical Surgery (MARS) randomised feasibility study. *Lancet Oncol*. 2011;12(8):763-772.

14. Rusch VW, Rosenzweig K, Venkatraman E, et al. A phase II trial of surgical resection and adjuvant high-dose hemithoracic radiation for malignant pleural mesothelioma. *J Thorac Cardiovasc Surg*. 2001;122(4):788-795.
15. Gupta V, Mychalczak B, Krug L, et al. Hemithoracic radiation therapy after pleurectomy/decortication for malignant pleural mesothelioma. *Int J Radiat Oncol Biol Phys*. 2005;63(4):1045-1052.
16. Stahel RA, Riesterer O, Xyrafas A, et al. Neoadjuvant chemotherapy and extrapleural pneumonectomy of malignant pleural mesothelioma with or without hemithoracic radiotherapy (SAKK 17/04): a randomised, international, multicentre phase 2 trial. *Lancet Oncol*. 2015;16(16):1651-1658.
17. Krug LM, Pass HI, Rusch VW, et al. Multicenter phase II trial of neoadjuvant pemetrexed plus cisplatin followed by extrapleural pneumonectomy and radiation for malignant pleural mesothelioma. *J Clin Oncol*. 2009;27(18):3007-3013.
18. Weder W, Stahel RA, Bernhard J, et al. Multicenter trial of neoadjuvant chemotherapy followed by extrapleural pneumonectomy in malignant pleural mesothelioma. *Ann Oncol*. 2007;18(7):1196-1202.
19. Sugarbaker DJ, Flores RM, Jaklitsch MT, et al. Resection margins, extrapleural nodal status, and cell type determine postoperative long-term survival in trimodality therapy of malignant pleural mesothelioma: results in 183 patients. *J Thorac Cardiovasc Surg*. 1999;117(1):54-63.
20. Muers MF, Stephens RJ, Fisher P, et al. Active symptom control with or without chemotherapy in the treatment of patients with malignant pleural mesothelioma (MS01): a multicentre randomised trial. *Lancet*. 2008;371(9625):1685-1694.
21. Vogelzang NJ, Rusthoven JJ, Symanowski J, et al. Phase III study of pemetrexed in combination with cisplatin versus cisplatin alone in patients with malignant pleural mesothelioma. *J Clin Oncol*. 2003;21(14):2636-2644.
22. van Meerbeeck JP, Gaafar R, Manegold C, et al. Randomized phase III study of cisplatin with or without raltitrexed in patients with malignant pleural mesothelioma: an intergroup study of the European Organisation for Research and Treatment of Cancer Lung Cancer Group and the National Cancer Institute of Canada. *J Clin Oncol*. 2005;23(28):6881-6889.
23. Zalcman G, Mazieres J, Margery J, et al. Bevacizumab for newly diagnosed pleural mesothelioma in the Mesothelioma Avastin Cisplatin Pemetrexed Study (MAPS): a randomised, controlled, open-label, phase 3 trial. *Lancet*. 2015;387:1405-1414.
24. Servais EL, Colovos C, Suzuki K, et al. Mesothelin is a biomarker of tumor aggressiveness and therapy response in malignant pleural mesothelioma (MPM). *J Am Coll Surg*. 2010;211(3):S36-S37.

25. Vogelzang NJ, Rusthoven JJ, Symanowski J, et al. Phase III study of pemetrexed in combination with cisplatin versus cisplatin alone in patients with malignant pleural mesothelioma. *J Clin Oncol.* 2003;21(14):2636-2644.
26. Ceresoli GL, Castagneto B, Zucali PA, et al. Pemetrexed plus carboplatin in elderly patients with malignant pleural mesothelioma: combined analysis of two phase II trials. *Br J Cancer.* 2008;99(1):51-56.
27. Castagneto B, Botta M, Aitini E, et al. Phase II study of pemetrexed in combination with carboplatin in patients with malignant pleural mesothelioma (MPM). *Ann Oncol.* 2008;19(2):370-373.
28. Santoro A, O'Brien ME, Stahel RA, et al. Pemetrexed plus cisplatin or pemetrexed plus carboplatin for chemonaive patients with malignant pleural mesothelioma: results of the International Expanded Access Program. *J Thorac Oncol.* 2008;3(7):756-763.
29. Jassem J, Ramlau R, Santoro A, et al. Phase III trial of pemetrexed plus best supportive care compared with best supportive care in previously treated patients with advanced malignant pleural mesothelioma. *J Clin Oncol.* 2008;26(10):1698-1704.
30. Stebbing J, Powles T, McPherson K, et al. The efficacy and safety of weekly vinorelbine in relapsed malignant pleural mesothelioma. *Lung Cancer.* 2009;63(1):94-97.
31. Kindler HL, van Meerbeeck JP. The role of gemcitabine in the treatment of malignant mesothelioma. *Semin Oncol.* 2002;29(1):70-76.
32. Calabro L, Morra A, Fonsatti E, et al. Tremelimumab for patients with chemotherapy-resistant advanced malignant mesothelioma: an open-label, single-arm, phase 2 trial. *Lancet Oncol.* 2013;14(11): 1104-1111.
33. Sartor O, Coleman R, Nilsson S, et al. Effect of radium-223 dichloride on symptomatic skeletal events in patients with castration-resistant prostate cancer and bone metastases: results from a phase 3, double-blind, randomised trial. *Lancet Oncol.* 2014;15(7):738-746.
34. Kindler HL, Scherpereel A, Calabrò L, et al. Tremelimumab as second- or third-line treatment of unresectable malignant mesothelioma (MM): Results from the global, double-blind, placebo-controlled DETERMINE study. *J Clin Oncol.* 2016;34(suppl; abstr 8502).
35. Alley EW, Molife LR, Santoro A, et al. Clinical safety and efficacy of pembrolizumab (MK-3475) in patients with malignant pleural mesothelioma: preliminary results from KEYNOTE-028. *AACR* 2015;75:103.
36. Hassan R, Thomas A, Patel MR, et al. Avelumab (MSB0010718C; anti-PD-L1) in patients with advanced unresectable mesothelioma from the JAVELIN solid tumor phase Ib trial: safety, clinical activity, and PD-L1 expression. *J Clin Oncol.* 2016;34(suppl; abstr 8503).
37. MacLeod N, Chalmers A, O'Rourke N, et al. Is radiotherapy useful for treating pain in mesothelioma? *J Thorac Oncol.* 2015;10(6):944-950.

15 Management of Thymic Tumors

Sukhmani K. Padda, Bryan M. Burt, and Heather A. Wakelee

INTRODUCTION

Epidemiology

Thymic epithelial tumors (TETs), including thymomas and thymic carcinomas, are derived from thymic epithelium and occur in the anterior mediastinum. The thymus is a critical organ that cultivates the immune system's T-cell repertoire (1). Because of the role of the thymus in the immune system, TETs (thymomas more so than thymic carcinomas) are associated with autoimmune paraneoplastic syndromes, and a higher risk of second malignancies (2,3). Thymomas are rare, with an estimated incidence of 0.13 per 100,000 person-years in the United States (2) and 1.4 million per year (1.7 million per year for all TETs) in Europe (4). Thymic carcinoma is even rarer than thymoma. The incidence of TETs is similar in both men and women. In the United States, thymoma is uncommon in children and young adults, but the incidence rises with age, peaking in the seventh decade (2).

Etiology

The etiology of TETs is unknown and their biology is complex. There are no known infectious or environmental risk factors.

International Thymic Malignancy Interest Group

The International Thymic Malignancy Interest Group (ITMIG) was formed to advance research in TETs and its inaugural meeting was held in August 2009 (5). The goals of the organization are to tackle research priorities for TETs (e.g., tissue banking), to provide standardized language among researchers (e.g., uniform staging system, standard outcome measures), and to develop and analyze the ITMIG worldwide retrospective and prospective patient databases (www.itmig.org). Throughout this chapter, ITMIG guidelines and policies are prioritized.

HISTOLOGY OF TETs

The *2015 WHO Classification of Tumors of the Thymus*, fourth edition, has recently been published (6,7). All thymomas have malignant potential and should not be categorized as benign, even if they appear to be noninvasive early stage tumors. The very rare exceptions are microscopic and micronodular thymomas, for which no tumor-related deaths have been reported. Updates in the classification of TETs from the new edition are detailed here.

WHO Classification

Thymomas are classified into the following categories: A, AB, B1, B2, and B3 (6,7). The *WHO* fourth edition has implemented "obligatory/indispensable" criteria and "optional" criteria for the classification of thymomas to make the system more reproducible (Table 15.1). The two major types of thymoma are type A and type B. They differ in the shape of the epithelial tumor cell (A—bland, spindle-shaped; B—polygonal or dendritic). Type B is further categorized by the degree of atypia of the epithelial cells and the relative abundance of the lymphocytic infiltrate. Thymomas that have features of both type A and type B1 are classified as type AB. In mixed tumors with more than one histologic subtype, all subtypes should be listed with the most prominent listed first and minor components quantified in 10% increments. The exceptions are type AB thymoma, which is its own distinct entity, and tumors containing both thymic carcinoma and thymoma, which are classified as combined thymic carcinoma. In the ITMIG retrospective database, the most common to least common histologic types are: B2 (28%), AB (23%), B3 (21%), B1 (17%), and A (11%) (8). The many subtypes of thymic carcinoma are listed in Table 15.1, with the most frequent being squamous cell carcinoma.

Immunohistochemistry to Assist in the Diagnosis of TETs

Immunohistochemistry (IHC) can be useful when the diagnosis of TET is not clear (6). Pan-cytokeratin antibodies stain epithelial cells of normal thymus, thymoma, and neuroendocrine tumors, although there are rare cytokeratin-negative thymomas. Cytokeratin 19 is expressed on epithelial cells of normal thymus, thymoma, and thymic carcinoma, while cytokeratin 20 is *not* expressed in normal thymus and thymoma, but may be found in thymic adenocarcinoma. P63 and P40 antibodies stain the nuclei of normal and neoplastic thymic epithelial cells. TdT antibodies stain immature T cells in the normal thymus and in

Table 15.1 WHO Histologic Subtypes of Thymic Epithelial Tumors

WHO classification	Epithelial cells (shape and distribution)	TdT⁺ lymphocytes (quantity and distribution)	Other
Thymoma			
A	Bland, spindle-shaped At least focal	Paucity[a] or absence Throughout	
Atypical type A variant	Bland, spindle-shaped At least focal	Paucity or absence Throughout	Comedo-type tumor necrosis; high mitotic count (>4/2 mm^2); nuclear crowding
AB	Bland, spindle-shaped At least focal	Abundance[a] Focal or Throughout	
B1	Paucity of polygonal or dendritic epithelial cells without clustering (<3 contiguous)	Abundance	Thymus-like architecture and cytology; areas of medullary differentiation (medullary islands)
B2	More polygonal or dendritic shaped, single or clustered	Abundance Intermingled	
B3	Polygonal slight to moderate atypia, sheets	Paucity or absence Intermingled	Absent or rare intercellular bridges
MNT (micronodular thymoma with lymphoid stroma)	Bland spindle or oval shaped, nodules	Epithelial cell-free lymphoid stroma	
Metaplastic thymoma	Biphasic tumor, solid area of epithelial cells in background of bland-spindle cells	Absence	

(continued)

Table 15.1 WHO Histologic Subtypes of Thymic Epithelial Tumors (*continued*)

WHO classification	Epithelial cells (shape and distribution)	TdT+ lymphocytes (quantity and distribution)	Other
Thymoma			
Rare others	Microscopic thymoma, sclerosing thymoma, lipofibroadenoma		
Thymic carcinoma	**Subtypes**		
	Squamous cell carcinoma Basaloid carcinoma Mucoepidermoid carcinoma Lymphoepithelioma-like carcinoma Clear cell carcinoma Sarcomatoid carcinoma Adenocarcinomas *—Papillary adenocarcinoma* *—Thymic carcinoma with adenoid cystic carcinoma-like features* *—Mucinous adenocarcinoma* *—Adenocarcinoma NOS* NUT carcinoma Undifferentiated carcinoma Other rare thymic carcinomas *—Adenosquamous carcinoma* *—Hepatoid carcinoma* *—Thymic carcinoma, NOS*		

Source: Adapted from Ref. (6). Marx A, Chan JK, Coindre JM, et al. The 2015 World Health Organization Classification of Tumors of the Thymus: continuity and changes. *J Thorac Oncol*. 2015;10:1383-1395.
[a]Abundance = "any area of crowded immature T cells or moderate numbers of immature T cells in more than 10% of the investigated tumor"; TdT, marker of immature T lymphocytes.

greater than 90% of thymomas. CD5 is found on immature and mature T cells of the thymus and greater than 90% of thymomas, and on epithelial cells in 70% of thymic carcinomas. CD20 antibodies stain normal and neoplastic B-cells, and epithelial cells in 50% of type A and AB thymomas. CD117 (c-kit) is expressed on the epithelial cells in 80% of thymic carcinomas.

PROGNOSTIC FACTORS

Masaoka and Masaoka-Koga Stage

Stage, as defined by the Masaoka and Masaoka-Koga classification systems, is an independent prognostic factor for thymoma (8). These staging systems are discussed in more detail in the following and in Table 15.2. In the ITMIG retrospective database, overall survival and cumulative incidence of recurrence (CIR) progressively worsened in patients who underwent R0 (complete) resection as stage increased from stages I/II to III to IVA to IVB. The prognostic significance of stage was also validated in a multivariate analysis.

WHO Histologic Classification

The prognostic impact of the WHO histologic classification is controversial (8). In a broad review of the literature, patients with thymic carcinoma consistently had worse clinical outcomes than those with thymoma, and those with type B3 thymoma appeared to have intermediate outcomes (13). However, the association of the other WHO subtypes with clinical outcome is less consistent. In the ITMIG retrospective database, there was a significant association between histology and stage, with relatively equivalent early stage distribution in types A and AB thymoma, but increasingly higher stage representation in B1, B2, and B3 thymoma (8). After adjusting for age, stage, and resection status, histology was not an independent factor associated with overall survival. However, histology was an independent factor associated with CIR, and histology may be more prognostic in earlier stage disease.

Resection Status

The prognostic significance of stage and histology can be overcome by achieving a complete (R0) resection. In a multivariate analysis of the ITMIG retrospective database, resection status was an independent prognostic factor (8). In a report from Japan, the 5-year survival rates for patients who underwent total resection or subtotal resection, or were inoperable 93%, 64%, and 36%, respectively, in stage III and IV thymoma, and 67%, 30%, and 24%, respectively, in thymic carcinoma (14).

DIAGNOSIS

History and Physical Exam

TETs are commonly found incidentally as an anterior mediastinal mass on imaging studies performed for other reasons. However, one-third of patients with TETs present with local symptoms, including pain, superior vena cava syndrome, dyspnea, cough, or tachycardia, or systemic symptoms including weight loss or fever.

Table 15.2 Masaoka-Koga staging and newly proposed IASLC/ITMIG TNM staging

Masaoka-Koga staging (9,10,12)			10-y OS (R0) ALL[d]	10-y CIR (R0) Thymoma[e]	10-y CIR (R0) TC[e]
I	Grossly and microscopically completely encapsulated tumor[a]		84%	8% (I/II)	25% (I/II)
IIa	Microscopic transcapsular invasion		83% (IIA/B)	–	–
IIb	Macroscopic invasion into thymic or surrounding fatty tissue[b], or grossly adherent to but not breaking through mediastinal pleura or pericardium		–	–	–
III	Macroscopic invasion into neighboring organs (i.e., great vessel, lung, pericardium)[c]		70%	29%	60%
IVa	Pleural or pericardial metastases		42%	71%	76%
IVb	Lymphogenous or hematogenous metastasis		53%	57%	61%
Stage (11)	**TNM**	**Details**			
I	**T1**N0M0	T1, tumor limited to the thymus with or without encapsulation, directly invades into the mediastinal fat only or directly invades the mediastinal pleura -T1a (no mediastinal pleural involvement) -T1b (direct invasion of the mediastinal pleura)	88% T: 88% TC: 72%	8%	26%

(*continued*)

Table 15.2 Masaoka-Koga staging and newly proposed IASLC/ITMIG TNM staging (*continued*)

IASLC/ITMIG TNM stage (11)			10-y OS (R0)	10-y CIR (R0)	10-y CIR (R0)
Stage	TNM	Details	ALL	Thymoma	TC
II	**T2**N0M0	T2, tumor directly invading pericardium	73% T: 77% TC: 60%	22%	46%
IIIa	**T3**N0M0	T3, tumor directly invading into any of the following: lung, brachiocephalic vein, superior vena cava, phrenic nerve, chest wall, or extrapericardial pulmonary artery or vein	73% T: 78% TC: 50%	36%	60%
IIIb	**T4**N0M0	T4, tumor invading into any of the following: aorta (ascending, arch, or descending), arch vessels, intrapericardial pulmonary artery, myocardium, trachea, esophagus	68% T: 77% TC: 48%	40%	50%
IVa	-T any **N1** M0 -T any N0,1 **M1a**	-N0, no nodal involvement -N1, anterior (perithymic) nodes -M0, no metastatic pleural, pericardial, or distant sites -M1a, separate pleural or pericardial nodule(s)	50% T: 60% TC: 31%	71%	74%

(*continued*)

Table 15.2 Masaoka-Koga staging and newly proposed IASLC/ITMIG TNM staging (*continued*)

IASLC/ITMIG TNM stage (11)					
Stage	TNM	Details	10-y OS (R0) ALL	10-y CIR (R0) Thymoma	10-y CIR (R0) TC
IVb	-T any **N2** M0,1a -T any N any **M1b**	-N2, deep intrathoracic or cervical nodes -M1b, pulmonary intraparenchymal nodule or distant organ metastasis	56% T: 76% TC: 31%	45%	59%

CIR, cumulative incidence of recurrence; OS, overall survival; T, thymoma; TC, thymic carcinoma; R0, completely resected.

[a]Invasion into but not through the capsule is classified as stage I and a partially absent capsule is not necessarily consistent with invasion.

[b]Macroscopic invasion must also be microscopically confirmed.

[c]Any involvement (either partial or penetrating) of mediastinal pleura or pericardium classified as stage III; also includes invasion into phrenic or vagus nerves.

[d]Overall survival analysis defined by pathologic Masaoka-Koga stage.

[e]Masaoka-Koga stage and Masaoka stage combined for analysis.

Source: Adapted from: Girard N, Ruffini E, Marx A, et al. Thymic epithelial tumours: ESMO clinical practice guidelines. Ann Oncol. 2015;26 (suppl 5): v40-v55 (12); Detterbeck FC, Nicholson AG, Kondo K, et al. The Masaoka-Koga stage classification for thymic malignancies: clarification and definition of terms. *J Thorac Oncol*. 2011;6:S1710-S1716 (9); and Detterbeck FC, Stratton K, Giroux D, et al. The IASLC/ITMIG Thymic Epithelial Tumors Staging Project: proposal for an evidence-based stage classification system for the forthcoming (8th) edition of the TNM classification of malignant tumors. *J Thorac Oncol*. 2014;9:S65-S72 (11); Detterbeck F. MS16.2—Towards a TNM-based prognostic classification for thymic tumours. 15th World Conference on Lung Cancer. Sydney, Australia, October 27-30, 2013 (10).

Thymomas are associated with a variety of autoimmune paraneoplastic syndromes, most commonly myasthenia gravis, which occurs in up to 40% of patients (15,16). Thus, special attention should be paid to the neurologic exam. Hypogammaglobulinemia (Good's syndrome) and pure red cell aplasia are observed in less than 1% of patients as reported in the ITMIG retrospective database.

Laboratory

Routine laboratory evaluation should include a complete blood count and a reticulocyte count (12,17). A serum anti-acetylcholine receptor (AChR) antibody level should be sent to evaluate for myasthenia gravis. Serum immunoglobulins and additional immunologic tests (e.g., flow cytometry for B-cell and T-cell subsets) may be evaluated, especially if there is a suspicion of Good's syndrome. Tumor markers to rule out germ cell tumors, such as serum beta-human chorionic gonadotropin (β-hCG) and alpha-fetoprotein (AFP) may be sent if clinically appropriate.

Imaging

Differential Diagnosis of Mediastinal Masses

Primary anterior mediastinal tumors comprise 50% of all mediastinal masses (18,19). Although thymoma is the most common tumor of the anterior mediastinum, additional malignant considerations include thymic carcinoma, thymic neuroendocrine tumor, mediastinal germ cell tumor (10%–15% of anterior mediastinal masses), lymphoma, and metastases from other primary sites. The presence of a paraneoplastic syndrome with an anterior mediastinal mass essentially clinches the diagnosis of thymoma (20). Benign conditions that can cause abnormal mediastinal masses include thymic hyperplasia, thymic cyst (3% of anterior mediastinal masses), mediastinal goiter, mediastinal parathyroid adenoma, aortic aneurysm, granulomatous disease, and pericardial cyst (18,19). It is important to differentiate between TETs and other entities, both benign and malignant, since management can be drastically different.

Chest Radiography

On chest radiography, thymoma appears as a smooth, ovoid mass with well-defined margins, located anywhere from the thoracic inlet to the cardiophrenic angle (21). An irregular pulmonary border suggests invasiveness into the lung, while an elevated hemidiaphragm indicates invasion of the phrenic nerve. Metastatic pleural nodules may also be seen on chest radiography.

Computed Tomography

The initial workup for a mediastinal mass must include a CT chest with contrast (12,17,21,22). Contrast should be given if there are no contraindications since it is critical for clinical staging. Although formal staging is based on pathologic findings, CT imaging and clinical staging are essential in guiding therapy. The diagnosis of thymoma is strongly suggested by a CT scan demonstrating a well-circumscribed, solid, anterior mediastinal mass without low-density areas representing the cystic and fatty components of a teratoma (20). Most thymomas appear solid and homogeneous, but up to a third may be necrotic, hemorrhagic, or cystic. CT scan has been shown to be equal or superior to MRI in diagnosing anterior mediastinal masses, except thymic cysts for which MRI is superior (diagnostic accuracy CT 46% vs. MRI 71%) (22).

ITMIG has formulated "standard report terms" that should be used to describe the characteristics of an anterior mediastinal mass that is suspicious for thymoma on CT (Table 15.3) (23).

Table 15.3 ITMIG "Standard Report Terms" for an anterior mediastinal mass suspicious for thymoma on computed tomography
Primary tumor size: *X*-axis (longest dimension on axial slice), *Y*-axis (perpendicular to longest dimension), and *Z*-axis (craniocaudal dimension)
Location
Contour: smooth vs. lobulated
Attenuation: heterogeneous vs. homogeneous vs. cystic
Presence of calcifications: yes vs. no
Infiltration of surrounding mediastinal fat: yes vs. no
Tumor abutting ≥50% mediastinal structures with loss of fat plane: yes (list structures) vs. no
Direct vascular invasion: yes (list blood vessels) vs. no
Mediastinal lymph node enlargement (short axis >1 cm on axial image): yes (list location) vs. no
Presence of adjacent lung abnormalities: yes vs. no
Pleural effusion: yes (unilateral/bilateral) vs. no
Diaphragm elevation: yes vs. no
Pleural nodules: yes (unilateral/bilateral) vs. no
Pulmonary nodules: yes vs. no
Distant extrathoracic metastases: yes (location) vs. no

Source: From Ref. (23). Marom EM, Rosado-de-Christenson ML, Bruzzi JF, et al. Standard report terms for chest computed tomography reports of anterior mediastinal masses suspicious for thymoma. *J Thorac Oncol.* 2011;6 (7 suppl 3):S1717-S1723.

CT Factors Associated With Invasiveness and Resectability

Many studies have examined the association of CT features with the invasiveness of thymoma. In one study of 99 patients, a multivariate analysis found that tumor size ≥7 cm, lobulated contour, and infiltration of mediastinal fat were associated with invasive thymoma (Masaoka stage III–IV) (24). In another study of 133 patients who underwent surgery, the degree of abutment of adjacent vessels and pleural nodularity was associated with an incomplete resection (25). These studies emphasize the importance of the radiologist in the management of TETs as some of these features may help in deciding whether or not to administer preoperative chemotherapy or to proceed directly to surgery.

Magnetic Resonance Imaging

MRI of the chest should be performed in patients in whom a CT with contrast is contraindicated, such as those with iodine allergy or renal insufficiency, for adequate evaluation of mediastinal vessels and clinical staging (21). MRI also has an advantage over CT as a follow-up exam, because of the lack of cumulative radiation. A variety of MRI techniques, such as chemical shift imaging, dynamic imaging, and multishot spiral sequencing, can be used to differentiate normal thymus from tumor or thymoma from other mediastinal tumors and to identify phrenic nerve involvement. The major disadvantage of MRI is that nonradiologists are more comfortable interpreting CT images than MRI images.

Positron Emission Tomography-CT

Positron emission tomography-CT (PET-CT) is optional in the workup of TETs (12,17). On ^{18}F-fluorodeoxyglucose (FDG)–PET, thymomas have a variable standard uptake value (SUV), but it is generally low, while thymic carcinomas tend to have a higher SUV. However, benign lesions (e.g., thymic hyperplasia) and other malignant lesions in the mediastinum (e.g., lymphoma) may also be highly FDG-avid. PET may be most useful in patients with aggressive thymic tumors (type B3 thymoma or thymic carcinoma), in advanced disease, and in recurrent disease. Several reports have correlated the level of metabolic PET activity (i.e., SUV) with histology, but the association with stage is less robust (26,27). Although the hope was that PET would improve identification of stage III disease, it has not been able to reliably differentiate early stage from more advanced stage disease (21).

Octreotide Scan

Indium-111 octreotide scan is used to help identify patients with unresectable/metastatic tumors who may respond to treatment with octreotide after failure of conventional chemotherapy (12). An octreotide scan is not generally indicated at initial diagnosis.

Biopsy

TETs do not need to be biopsied if the clinical and radiographic characteristics are highly suspicious and the mass is deemed primarily resectable (28). If a biopsy is necessary, then a variety of approaches can be employed depending on the location of the mass, including fine needle aspiration (FNA), core needle biopsy, and surgical biopsy (video-assisted thoracoscopic surgery [VATS], anterior mediastinotomy, mini-thoracotomy, Chamberlain procedure). Caution should be taken when biopsying mediastinal cystic lesions given the potential for infection. For the most common location of thymoma in the anterior mediastinum, transthoracic ultrasound or CT-guided FNA and biopsy are generally used. The sensitivity and specificity of mediastinal biopsy are 71% to 100% and 77% to 100%, respectively, for transthoracic FNA, and 40% to 93% and 76% to 90%, respectively, for percutaneous core biopsy (28). The sensitivity for surgical biopsy is much higher (>90%). Surgical dogma dictates that a biopsy will disrupt the capsule of an early stage thymoma, resulting in tumor seeding of the biopsy tract. However, reports of such outcomes are exceedingly rare (29–31). For example, there is a case report in which CT-guided biopsy of a stage I thymoma resulted in seeding of the chest wall with recurrence 12 years later (29). VATS biopsy of an anterior mediastinal mass in which thymoma is on the differential should be avoided due to the potential for spread into the pleural space, which has been reported in the literature (32,33). If core needle biopsy fails and a diagnosis is required, a Chamberlain procedure (anterior mediastinotomy) could be performed. FNAs and biopsies should be interpreted carefully given the heterogeneity of TETs and the limited tissue specimen obtained. Pathologic findings should always be correlated with clinical findings.

STAGING

Masaoka-Koga Staging

Despite the malignant potential of thymoma and thymic carcinoma, there is no official American Joint Committee on Cancer (AJCC) or Union for International Cancer Control (UICC) staging system. Many staging systems have been proposed for thymoma. ITMIG has stated that the Masaoka-Koga staging system should be used until a validated tumor-node-metastasis (TNM) system is defined for the 2017 edition of the AJCC/UICC staging manuals (Table 15.2) (6,9). In summary, the Masaoka-Koga staging system describes the primary tumor (encapsulated or not), degree of involvement of surrounding structures (adherence or invasion), and the presence or absence of metastases (pleural/pericardial or distant). Some of the criticisms of this system include the lack of a survival difference between stage I and II disease, the heterogeneity of stage III disease, and heavy reliance on pathologic information making it poorly applicable to clinical staging.

Nuances of Masaoka-Koga Staging

The Capsule: The emphasis on the tumor capsule is not consistent with other staging systems, since the capsule is not an anatomic landmark, but rather a desmoplastic reaction caused by the tumor (9). Invasion into the capsule, but not through the capsule, is considered stage I. In tumors where the capsule is partially absent, the pathology report should explain that capsular invasion cannot be fully assessed, but the tumor should not be categorized as stage II. An unencapsulated tumor interfacing with adjacent tissue is also still considered stage I, not invasive stage IIA disease.

Microscopic Confirmation Essential: A significant ITMIG clarification is that the final Masaoka-Koga stage assignment is based only on the confirmation of *microscopic* invasion, and not on suspected macroscopic invasion.

Pleura and Pericardium—Differentiating Stages IIB and III Disease: Stage IIB tumors are macroscopically invasive and can extend up to the mediastinal pleura and pericardium without involving these structures. However, it is difficult to discern stage IIB from stage III disease. If the tumor invades the mediastinal pleura or pericardium, even partially, it is considered stage III disease. The mediastinal pleura should be labeled since it is difficult to identify retrospectively. The term "adherence" is also difficult to define in relation to stage IIB disease; however, if the tumor is so close to the pleura or pericardium that it must be resected, it should be considered "adherent."

Masaoka-Koga Stage IVB Disease: Stage IVB disease includes distant metastases and any level of lymph node involvement, including nodes in the anterior mediastinal, intrathoracic, or low or anterior cervical regions. Since some distinction should be made for distant metastases (i.e., those outside the cervical/perithymic region), it has been proposed that these sites should be labeled "pulmonary and extrathoracic metastases" rather than hematogenous metastases in order to describe the anatomical site rather than a hypothetical mechanism of spread.

Distribution of Masaoka-Koga Stage and Outcome

In a study of 8,145 patients, the distribution of Masaoka and Masaoka-Koga stage was stage I 33%, stage II 27%, stage III 23%, stage IVA 7%, and stage IVB 5% (10). The 10-year overall survival rate and CIR per Masaoka-Koga stage are shown in Table 15.2.

IASLC/ITMIG Proposed Staging for the Eighth Edition of the TNM Classification

In 2009, ITMIG and the International Association for the Study of Lung Cancer (IASLC) partnered to redefine the TET staging classifications (11). The proposed staging system is based on 10,808 patients from the databases of ITMIG and the Chinese Alliance for Research of Thymoma. These were further supplemented by the databases from the Japanese Association for Research in the Thymus (JART) and the European Society of Thoracic Surgeons (ESTS). The purpose was to develop a TNM-based staging system that applies to both thymoma and thymic carcinoma, recognizing the biologic differences between these tumors, but realizing the benefit of having a consistent system. The separation of T, N, and M categories and stage groupings were based at least partly on the ability to separate groups prognostically, examining endpoints of CIR and overall survival (Table 15.2). However, the TNM categories were also chosen based on simplicity, applicability to clinical staging, and reliability.

This staging classification is meant to describe the anatomic extent of disease. T stage is based on level of involvement, with assignment based on the highest level of structures involved, even if lower structures are uninvolved (Table 15.2). The nodal groups are based on their proximity to the thymus, including N1, anterior perithymic nodes, and N2, deep intrathoracic or cervical nodes. The nodes outside of these regions are considered metastatic disease. Metastatic disease is subdivided into M1a, separate pleural or pericardial nodules, and M1b, intraparenchymal pulmonary nodules or distant metastases. Stage groupings for stages I to IIIB are primarily based upon the T component, while stage IVA disease is determined by the presence of N1 or M1a disease and stage IVB disease by the presence of N2 or M1b disease. Overall, as stage increases, the risk of recurrence and death also increases.

MANAGEMENT OF TETs

Guidelines

The National Comprehensive Cancer Network (NCCN) has recently published an updated guideline for thymoma and thymic carcinoma (17). The European Society of Medical Oncology (ESMO) also published guidelines for TETs in 2015 (12). An experienced multidisciplinary team that includes a radiologist, pathologist, thoracic surgeon, radiation oncologist, medical oncologist, and pulmonologist should evaluate all patients with TETs given the rarity of the disease and complexity of management.

Resectable Disease

The primary decision for treatment of TETs is whether or not the tumor is resectable. If primary complete resection is possible, the patient should go directly to surgery without the need for biopsy. This usually applies to Masaoka-Koga stage I/II and some stage III tumors (Table 15.2). Thereafter, depending on the resection status, stage, and histology, surgery may be followed by radiation therapy (RT) and/or infrequently chemotherapy (34). The schema for treatment per stage is given in Figure 15.1.

Preoperative Evaluation of Myasthenia Gravis

All patients with suspected thymoma should be evaluated for myasthenia gravis because of its potential perioperative complications (35). This evaluation usually begins with a careful assessment for ocular, bulbar, and/or limb muscle weakness. The diagnosis of myasthenia gravis requires two positive confirmatory tests among pharmacologic (Tensilon test), serologic (anti-AChR antibodies), and electrodiagnostic (EMG) studies. If there is any suggestion of myasthenia gravis on initial presentation, the patient should undergo preoperative evaluation by a neurologist. Medical optimization prior to surgery using a combination of cholinesterase inhibitors, intravenous immunoglobulin, plasmapheresis,

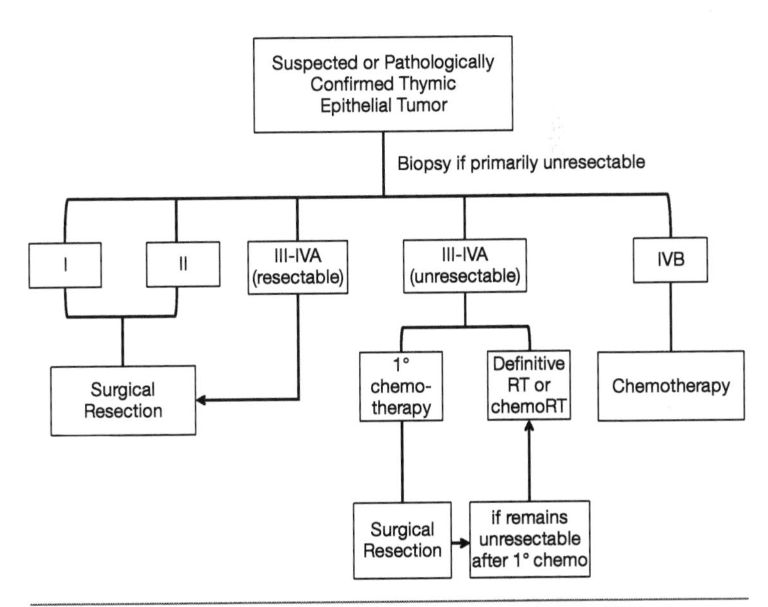

Figure 15.1 Management of Thymic Epithelial Tumors (ChemoRT, Chemoradiotherapy; RT, Radiation Therapy)

and/or corticosteroids, can help to avoid respiratory failure in the perioperative period.

Surgery for Thymoma

Masaoka-Koga stage I/II thymoma can be managed with complete resection alone. Stage III thymoma may require *en bloc* resection of lung, pericardium, innominate vein, superior vena cava, phrenic nerve, or even aorta. Depending upon the size of the tumor and its extent of invasion into such structures, stage III thymoma can be resected primarily or after a course of primary chemotherapy, which can significantly improve resectability. For a thymoma that is initially considered unresectable, primary chemotherapy followed by surgical resection can result in favorable rates of overall and disease-free survival (36). The treatment of stage IVA thymoma is controversial; however, in selected patients who are physiologically fit and have disease limited to an ipsilateral hemithorax, aggressive resections of the primary tumor and pleural metastases may be associated with favorable long-term survival. In a review of eight series of highly selected patients with stage IVA thymoma who underwent primary chemotherapy followed by surgical resection, Shapiro and Korst reported 5-year survival rates of 70% to 88%. A significant fraction of these patients had undergone either pleurectomy/decortication or extrapleural pneumonectomy (37). It is possible that intraoperative treatment of the pleural space with a local therapy (e.g., heated chemotherapy, heated betadine, photodynamic therapy) at the time of pleural resection, may improve recurrence-free survival (RFS). There is a limited role of surgery in patients with stage IVB thymoma.

Surgery for Thymic Carcinoma

While there is no standard approach for patients with thymic carcinoma, a multidisciplinary strategy is recommended since they tend to present with more advanced disease and many are only appropriate for a "subtotal" resection (14,38). In addition, thymic carcinoma has a higher incidence of nodal metastases than thymoma. Many patients with stage I to III disease and some with IVA disease are treated with a combination of surgical resection plus chemotherapy and/or RT in the postoperative setting, especially for stage III/IVA disease. For the rare thymic carcinoma patient with clearly resectable disease, surgery is considered as the primary therapeutic modality. For those with disease thought to be primarily unresectable or disease that appears to be invading one or more surrounding organs or major vascular structures, primary chemotherapy and/or RT can be administered in an attempt to improve operability and permit subsequent resection. This approach is discussed further in the section on locally advanced thymoma since the principles for management are similar for thymoma and thymic carcinoma.

Role of Debulking Surgery: "Subtotal Resection"

Debulking is utilized in some patients with thymoma in order to allow for the delivery of definitive RT (12). However, it is not recommended for thymic carcinoma. After debulking or grossly incomplete (R2) resection, postoperative chemoradiotherapy with cisplatin plus etoposide and RT of 60 Gy can be considered. In a quantitative meta-analysis of 314 patients with unresectable thymoma (stages III–IV), overall survival significantly favored patients who underwent debulking surgery over surgical biopsy (5 year, 64% vs. 35%; HR 0.45, 95% confidence interval [CI] 0.33–0.60; $P < .001$) (39). Most patients who underwent debulking surgery received postoperative RT.

Surgery for Recurrent Disease

Surgical resection plays an important role in the management of local-regional recurrence within the mediastinum and/or ipsilateral hemithorax, and complete resection of a recurrent tumor can result in improved overall survival (40).

Surgical Approach

Resection of even a small, stage I thymoma without myasthenia gravis should include removal of the entire thymus *en bloc* along with the tumor because: (a) myasthenia gravis can potentially develop postoperatively and total thymectomy is an appropriate treatment for myasthenia gravis; and (b) a second focus of tumor within the thymus is occasionally found. The traditional surgical approach for thymoma remains median sternotomy, but minimally invasive approaches, including VATS and robotic techniques, are likely equally effective for smaller tumors in experienced hands. For advanced tumors requiring extended resection, open approaches including sternotomy, thoracotomy, thoracosternotomy, and clamshell techniques can be utilized.

A number of single institution studies have suggested that minimally invasive thymectomy (MIT) using video-assisted and robotic-assisted thoracosopic approaches have improved short-term outcomes when compared with open thymectomy. Compared with open thymectomy, MIT has been associated with shorter hospital stays, shorter length of stay in the intensive care unit, lower operative blood loss, improved postoperative pulmonary function, decreased postoperative pain, and similar operating room time (41–43). The influence of MIT on oncologic outcomes, such as extent of resection and RFS, have not yet been fully determined; however, a recent meta-analysis suggested that similar oncologic outcomes can be achieved with MIT and open thymectomy (44).

Surgically Resectable Disease, But Not a Surgical Candidate

When a patient has a surgically resectable tumor, but is not medically fit to undergo surgery, definitive RT is recommended as part of a sequential chemoradiotherapy plan (12,45). As an alternative, concurrent chemotherapy with cisplatin plus etoposide and RT of 60 to 66 Gy may be offered.

Postoperative Radiation ± Chemotherapy

Postoperative treatment should be discussed in a multidisciplinary tumor board experienced in the care of patients with TETs. Resection status is a key factor in dictating administration of postoperative treatment. Additional factors like close margins, and high-risk features of advanced Masaoka-Koga stage and aggressive histology (B3 thymoma, thymic carcinoma) should also be taken into account.

Postoperative RT

Postoperative RT (PORT) after R0 resection is controversial, but PORT is recommended after R1 (microscopic) or R2 (macroscopic) incomplete resections and is typically administered within 3 months of surgery (46). Doses less than 40 Gy or greater than 64 Gy are not appropriate in the postoperative setting. Generally, a dose of 40 to 50 Gy is used for a close margin, 54 Gy for microscopically positive resection margins (R1), and 60 Gy for macroscopically positive resection margins (R2). The surgeon and pathologist must interact closely with the radiation oncologist to understand where microscopic residual disease remains. Elective nodal radiation is not recommended given the low risk for thymoma to metastasize to lymph nodes. The clinic target volume (CTV = gross tumor volume + microscopic spread) needs to encompass the region at risk as indicated by preoperative imaging and intraoperative findings, including the placement of surgical clips (17,46). The minimum RT field should include presurgically involved areas, surgical clips, and areas concerning for positive margins or residual microscopic disease. The field may also encompass pleural implants or involved lymph nodes. RT should be delivered with 3-D conformal techniques or intensity-modulated RT (IMRT) to reduce damage to surrounding normal tissues (e.g., heart, lungs, esophagus, spinal cord). Guidelines from lung cancer for tissue toxicity may be used; however, they should be applied more conservatively given that patients with thymoma are generally younger and have longer term survival. Potential RT-induced toxicities include esophagitis, pneumonitis, dermatitis, pericarditis, arrhythmias, and coronary artery disease.

There is continuing controversy about the potential benefit of PORT for resected stage III thymic malignancies and some stage II thymic carcinomas, and this has led to the design of specific clinical trials. Until a definitive trial is completed, the controversy will continue. PORT is being used less frequently in thymoma due to unfavorable reports from studies of large retrospective databases (47–50). PORT appears to have little benefit for patients with stage I to IIA disease, marginal benefit in stage IIB disease, and perhaps a more clear benefit in stage III to IV disease. There is no overall survival benefit for PORT in stage I thymoma or for R0/R1 resected stage II to III thymoma, and PORT has not been shown to decrease recurrence in thymoma after a complete resection. However, there may be a role for PORT in thymic carcinoma, since both an improvement in RFS and overall survival have been noted with PORT (12).

Most of the data regarding PORT comes from retrospective analyses, so there may be significant selection bias as to which patients undergo PORT and which do not. In a SEER database study of 901 patients, there was no benefit for PORT in Masaoka stage I thymoma or thymic carcinoma, but a possible benefit in stage II to III disease (47). In the JART database, including 155 patients with thymic carcinoma and 1,110 with thymoma with 71% having stage II disease and 29% stage III disease, PORT was associated with improved RFS, but not overall survival in thymic carcinoma (RFS HR 0.48, 95% CI 0.30–0.78; $P = .003$), but there was no associated improvement in RFS or overall survival for stage II to III thymoma (48). In a multivariate analysis of 1,042 cases of thymic carcinoma from the ITMIG database, R0 resection and PORT were associated with prolonged overall survival (49). In a meta-analysis and systematic review, PORT had no impact on recurrence in 592 completely resected stage II to III TETs (50). In addition, the most common sites of recurrence were outside the RT field, including lung, pleura, and diaphragm (50,51). This conflicting data emphasize that these cases should be discussed in a multidisciplinary tumor board with experience in the management of this disease.

Postoperative Chemotherapy

There is minimal data for the use of postoperative chemotherapy in the management of TETs. Postoperative chemotherapy is not recommended after R0/R1 resection for thymoma (52). According to the ESMO guidelines for thymic carcinoma, postoperative chemotherapy can be considered after an R1 resection of stage IIA/IIB or an R0/R1 resection of stage III to IVA disease, especially if it had not been given in the preoperative setting (12). Part of this consideration is due to the fact that thymic carcinoma is associated with early recurrences after incomplete surgery (9). Postoperative chemotherapy in combination with RT can be considered after an R2 resection of thymoma and should be considered after an R2 resection of thymic carcinoma.

Summary of Guidelines on Postoperative Treatment

Complete Resection (R0): The NCCN guideline states that PORT can be *considered* in stage II to IV thymoma or thymic carcinoma (17). The ESMO guideline takes into consideration the histologic subtype. Generally, PORT is not recommended in stage I to II thymoma. However, PORT can be *considered* in stage II disease with more aggressive histologies, including stage IIA type B3 and stage IIB type B2 to B3 thymoma. However, the risks of radiation should be weighed. PORT is generally recommended with boost to the areas of concern in stage III to IVA thymoma. PORT is optional for stage I thymic carcinoma; however, this is supported by the lowest level of evidence. PORT can be *considered* in stage II thymic carcinoma and is generally recommended for stage III to IVA thymic carcinoma. The addition of chemotherapy can also be considered postoperatively in stage III to IVA resected thymic carcinoma. There is considerable controversy given the lack of high-level evidence and these cases should be discussed in a multidisciplinary tumor board experienced in this disease.

Microscopic Incomplete Resection (R1): For patients who undergo a R1 resection, PORT is recommended. The NCCN guideline recommends PORT for R1 resected thymoma and PORT ± chemotherapy for R1 resected thymic carcinoma (17). The ESMO guidelines also recommend PORT for R1 resected thymoma and thymic carcinoma (12). Chemotherapy in addition to RT can be *considered* for stage II to IVA thymic carcinoma.

Macroscopic Incomplete Resection (R2): A definitive RT approach may be attempted with a total dose of at least 60 Gy in 1.8- to 2.0-Gy fractions (17,12). RT doses below 54 Gy are not adequate for treatment of gross residual disease (46), and a 10-Gy boost can be given to areas of residual disease. The NCCN guideline recommends definitive RT ± chemotherapy for thymoma, while definitive RT plus chemotherapy is recommended for thymic carcinoma. The ESMO guideline recommends definitive RT for thymoma or thymic carcinoma, with an option of chemoradiotherapy (12).

Locally Advanced, Primarily Unresectable Disease

Preoperative Therapy

Preoperative chemotherapy, RT, or the combination of both can be effective for locally advanced TETs, particularly in "down-staging" the tumor and improving resectability (46). Complete primary resection is not always possible for Masaoka-Koga stage III to IVA disease, but if an experienced thoracic surgeon deems that the tumor would be resectable with good response, then preoperative therapy is a favored option (12). After confirming the diagnosis of TET by biopsy, primary chemotherapy can be delivered as part of a curative intent treatment plan that involves sequential surgery or RT. If RT is administered preoperatively, doses below 40 Gy or above 64 Gy are not considered appropriate.

Primary Chemotherapy

The ITMIG term "primary chemotherapy" encompasses the common terms induction, neoadjuvant, and preoperative. It is usually reserved for patients with Masaoka-Koga stage III or IVA disease, and the objective is to increase the chances of achieving a complete resection (R0). Several primary chemotherapy regimens have been studied, as reviewed in the ITMIG chemotherapy definitions and policies statement (34). These regimens are platinum-based combinations, and an anthracycline may be incorporated to enhance the response rate. Cisplatin-based regimens are generally recommended, including the combinations of cyclophosphamide, doxorubicin, and cisplatin (CAP), or cisplatin plus etoposide. The regimens used for primary chemotherapy are similar to those used in the metastatic setting, which are described in more detail in the following and in Table 15.4. Primary chemotherapy is usually administered for two to four cycles and repeat imaging with contrast-enhanced CT is performed 3 to 4 weeks after the last cycle. Ideally, surgery should be performed within 8 weeks of completion of chemotherapy. In the largest studies, which enrolled at least 20 patients, the response rate with primary chemotherapy was 60% to 80% (34). If an R0 resection is not possible after primary chemotherapy, either due to tumor characteristics or poor performance status, then definitive RT can be delivered. RT should be started no later than 6 weeks after the last chemotherapy cycle. As reported in the literature, up to 50% of patients go on to definitive RT after receiving primary chemotherapy (34). If definitive RT or surgery is not possible, then the intent of chemotherapy is palliative.

The largest study examining primary chemotherapy was performed at M.D. Anderson with CAP plus prednisone for three

(text continues on page 332)

Table 15.4 Chemotherapy regimens for thymic epithelial tumors

Acronym	Details of regimen	Number of patients	Efficacy data
First-line anthracycline based			
CAP (53) **(Preferred)**	Cisplatin 50 mg/m^2 (d1) Doxorubicin 50 mg/m^2 (d1) Cyclophosphamide 500 mg/m^2 (d1) *Q3 wk*	30 (29 T, 1 TC)	ORR 50% mDOR 11.8 mo mTTF 18.4 mo mOS 37.7 mo 2-y OS 64.5% 5-y OS 32%
ADOC (54)	Doxorubicin 40 mg/m^2 (d1) Cisplatin 50 mg/m^2 (d1) Vincristine 0.6 mg/m^2 (d3) Cyclophosphamide 700 mg/m^2 (d4) *Q3 wk*	37 T	ORR 91.8% mDOR 12 mo mOS 15 mo
First-line nonanthracycline based			
PE (55) **(Reasonable Alternative)**	Cisplatin 60 mg/m^2 (d1) Etoposide 120 mg/m^2 (d1–3) *Q 3 wk*	16 T	ORR 56% mDOR 3.4 y mPFS 2.2 y mOS 4.3 y 3-y OS 69%

(*continued*)

Table 15.4 Chemotherapy regimens for thymic epithelial tumors (*continued*)

First-line nonanthracycline based			
Acronym	**Details of regimen**	**Number of patients**	**Efficacy data**
VIP (56,57)	Etoposide 75 mg/m^2 (d1–4) Ifosfamide 1.2 g/m^2 (d1–4) Cisplatin 20 mg/m^2 (d1–4) *Q 3 wk*	28 (20 T, 8 TC)	ORR 32% mDOR 11.9 mo mOS 31.6 mo 1-y OS 89% 2-y OS 70%
Carbo-Pac (58,59)	Carboplatin AUC 5–6 (d1) Paclitaxel 200–225 mg/m^2 (d1) *Q 3 wk*	US: 44 (21 T, 23 TC/ B3 T) Japan: 39 TC	T: ORR 42.9% mDOR 16.9 mo mPFS 16.7 mo mOS NR TC: ORR 21.7% mDOR 4.5 mo mPFS 5 mo mOS 20.0 mo ORR 36% mPFS 7.5 mo mOS NR 1-y OS 85% 2-y OS 71%

(*continued*)

Table 15.4 Chemotherapy regimens for thymic epithelial tumors (*continued*)

Second-line			
Acronym	**Details of regimen**	**Number of patients**	**Efficacy data**
CAPGEM (60)	Capecitabine 650 mg/m^2 twice daily day 1–14 Gemcitabine 1,000 mg/m^2 days 1 and 8 *Q 3 wk* until progressive disease	30 (22T, 8 TC)	ORR 40% mPFS 11 mo (T 11 mo, & TC 6 mo) 1-y OS 90% 2-y OS 66%
Pemetrexed (61)	500 mg/m^2 every 3 wk up to six cycles or until progressive disease *Q 3 wk*	23 T/TC	ORR 17.4% mTTP 45 wk (T 45.4 wk, TC 5.1 wk)
Sunitinib (62)	Sunitinib 50 mg once a day 4 wk on/2 wk off *Q 6 wk* until progressive disease	41 (16 T, 25 TC)	TC: ORR 26% mTTR 5.6 mo mDOR 16.4 mo DCR 91% mPFS 7.2 mo mOS NR 1-y OS 78% T: ORR 6% DCR 81% mPFS 8.5 mo mOS 15.5 mo 1-y OS 86%

(*continued*)

Table 15.4 Chemotherapy regimens for thymic epithelial tumors (*continued*)

Second-line			
Acronym	**Details of regimen**	**Number of patients**	**Efficacy data**
Octreotide ± prednisone (63,64)	Octreotide 0.5 mg SQ TID for up to 1 y ± prednisone 0.6 mg/kg day All patients had a positive octreotide scan	38 (32 T, 5 TC, 1 carcinoid)	ORR 31.6% (all T) octreotide alone 10.5% T: mPFS 8.8 mo mOS NR TC: mPFS 4.5 mo mOS 24.3 mo
Everolimus (65)	Everolimus 10 mg once daily until progressive disease	50 (30 T, 19 TC, 1 unknown)	ORR 22% (not stratified by T or TC) T: DCR 93.3% mPFS NR 1-y PFS 70.2% mOS NR 1-y OS 82.3% TC: DCR 73.7% mPFS 5.5 mo 1-y PFS 16.6% mOS 18.6 mo 1-y OS 62.3%

d, day; DCR, disease control rate; DOR, duration of response; m, median; mo, month; NR, not reached; ORR, overall response rate; OS, overall survival; PFS, progression-free survival; SQ, subcutaneous; T, thymoma; TC, thymic carcinoma; TID, three times a day; TTF, time to treatment failure; TTP, time to progression; TTR, time to response; wk, week; y, year.

cycles, followed by surgery and then postoperative RT and consolidation chemotherapy in patients with stage III to IVB thymoma. Of the 22 patients, 17 had an objective response and 76% underwent a complete resection (66). In a Japan Clinical Oncology Group study of preoperative cisplatin-based, dose-dense chemotherapy in 21 patients with stage III thymoma, there were 13 partial responses and 39% underwent a complete resection (67). Primary chemotherapy followed by definitive RT was highlighted in a study of CAP chemotherapy followed by 54 Gy of RT in patients with unresectable TET (45). Of the 23 assessable patients, the objective response rate was 70%, including five complete responses, and the addition of RT enhanced the response rate.

Concurrent Chemoradiotherapy

Concurrent chemoradiotherapy without subsequent resection is a definitive treatment option for patients with unresectable thymoma or thymic carcinoma, with the use of platinum plus etoposide along with concurrent RT to 60 Gy (68,69). Concurrent chemoradiotherapy can also be used in a preoperative manner for primarily unresectable tumors in order to maximally attempt to achieve tumor shrinkage and surgical resection. A pilot trial showed that preoperative chemoradiotherapy with cisplatin plus etoposide for two cycles and 45 Gy RT is feasible in patients with TET (68). Of 21 patients (seven with thymic carcinoma), there were 10 partial responses and 81% were able to undergo a complete resection. If RT is incorporated, repeat CT thorax should be performed 3 to 6 weeks after completion of RT to determine resectability (46). If the tumor is still not deemed resectable, RT doses can go higher to 60 to 66 Gy.

Locally Advanced or Metastatic Disease Not Amenable to Surgery or Radiation

First-Line Chemotherapy

In patients who have unresectable disease that is not amenable to definitive surgery or RT or a Masaoka-Koga stage IVB tumor, the goal of therapy is palliative, with the aims of improving tumor-related symptoms, prolonging survival, and preventing worsening of paraneoplastic symptoms. Platinum-based regimens are recommended, but no randomized studies have been published in this setting (12,17). Although individual trials have reported similar response rates with CAP (53) and with nonanthracycline-based regimens (e.g., cisplatin plus etoposide) (55), a pooled analysis with large patient numbers showed that anthracycline-based approaches appear to improve the response rate (34).

In a systematic review and pooled analysis by Okuma et al. of 314 patients with thymoma from 15 studies, the response rate was higher with anthracycline-based therapy (69.4% vs. 37.8%; $P < .0001$) (70). Therefore, the preferred first-line regimen for both thymoma and thymic carcinoma is CAP (12, 34) (Table 15.4). Prednisone can be added to CAP for patients with thymoma if there are significant tumor-related symptoms and rapid response is required, since corticosteroids can decrease the lymphocytic component of thymoma. Cisplatin plus etoposide is a reasonable alternative regimen (Table 15.4). For patients with thymic carcinoma, carboplatin plus paclitaxel is listed in the NCCN guideline as the preferred regimen based on higher level prospective phase II data (17). Carboplatin plus paclitaxel is also an option for patients who can't tolerate an anthracycline or cisplatin. The addition of vincristine to CAP resulted in a response rate of greater than 90%, but was associated with higher toxicity. The addition of ifosfamide to cisplatin plus etoposide was inferior to cisplatin–doxorubicin regimens, did not offer a significant advantage over cisplatin plus etoposide alone, had a more difficult administration schedule, and resulted in greater side effects.

Chemotherapy should be administered for three to six cycles. If the patient has recurrent, unresectable disease, reuse of a previously efficacious regimen used in the preoperative setting can be considered, especially if the recurrence is late. Anthracyclines may be readministered if the target cumulative dose has not been exceeded. Caution should be taken in patients who received prior mediastinal RT, since this increases the risk of cardiac toxicity with anthracyclines. The efficacy of common first-line regimens used for TETs is detailed in Table 15.4 (53–59).

Subsequent Chemotherapy

Depending on the first-line therapy delivered, the chemotherapy regimens available for second-line treatment include carboplatin plus paclitaxel (58), platinum plus etoposide (55), capecitabine plus gemcitabine (60), and various single-agents including pemetrexed (61) (Table 15.4). Several targeted therapies can be used beyond the second-line setting, including octreotide (63,71), c-KIT targeted agents (e.g., imatinib) since c-KIT mutations occur in less than 10% of thymic carcinomas (12), sunitinib in thymic carcinoma (62), and everolimus (65). Sunitinib can also be considered as second-line therapy for thymic carcinoma given the relatively high response rate. Octreotide has limited single-agent activity, which is increased by the addition of corticosteroids, but can be considered in patients with autoimmune diarrhea or refractory tumors, especially if they are positive by octreotide scan (63,71).

As we learn more about the molecular characteristics of thymic tumors, targeted therapy may play more of a role. In addition, there may be a role for immunotherapy, like programmed-death receptor-1 (PD1) inhibitors, although caution will need to be taken given the risk of autoimmune adverse events in a population that is already at high risk for such occurrences.

FOLLOW-UP EVALUATION

In a consensus statement, ITMIG recommends at minimum, yearly CT scans of the thorax for 5 years after surgical resection, followed by annual CT chest alternating with chest radiography until year 11, followed by annual chest radiography alone (72). Higher risk tumors, including resected stage III to IVA thymoma, resected thymic carcinoma, or incompletely resected TETs, should undergo more frequent CT imaging every 6 months for the first 3 years. It is useful to obtain a new baseline CT 4 to 12 weeks postoperatively. MRI may also be useful for surveillance to minimize the cumulative radiation dose, particularly in young patients. PET scans are currently not recommended for surveillance. The NCCN guideline recommends CT surveillance every 6 months for 2 years then annually for 5 years for thymic carcinoma and 10 years for thymoma (17). The ESMO guideline recommends annual CT for 5 years, then every 2 years up to 10 to 15 years for completely resected stage I/II thymoma (12). For higher risk stage, histology, and resection status, ESMO recommends a CT scan every 6 months for 2 years, then annually for 10 to 15 years.

KEY POINTS

- TETs are rare tumors of the thymus that include thymoma and thymic carcinoma. The majority of TETs occur in the anterior mediastinum and can be associated with paraneoplastic autoimmune syndromes, most commonly myasthenia gravis.
- TETs do not need to be biopsied prior to resection if the clinical and radiographic characteristics are highly suspicious of TET and the mass is deemed primarily resectable.
- The most important prognostic factors in TETs include Masaoka-Koga stage and completeness of resection. Therefore, the mainstay of treatment is to obtain a complete (R0) resection.
- The role of postoperative RT (PORT) is controversial, especially after a complete (R0) resection. All patients,

especially if they have higher risk stage or histology, should be discussed in a multidisciplinary tumor board with experience in the management of TETs. PORT should be delivered for patients who underwent a microscopic (R1) or macroscopic (R2) incomplete resection. There is little data to support postoperative chemotherapy, though it may be used for more aggressive histologies, such as thymic carcinoma.

- TETs are frequently managed in a multidisciplinary fashion. If a TET is considered primarily unresectable (e.g., invasion into adjacent structures or organs), cisplatin (± anthracycline)-based preoperative chemotherapy can be given for two to four cycles to improve resectability. If the tumor is still unresectable, then definitive RT to 60 Gy can be administered.
- If TETs are primarily unresectable and unlikely to be resectable after chemotherapy, concurrent definitive chemoradiotherapy with platinum plus etoposide and radiation to 60 Gy should be administered.
- If resection or definitive radiation is not possible, platinum-based palliative chemotherapy should be administered for three to six cycles. Preferred regimens include cyclophosphamide, cisplatin, and doxorubicin (CAP) or cisplatin plus etoposide. The goals of treatment are to improve tumor-related symptoms and prolong survival. Chemotherapy produces a high objective response rate (>60%), which is often durable.

REFERENCES

1. Klein L, Kyewski B, Allen PM, et al. Positive and negative selection of the T cell repertoire: what thymocytes see (and don't see). *Nat Rev Immunol*. 2014;14(6):377-391.
2. Engels EA. Epidemiology of thymoma and associated malignancies. *J Thorac Oncol*. 2010;5(10 suppl 4):S260-S265.
3. Filosso PL, Galassi C, Ruffini E, et al. Thymoma and the increased risk of developing extrathymic malignancies: a multicentre study. *Eur J Cardiothorac Surg*. 2013;44(2):219-224; discussion 224.
4. Siesling S, van der Zwan JM, Izarzugaza I, et al. Rare thoracic cancers, including peritoneum mesothelioma. *Eur J Cancer*. 2012;48(7):949-960.
5. Detterbeck F, Giaccone G, Loehrer P, et al. International thymic malignancy interest group. *J Thorac Oncol*. 2010;5(1):1-2.

6. Marx A, Chan JK, Coindre JM, et al. The 2015 World Health Organization classification of tumors of the thymus: continuity and changes. *J Thorac Oncol*. 2015;10(10):1383-1395.
7. Travis WD, Brambilla E, Muller-Hermelink HP. *Pathology and Genetics of Tumors of the Lung, Pleura, Thymus and Heart.* Lyon, France: IARC Press; 2004.
8. Weis CA, Yao X, Deng Y, et al. The impact of thymoma histotype on prognosis in a worldwide database. *J Thorac Oncol*. 2015;10(2): 367-372.
9. Detterbeck FC, Nicholson AG, Kondo K, et al. The Masaoka-Koga stage classification for thymic malignancies: clarification and definition of terms. *J Thorac Oncol*. 2011;6(7 suppl 3):S1710-S1716.
10. Detterbeck F. MS16.2—Towards a TNM-based prognostic classification for thymic tumours. *15th World Conference on Lung Cancer.* Sydney, Australia, October 27-30, 2013.
11. Detterbeck FC, Stratton K, Giroux D, et al. The IASLC/ITMIG Thymic Epithelial Tumors Staging Project: proposal for an evidence-based stage classification system for the forthcoming (8th) edition of the TNM classification of malignant tumors. *J Thorac Oncol*. 2014;9 (9 suppl 2):S65-S72.
12. Girard N, Ruffini E, Marx A, et al. Thymic epithelial tumours: ESMO Clinical Practice Guidelines. *Ann Oncol*. 2015;26 (suppl 5): v40-v55.
13. Detterbeck FC. Clinical value of the WHO classification system of thymoma. *Ann Thorac Surg*. 2006;81(6):2328-2334.
14. Kondo K, Monden Y. Therapy for thymic epithelial tumors: a clinical study of 1,320 patients from Japan. *Ann Thorac Surg*. 2003;76(3): 878-884; discussion 884-875.
15. Evoli A, Lancaster E. Paraneoplastic disorders in thymoma patients. *J Thorac Oncol*. 2014;9(9 suppl 2):S143-S147.
16. Huang J, Ahmad U, Antonicelli A, et al. Development of the international thymic malignancy interest group international database: an unprecedented resource for the study of a rare group of tumors. *J Thorac Oncol*. 2014;9(10):1573-1578.
17. Thymomas and thymic carcinomas. *National Comprehensive Cancer Network, NCCN Practice Guidelines in Oncology,* 2016; version 1.2016.
18. Strollo DC, Rosado de Christenson ML, Jett JR. Primary mediastinal tumors. Part 1: tumors of the anterior mediastinum. *Chest*. 1997;112(2):511-522.
19. Strollo DC, Rosado-de-Christenson ML, Jett JR. Primary mediastinal tumors: part II. Tumors of the middle and posterior mediastinum. *Chest*. 1997;112(5):1344-1357.
20. Hoerbelt R, Keunecke L, Grimm H, et al. The value of a noninvasive diagnostic approach to mediastinal masses. *Ann Thorac Surg*. 2003;75(4):1086-1090.
21. Marom EM. Advances in thymoma imaging. *J Thorac Imaging*. 2013;28(2):69-80; quiz 81-63.

22. Tomiyama N, Honda O, Tsubamoto M, et al. Anterior mediastinal tumors: diagnostic accuracy of CT and MRI. *Eur J Radiol*. 2009;69(2):280-288.

23. Marom EM, Rosado-de-Christenson ML, Bruzzi JF, et al. Standard report terms for chest computed tomography reports of anterior mediastinal masses suspicious for thymoma. *J Thorac Oncol*. 2011;6 (7 suppl 3):S1717-S1723.

24. Marom EM, Milito MA, Moran CA, et al. Computed tomography findings predicting invasiveness of thymoma. *J Thorac Oncol*. 2011;6(7):1274-1281.

25. Hayes SA, Huang J, Plodkowski AJ, et al. Preoperative computed tomography findings predict surgical resectability of thymoma. *J Thorac Oncol*. 2014;9(7):1023-1030.

26. Viti A, Terzi A, Bianchi A, et al. Is a positron emission tomography-computed tomography scan useful in the staging of thymic epithelial neoplasms? *Interact Cardiovasc Thorac Surg*. 2014;19(1): 129-134.

27. Treglia G, Sadeghi R, Giovanella L, et al. Is (18)F-FDG PET useful in predicting the WHO grade of malignancy in thymic epithelial tumors? A meta-analysis. *Lung Cancer*. 2014;86(1):5-13.

28. Marchevsky A, Marx A, Strobel P, et al. Policies and reporting guidelines for small biopsy specimens of mediastinal masses. *J Thorac Oncol*. 2011;6(7 suppl 3):S1724-S1729.

29. Kattach H, Hasan S, Clelland C, et al. Seeding of stage I thymoma into the chest wall 12 years after needle biopsy. *Ann Thorac Surg*. 2005;79(1):323-324.

30. Nagasaka T, Nakashima N, Nunome H. Needle tract implantation of thymoma after transthoracic needle biopsy. *J Clin Pathol*. 1993;46(3):278-279.

31. Detterbeck FC. Does an anecdote substantiate dogma? *Ann Thorac Surg*. 2006;81(3):1182; author reply 1182-1183.

32. Vannucci J, Pecoriello R, Ragusa M, et al. Multiple pleuropericardial implants of thymoma after videothoracoscopic resection. *Interact Cardiovasc Thorac Surg*. 2010;11(5):696-697.

33. Xie A, Tjahjono R, Phan K, et al. Video-assisted thoracoscopic surgery versus open thymectomy for thymoma: a systematic review. *Ann Cardiothorac Surg*. 2015;4(6):495-508.

34. Girard N, Lal R, Wakelee H, et al. Chemotherapy definitions and policies for thymic malignancies. *J Thorac Oncol*. 2011;6(7 suppl 3): S1749-S1755.

35. Detterbeck FC, Parsons AM. Management of stage I and II thymoma. *Thorac Surg Clin*. 2011;21(1):59-67, vi-vii.

36. Riely GJ, Huang J. Induction therapy for locally advanced thymoma. *J Thorac Oncol*. 2010;5(10 suppl 4):S323-S326.

37. Shapiro M, Korst RJ. Surgical approaches for stage IVA thymic epithelial tumors. *Front Oncol*. 2014;3:332.

38. Kondo K, Monden Y. Lymphogenous and hematogenous metastasis of thymic epithelial tumors. *Ann Thorac Surg*. 2003;76(6):1859-1864; discussion 1864-1855.

39. Hamaji M, Kojima F, Omasa M, et al. A meta-analysis of debulking surgery versus surgical biopsy for unresectable thymoma. *Eur J Cardiothorac Surg*. 2015;47(4):602-607.
40. Hamaji M, Ali SO, Burt BM. A meta-analysis of surgical versus nonsurgical management of recurrent thymoma. *Ann Thorac Surg*. 2014;98(2):748-755.
41. Jurado J, Javidfar J, Newmark A, et al. Minimally invasive thymectomy and open thymectomy: outcome analysis of 263 patients. *Ann Thorac Surg*. 2012;94(3):974-981; discussion 981-972.
42. Ruckert JC, Walter M, Muller JM. Pulmonary function after thoracoscopic thymectomy versus median sternotomy for myasthenia gravis. *Ann Thorac Surg*. 2000;70(5):1656-1661.
43. Toker A, Eroglu O, Ziyade S, et al. Comparison of early postoperative results of thymectomy: partial sternotomy vs. videothoracoscopy. *Thorac Cardiovasc Surg*. 2005;53(2):110-113.
44. Friedant AJ, Handorf EA, Su S, et al. Minimally invasive versus open thymectomy for thymic malignancies: systematic review and meta-analysis. *J Thorac Oncol*. 2016;11(1):30-38.
45. Loehrer PJ Sr., Chen M, Kim K, et al. Cisplatin, doxorubicin, and cyclophosphamide plus thoracic radiation therapy for limited-stage unresectable thymoma: an intergroup trial. *J Clin Oncol*. 1997;15(9): 3093-3099.
46. Gomez D, Komaki R, Yu J, et al. Radiation therapy definitions and reporting guidelines for thymic malignancies. *J Thorac Oncol*. 2011;6 (7 suppl 3):S1743-S1748.
47. Forquer JA, Rong N, Fakiris AJ, et al. Postoperative radiotherapy after surgical resection of thymoma: differing roles in localized and regional disease. *Int J Radiat Oncol Biol Phys*. 2010;76(2):440-445.
48. Omasa M, Date H, Sozu T, et al. Postoperative radiotherapy is effective for thymic carcinoma but not for thymoma in stage II and III thymic epithelial tumors: the Japanese Association for Research on the Thymus Database Study. *Cancer*. 2015;121(7):1008-1016.
49. Ahmad U, Yao X, Detterbeck F, et al. Thymic carcinoma outcomes and prognosis: results of an international analysis. *J Thorac Cardiovasc Surg*. 2015;149(1):95-100, 101, e101-e102.
50. Korst RJ, Kansler AL, Christos PJ, et al. Adjuvant radiotherapy for thymic epithelial tumors: a systematic review and meta-analysis. *Ann Thorac Surg*. 2009;87(5):1641-1647.
51. Rimner A, Gomez DR, Wu AJ, et al. Failure patterns relative to radiation treatment fields for stage II-IV thymoma. *J Thorac Oncol*. 2014;9(3):403-409.
52. Attaran S, McCormack D, Pilling J, et al. Which stages of thymoma benefit from adjuvant chemotherapy post-thymectomy? *Interact Cardiovasc Thorac Surg*. 2012;15(2):273-275.
53. Loehrer PJ Sr., Kim K, Aisner SC, et al. Cisplatin plus doxorubicin plus cyclophosphamide in metastatic or recurrent thymoma: final

results of an intergroup trial. The Eastern Cooperative Oncology Group, Southwest Oncology Group, and Southeastern Cancer Study Group. *J Clin Oncol*. 1994;12(6):1164-1168.

54. Fornasiero A, Daniele O, Ghiotto C, et al. Chemotherapy for invasive thymoma. A 13-year experience. *Cancer*. 1991;68(1):30-33.
55. Giaccone G, Ardizzoni A, Kirkpatrick A, et al. Cisplatin and etoposide combination chemotherapy for locally advanced or metastatic thymoma. A phase II study of the European Organization for Research and Treatment of Cancer Lung Cancer Cooperative Group. *J Clin Oncol*. 1996;14(3):814-820.
56. Loehrer PJ Sr., Jiroutek M, Aisner S, et al. Combined etoposide, ifosfamide, and cisplatin in the treatment of patients with advanced thymoma and thymic carcinoma: an intergroup trial. *Cancer*. 2001;91(11):2010-2015.
57. Grassin F, Paleiron N, Andre M, et al. Combined etoposide, ifosfamide, and cisplatin in the treatment of patients with advanced thymoma and thymic carcinoma. A French experience. *J Thorac Oncol*. 2010;5(6):893-897.
58. Lemma GL, Lee JW, Aisner SC, et al. Phase II study of carboplatin and paclitaxel in advanced thymoma and thymic carcinoma. *J Clin Oncol*. 2011;29(15):2060-2065.
59. Hirai F, Yamanaka T, Taguchi K, et al. A multicenter phase II study of carboplatin and paclitaxel for advanced thymic carcinoma: WJOG4207L. *Ann Oncol*. 2015;26(2):363-368.
60. Palmieri G, Buonerba C, Ottaviano M, et al. Capecitabine plus gemcitabine in thymic epithelial tumors: final analysis of a Phase II trial. *Future Oncol*. 2014;10(14):2141-2147.
61. Loehrer PJ, Yiannoutsos CT, Dropcho S, et al. A phase II trial of pemetrexed in patients with recurrent thymoma or thymic carcinoma *J Clin Oncol. (Meeting Abstracts)* 2006;24(18 suppl 7079): 2006.
62. Thomas A, Rajan A, Berman A, et al. Sunitinib in patients with chemotherapy-refractory thymoma and thymic carcinoma: an open-label phase 2 trial. *Lancet Oncol*. 2015;16(2):177-186.
63. Loehrer PJ, Sr., Wang W, Johnson DH, et al. Octreotide alone or with prednisone in patients with advanced thymoma and thymic carcinoma: an Eastern Cooperative Oncology Group Phase II Trial. *J Clin Oncol*. 2004;22(2):293-299.
64. Palmieri G, Montella L, Martignetti A, et al. Somatostatin analogs and prednisone in advanced refractory thymic tumors. *Cancer*. 2002;94(5):1414-1420.
65. Zucali PA, Martino De Pas T, Palmieri G, et al. Phase II study of everolimus in patients with thymoma and thymic carcinoma previously treated with cisplatin-based chemotherapy. *J Clin Oncol*. 2014;32:5s (suppl; abstr 7527).
66. Kim ES, Putnam JB, Komaki R, et al. Phase II study of a multidisciplinary approach with induction chemotherapy, followed by

surgical resection, radiation therapy, and consolidation chemotherapy for unresectable malignant thymomas: final report. *Lung Cancer*. 2004;44(3):369-379.

67. Kunitoh H, Tamura T, Shibata T, et al. A phase II trial of dose-dense chemotherapy, followed by surgical resection and/or thoracic radiotherapy, in locally advanced thymoma: report of a Japan Clinical Oncology Group trial (JCOG 9606). *Br J Cancer*. 2010;103(1):6-11.
68. Korst RJ, Bezjak A, Blackmon S, et al. Neoadjuvant chemoradiotherapy for locally advanced thymic tumors: a phase II, multi-institutional clinical trial. *J Thorac Cardiovasc Surg*. 2014;147(1):36-44, 46.e31.
69. Wright CD, Choi NC, Wain JC, et al. Induction chemoradiotherapy followed by resection for locally advanced Masaoka stage III and IVA thymic tumors. *Ann Thorac Surg*. 2008;85(2):385-389.
70. Okuma Y, Saito M, Hosomi Y, et al. Key components of chemotherapy for thymic malignancies: a systematic review and pooled analysis for anthracycline-, carboplatin- or cisplatin-based chemotherapy. *J Cancer Res Clin Oncol*. 2015;141(2):323-331.
71. Ottaviano M, Damiano V, Nappi L, et al. Effectiveness of somatostatin analogs plus prednisone in aggressive histotype and advanced stage of thymic epithelial tumors. *J Clin Oncol*. 2015;33(suppl; abstr 7582): 2015.
72. Huang J, Detterbeck FC, Wang Z, et al. Standard outcome measures for thymic malignancies. *J Thorac Oncol*. 2011;6(7 suppl 3):S1691-S1697.

Palliative Care in Thoracic Oncology 16

Susan Urba and Joseph A. Bovi

MANAGEMENT OF COMMON SYMPTOMS

Patients with lung cancer commonly present with symptoms from their cancer or its treatment. Sixty-five percent of patients with early stage cancer, and 74% of patients with late-stage cancer experience moderate-to-severe symptoms (1). The most common symptoms include cough, dyspnea, and pain. The medical oncologist is called upon to manage these problems, while simultaneously coordinating cancer-directed therapy.

Airway Symptoms

Cough

Cough is present in 47% to 86% of lung cancer patients (2). Tumor-related etiologies for cough include direct stimulation of the central airway mucosa by tumor, sputum accumulation, lymphangitic spread of disease, and pleural or pericardial effusion. Pneumonitis may occur in patients treated with localized radiation therapy (RT), and cough may result from this inflammatory response. Unrelenting cough is a major impediment to quality-of-life. The cough can annoy both patients and those around them to the point that they withdraw from social activities. It can interfere with sleep, preventing patients from falling asleep or staying asleep. This can exacerbate fatigue, which is already frequently a problem.

The underlying principle of therapy is to treat any reversible cause of the cough: chemotherapy or RT for the cancer, antimicrobials for infection, or thoracentesis for a pleural effusion. However, other measures can be used simultaneously to try to give the patient relief. There is a paucity of randomized clinical trial data comparing cough suppressants in patients with lung cancer. As a matter of fact, a meta-analysis of 17 trials assessing cough interventions concluded that no practice recommendations could be drawn from its review, and that there is an urgent need to increase the number and quality of studies evaluating the effects of interventions for the management of cough in cancer (3). Therefore, agents that have been developed as antitussives for the general population are most often used for patients with lung cancer.

Benzonatate: This is an oral, nonopiate, peripherally acting antitussive. It is dosed at 100 mg orally three times a day. There is evidence that when added to opiates, there may be additional improvement in cough suppression (4).

Dextromethorphan: A meta-analysis has been reported of six randomized, double-blind studies of single-dose dextromethorphan 30 mg versus placebo, utilizing a 3-hour postdose cough evaluation (5). It demonstrated significantly greater overall reductions in cough bouts, cough components, and cough effort, and an increase in cough latency for patients treated with dextromethorphan versus those treated with placebo.

Guaifenesin: Expectorants such as guaifenesin are used for patients who have thick mucus secretions, in order to allow thinning of the secretions so that the cough may be more productive, which may make the patient more comfortable. However, it does little to actually stop the coughing.

Opiates: Opiates are thought to act on μ-receptors in the central cough center, and they often become the mainstay of treatment for lung cancer patients with chronic cough. Codeine is the oldest cough suppressant and is often combined with other peripherally acting agents, such as dextromethorphan. A meta-analysis of 49 studies that included 3,067 patients reviewed opiate and nonopiate agents used for cough suppression (6). In studies that had an active or placebo comparison, codeine and dextromethorphan were found to reduce the frequency and severity of chronic cough. In 11 comparisons of opioids versus placebo, eight showed that opioids were more effective for decreasing cough frequency and severity and improving quality of life. Combination products are available that include both an opiate and another type of cough suppressant in one product, such as Robitussin AC (guaifenesin and codeine) and Tussionex (chlorpheniramine and hydrocodone).

Corticosteroids: Some patients have bronchospasm either from chronic obstructive pulmonary disease (COPD) or as part of the clinical scenario related to their lung cancer. For this group, dexamethasone 4 mg one to three times a day may be useful. Patients who develop radiation pneumonitis leading to a severe cough as the result of a relatively large radiation port may benefit from steroids. The data guiding dosing of steroids is very old, and mostly based on animal models. A typical approach would include prednisone 60-mg daily × 1 to 2 weeks, followed by a slow taper over several weeks (7).

Dyspnea

One of the most frightening symptoms that lung cancer patients may have to face is dyspnea. The crucial first step is to make a thorough evaluation of the cause. Some of the problems that cause cough are also responsible for dyspnea, including the tumor compressing or blocking a bronchus, pleural effusion, pneumonia, lymphangitic spread of cancer, radiation pneumonitis, or pulmonary embolism. Besides trying to relieve the cause of the dyspnea, there are several mainstays of symptomatic treatment that can also be implemented.

Oxygen: Many patients complain of shortness of breath, despite the fact that their oxygen saturation is greater than 90%. Unfortunately, most insurance companies will not pay for supplemental oxygen if the oxygen saturation is not in the 80s, even though some patients with a "normal" oxygen level do find some relief with supplemental oxygen.

Opiates: Opiate medications are a mainstay for the management of dyspnea. For patients who are opiate naïve, starting doses are similar to starting doses for pain management. Morphine would be started at 2.5 to 10 mg orally every 2 hours (8). Oxycodone would be started at 5 mg every 3 to 4 hours. For elderly patients, these doses should be even lower. If the patient is already on chronic opiates for pain control, consideration can be given to increasing the dose by 25%.

Nebulized morphine has been studied because of its potentially rapid onset of action and ease of administration, and because if less of the opiate is absorbed systemically, adverse reactions might be minimized. A systematic review of 18 randomized, double-blind, controlled trials of opiates (nine of these trials used nebulized opiates) for relief of dyspnea in terminally ill patients concluded that there was no evidence to support nebulized opiate administration. However, there was evidence to support the use of oral or intravenous opiates (9).

Benzodiazepines: Opiates may not be sufficient to relieve dyspnea in some patients. If there is a substantial anxiety component, then a benzodiazepine such as lorazepam 0.5 to 1 mg every 4 hours as needed is helpful. Elderly patients may not tolerate a benzodiazepine, because they may experience paradoxical agitation from it. In that case, gentle titration of the opiate may be preferable to the addition of a benzodiazepine.

Nonpharmacologic measures: Several changes can be made to the patient's local environment to help relieve the sensation of dyspnea. Even though there is little randomized data to support these measures, anecdotally they may improve patient comfort. A bedside fan should be kept on, at a comfortable distance from the patient, to give the sensation of movement of cool air. The room should not be kept dark and close, but rather as airy as possible, with an open window or open door to reduce the sensation of "smothering." The patient may need to sleep in a semi-upright position in a recliner chair or propped up in bed with several pillows.

Anxiety and stress related to dyspnea can aggravate breathlessness, so it is important to consider relaxation techniques or guided imagery as an adjunct to symptom management. Often, the family can be educated in a few simple techniques of relaxed deep breathing in order to help the patient at home in a time of crisis.

Radiation for Airway Symptoms

Symptoms that originate from advanced cancer within the thoracic cavity can be palliated with a number of therapeutic modalities, such as external beam RT, brachytherapy, chemotherapy, surgical procedures, and/or supportive care. In this section, we concentrate on the radiotherapeutic options (10).

External beam RT: Palliative RT continues to play a pivotal role in the management of thoracic symptoms from lung cancer. It is particularly beneficial for endobronchial or extrinsic lesions causing atelectasis, postobstructive pneumonia, shortness of breath, cough, hemoptysis, pain, and large airway obstruction. RT cannot be expected to relieve shortness of breath that results from other cancer-related causes such as widespread parenchymal tumor involvement, pleural effusion, or lymphangitic tumor dissemination. Careful evaluation of the source of the patient's dyspnea must be paid attention to.

Numerous randomized trials have compared different palliative thoracic RT schedules for non–small-cell lung cancer (NSCLC). Many, but not all studies, have suggested that a less extensive course of RT consisting of 17 Gy (8.5 Gy × 2, delivered 1 week apart) or 10 Gy in a single fraction provide better palliation. In a Medical Research Council (MRC) study, shorter treatment regimens resulted in 80% to 85% of patients reporting an improvement in hemoptysis, 60% reporting an improvement in cough, and two-thirds reporting improvement in pain (11). An additional MRC study randomized 369 patients to 17 Gy (8.5 Gy × 2, delivered 1 week apart) versus 30 Gy in 10 fractions, with 81% of patients achieving improvement in hemoptysis with the short course of therapy compared to 86% in the longer treatment arm. These results were not statistically different from one another. Cough was improved in 65% of patients in the short course arm and in 56% of patients in the longer treatment arm, and again no statistical difference was detected. These results support the use of shorter treatment regimens in these patients (12). An additional study by Teo et al. randomized 291 patients to 45 Gy in 18 fractions over 4½ weeks versus 31.2 Gy in four fractions over 4 weeks

(7.8 Gy once per week). There was better symptom palliation with the 18-fraction treatment regimen, (71% vs. 54%) (13). Finally, Simpson et al., in Radiation Therapy Oncology Group (RTOG) 73-02, published on 409 patients randomized to 40 Gy in 10 fractions over 5 weeks versus 40 Gy in 20 fractions over 4 weeks versus 30 Gy in 10 fractions over 2 weeks. This study did not show superiority of one-fractionation regimen over another in terms of symptom control, again suggesting that a shorter fractionation schedule is as effective as a more protracted treatment schedule (14).

The third in a series of MRC studies on NSCLC was intriguing in that it suggested that a higher RT dose, 39 Gy in 13 fractions, may result in prolonged survival in good performance status patients as compared to 17 Gy (8.5 Gy × 2, delivered 1 week apart) (15). Subsequent to this MRC trial, a Canadian randomized trial of 10 Gy in a single fraction versus 20 Gy in five fractions revealed a 2-month longer median survival in patients in the multifraction arm, 6 months with 20 Gy versus 4.2 months with 10 Gy (16). To date, no dose fractionation schedule has demonstrated clear superiority in terms of palliation.

It is unclear if external beam RT should be recommended in patients who have minimal or no thoracic symptoms. This was examined by an additional MRC study (17). In this randomized, controlled trial, 230 patients with previously untreated incurable NSCLC, but no symptoms that would require immediate thoracic RT were randomized to either immediate RT (8.5 Gy × 2, delivered 1 week apart or a single 10 Gy fraction) delivered to their thoracic primary tumor or delayed RT as required at the time of symptom occurrence. The primary endpoint was the proportion of patients alive and free of moderate or severe thoracic symptoms at 6 months. This proportion was also examined at 1, 2, and 4 months. At no point was there a difference observed between the two study arms, with 28% of patients in the immediate RT arm and 26% of patients in the delayed RT arm remaining alive and free of moderate or severe symptoms at 6 months. In the delayed RT arm, 42% of patients received subsequent RT to their thoracic primary tumor and 56% died without receiving RT. Survival was similar with immediate or delayed RT. This study suggests that in patients who are candidates for radical treatment, prophylactic palliative RT should not be routinely used.

Endobronchial brachytherapy: In patients who have already received a prior course of external beam RT or in cases where an endobronchial tumor is causing obstruction of a major airway, direct insertion of radioactive sources into the bronchial lumen may be considered. This is called endobronchial brachytherapy.

The most commonly used source is iridium-192 delivered through a high dose-rate after-loading device. Reported response rates have varied between 70% and 90% in appropriately selected patients (18). Small tumors less than 2 cm in size may be effectively palliated for long periods of time with a recommended dose of 15 Gy (19). A randomized trial compared endobronchial brachytherapy (15 Gy at 1-cm distance) to external beam RT (30 Gy in 10 fractions) in palliative treatment of patients with NSCLC (20). In 99 previously untreated patients, symptom relief was comparable although fewer retreatments were needed in the external beam RT arm. Survival was also statistically better in patients treated on the external beam RT arm (9.5 vs. 8.3 months).

Conclusion: RT is an extremely effective palliative treatment in advanced lung cancer. It is most appropriately utilized if symptoms are localized and can often achieve urgent palliation of symptoms such as hemoptysis, airway obstruction, or superior vena cava (SVC) syndrome. There is little evidence to support combining chemotherapy and RT in the palliative setting. Therefore, one modality or the other should be utilized at one time to avoid the combined side effects of both modalities.

SVC Syndrome

SVC syndrome is a group of signs and symptoms resulting from compression or occlusion of the SVC. SVC syndrome is the manifestation of impaired return of venous blood from the face, neck, upper extremities, and upper thorax. This impaired venous drainage results in venous hypertension and subsequent venous congestion. Treatment aims to provide relief of symptoms based on the underlying cause (21).

SVC obstruction may be caused by direct invasion and compression of the SVC by the primary tumor or by nodal compression of the SVC. The distinction is important because resection of the SVC directly invaded by NSCLC can result in cures, whereas resection of the SVC compressed by paratracheal nodal metastases results in no 5-year survivors (22).

The goals of treatment for SVC syndrome are relief of the obstruction and improvement in symptoms. Steroids and diuretics are often given to decrease edema and inflammation. There are no controlled studies that document the efficacy of this intervention, which remains controversial (21). RT will relieve symptoms; however, it may take weeks. About 85% to 90% of patients report symptomatic relief within 3 weeks (23,24). Chemotherapy may be the treatment of choice if the maximum RT dose has been reached or the tumor is very chemosensitive, like lymphoma or small-cell lung cancer (25).

Stenting provides the most rapid resolution of symptoms. Angioplasty may be performed in conjunction with venography and stenting. Preprocedure venography identifies the site of stenosis or occlusion and the presence of any thrombi, while postprocedure venography documents successful deployment and placement of the stent (23,26).

Pain

Pain is very prevalent in many types of advanced cancer, and more than one-third of patients report their pain as moderate to severe. In a meta-analysis of 52 studies, 55% of 1,546 patients with lung cancer reported pain (27). Other than chest wall pain from direct tumor invasion, common pain syndromes in these patients include bone metastases and Pancoast tumors.

Bone Pain

Bone metastases will occur in 30% to 65% of patients with lung cancer (28). Bone metastases occur in various forms that can have a significant impact on the patients' quality of life. Complications from bone metastases can include pathologic fracture, spinal cord compression, and hypercalcemia. Bone pain often requires multimodality management with opioid narcotics, bone radiation, and possible surgical intervention. Orthopedic surgery consultation should be obtained when there is a bone fracture or an impending fracture of a weight-bearing bone as defined by erosion of 30% or more of cortical thickness as seen on plain radiographs.

Radiation therapy: External beam RT can provide significant palliation of painful bone metastases in 50% to 80% of patients with up to one-third of patients achieving complete pain relief at the treated site (29). There is significant variation worldwide in dose fractionation schedules (30). There have been numerous prospective randomized and retrospective trials that have shown similar pain relief outcomes with single-fraction schedules compared to longer courses of palliative RT for previously unirradiated bone metastases. The greatest advantages of a single-fraction treatment are increased convenience and lower cost.

There is also a wide range of radiotherapeutic options for pain that recurs after standard RT. Painful bone lesions at several anatomic sites can be treated with injectable radiopharmaceutical agents or hemibody RT depending on tumor histology and the distribution of the metastases. There has also been significant interest devoted to technological advances in RT delivery, such as stereotactic body radiation (SBRT), which can improve the results of primary or repeated treatment of metastatic spinal lesions. Although clinical trials with bisphosphonates initially consider the need for external beam RT as a failure of therapy, external beam RT to the index lesion may symptomatically provide more prompt and durable symptom relief (31).

Clinical trials: Many clinical trials have evaluated different dose and fractionation schemes for treatment of painful bone metastases. One of the largest trials was performed in 1999 by the Bone Pain Trial Working Party. This trial enrolled 775 patients with various cancer types, the majority of whom had lung cancer, and randomized them to receive 8 Gy in a single fraction versus 20 Gy in five fractions or 30 Gy in 10 fractions. Overall pain relief was equivalent in both arms at 78% and the complete response rate was also equivalent at 57% in the 8-Gy arm and 58% in the multifractionation arm. In addition, acute toxicity was similar in both arms and late toxicity was minimal. There was a higher retreatment rate in the single-fraction arm with 23% of the patients necessitating repeat treatment compared to 10% of patients in the multifractionation arm (32). Another large trial performed by Steenland et al. included 1,171 patients with various cancer subtypes who were randomized to receive either 8 Gy in a single fraction or 24 Gy in 6 fractions. Overall pain relief was similar in both arms (72% vs. 69%, respectively). Twenty-five percent of patients required retreatment in the single-fraction arm compared to 7% in the multifraction arm (33).

As is seen in Table 16.1, multiple other trials have demonstrated similar rates of complete response to pain with single-fraction treatments compared to multifraction regimens. However, there is also a significantly higher retreatment rate in the single-fraction arms. Care must be taken to appropriately select patients for single-fraction treatments. If survival is thought to be limited, then a single-fraction course might be reasonable. If survival is expected to be relatively long, a multifraction treatment schema might be better suited for the patient. As part of ASTRO's *Choosing Wisely* campaign, clinicians are asked to consider a shorter fractionation course for patients with painful bone metastases based on the evidence described earlier (41).

Radiopharmaceutical therapy: Since multiple sites of osseous metastases are common and some patients have multifocal bone pain, systemic-targeted treatment offers the potential for pain relief with minimal side effects. Radiopharmaceuticals developed for the treatment of painful bone metastases include phosphorus 32 (P32), strontium 89, and samarium 153. All of these agents have specific advantages and toxicities, and they differ in terms of mechanism of action, efficacy, duration, palliation, side effects, and the ability to repeat treatment. Phosphorus and strontium distribute more widely throughout the bone.

Table 16.1 Randomized trials comparing single-fraction to multiple-fraction RT for painful bone metastases

Study	Patient number	Dose and fractionation	Overall pain relief (%)	Complete response (%)	Acute toxicity (%)	Late toxicity (%)	Repeat treatment rate (%)
Bone Pain Trial Working Party (32)	775	8 Gy/1 Fx	78	57	30	2	23
		20 Gy/5 Fx or 30 Gy/10 Fx	78	58	32	1	10
Foro (34)	160	8 Gy/1 Fx	75	15	13	NR	28
		30 Gy/10 Fx	86	13	18	NR	2
Hartsell (35)	898	8 Gy/1 Fx	66	15	10	4	18
		30 Gy/10 Fx	66	18	17	4	9
Jeremic (36)	327	4 Gy/1 Fx	59	21	32	6	42
		6 Gy/1 Fx	73	27	29	7	44
		8 Gy/1 Fx	78	32	37	7	48
Kaasa (37)	376	8 Gy/1 Fx	Equivalent	NR	NR	4	4
		30 Gy/10 Fx	Equivalent	NR	NR	11	
Nielsen (38)	241	8 Gy/1 Fx	62	15	35	5	21
		20 Gy/4 Fx	71	15	35	5	12
Roos (39)	272	8 Gy/1 Fx	53	26	5	5	29
		20 Gy/5 Fx	61	27	11	4	24
Sande (40)	188	8 Gy/1 Fx	*			5	27
		30 Gy/10 Fx	*			5	5
Steenland (33)	1,171	8 Gy/1 Fx	72	37	Equivalent	4	25
		24 Gy/6 Fx	69	33	Equivalent	2	7

Equivalent, equivalent outcome between treatment arms; Fx, radiotherapy fractions; NR, not reported.
*Previously reported in Ref. (37). Kaasa S, Brenne E, Lund JA, et al. Prospective randomised multicenter trial on single-fraction radiotherapy (8 Gy × 1) versus multiple fractions (3 Gy × 10) in the treatment of painful bone metastases. *Radiother Oncol*. 2006;79(3):278-284.

P32 is a reactor-produced, pure beta-emitting radionucleotide with a physical half-life of 14.3 days. The maximum and mean beta particle energies are 1.71 and 0.695 MeV, respectively, where the mean and maximum particle ranges in tissue are 3 and 8 mm, respectively. P32 was one of the first radiopharmaceuticals used to reduce pain from bone metastases, being widely used until the 1980s (42). Pain palliation typically occurs within 14 days with a range of 2 days to 4 weeks. The major side effects of P32 are myelosuppression and pancytopenia.

Strontium is an element that behaves biologically like calcium. It localizes in bone, primarily in areas of osteoblastic activity. Strontium 89 has a physical half-life of 50.5 days, a maximum beta particle energy of 1.46 MeV, and a soft tissue range of 2.4 mm. After IV administration, strontium 89 is concentrated in bone in proportion to osteoblastic activity with a biological half-life of 4 to 5 days (43). Strontium 89 can relieve bone pain for up to 14 months and is recommended for use in patients with moderate pain with a reasonable life expectancy. Response rates range from 60% to 84% with an onset of pain relief of 7 to 21 days and a mean duration of relief of about 6 months (44). However, a transient increase in bone pain can occur within the first 2 to 3 days of treatment. This flare is usually mild, can be controlled with over the counter analgesics, and usually indicates a good response to treatment.

The final radionucleotide worth mentioning is samarium 153, which has a physical half-life of 1.9 days, a maximum beta particle energy of 0.81 MeV, and an average soft tissue range of 0.6 mm. This agent works by forming a phosphonate complex that concentrates in bones in areas of osteoblastic activity. Approximately 65% of the dose remains in the skeleton. Effective palliation occurs in about 62% to 74% of patients (45–47). Samarium 153 is the most widely used pain palliation radiopharmaceutical agent in the United States. Its ease of use, the ability to image its distribution, and its clinical results make it attractive, while issues with availability, radiation safety, and potentially irreversible myelosuppression limit wider use.

Medical Management of Bone Pain

The primary treatment for the source of bony pain is RT. However, other measures should be taken for pain relief while waiting for the treatment to take effect, which could be days to weeks.

Nonsteroidal anti-inflammatory drugs (NSAIDs): NSAIDs block biosynthesis of prostaglandins, the inflammatory mediators that cause and intensify pain. NSAIDs are a mainstay in the treatment of bony metastases, although all patients (and elderly patients in particular) should be watched closely for gastric irritation and renal insufficiency.

Bisphosphonates and RANKL inhibitors: Bisphosphonates, such as zoledronic acid and ibandronate, and RANKL inhibitors, such as denosumab, have demonstrated effectiveness in preventing skeletal related events and have been shown to palliate existing bone pain. In a randomized trial comparing denosumab to zoledronic acid in breast cancer patients with bony metastases, 26% of patients in both arms experienced meaningful pain relief. Fewer patients receiving denosumab complained of worsening of pain and there was also a longer time to worsening of pain in the denosumab group (48).

Opiates: Opiates are useful for most types of moderate to severe pain, although bony pain usually requires the addition of other adjuvant analgesics, such as an NSAID. When opiates are used, the basic principles of opiate therapy should be followed:

- The lowest effective dose should be used, to minimize the risk of side effects. Typically, an opiate-naïve patient should be started on a mild opiate, such as hydrocodone or codeine on an as-needed basis (49).
- If pain is chronic and requires numerous doses of immediate-release medication, then an extended-release opiate should be added. This can be started at the lowest dose available, or if information is available from the patient's use of opiates for breakthrough pain, then the extended-release dose should reflect the total amount that the patient has been taking in an average 24-hour period.
- Opiate toxicities should be carefully monitored. Constipation is the most common side effect, so a laxative should be routinely prescribed when an opiate is started. Nausea and sedation are other possible negative effects, but they may subside over a period of days.

Chest Wall Pain and Pancoast Tumors

Pancoast tumors involve the superior pulmonary sulcus and were described by Henry Pancoast in the early 1900s. Typically pain is experienced in the shoulder and arm, in the distribution of the C8, T1, and T2 dermatomes, and can be associated with muscle weakness and atrophy. The tumor can invade the brachial plexus, and therefore pain is often neuropathic in nature. Patients may experience prickling, burning, and numbness. Medications that may be helpful to relieve the neuropathic aspect of the pain include antidepressants and anticonvulsants (50). Much of the data supporting these agents are extrapolated from nonmalignant neuropathic pain management studies, such as those for diabetic neuropathy.

These adjuvant agents are frequently used in combination with opiates for moderate to severe neuropathic pain.

In situations where the tumor is unresectable and palliative RT is either not feasible or ineffective, some pain relief interventions have been used successfully. These include continuous interscalene brachial plexus block via catheter, selective cervical nerve root blocks, dorsal rhizotomy, and cordotomy. The best treatment depends on the size of the tumor, the extent of local invasion, and the specific structures involved. An intercostal nerve block can be very useful for localized chest wall pain. If the pain remains difficult to control despite the best efforts at medical management, then the Anesthesia Pain Service should be consulted for their input.

Tricyclic antidepressants and serotonin–norepinephrine reuptake inhibitors (SNRIs)

- Start with a low dose to make sure that the medication is tolerated; then titrate upward every 3 to 5 days, as tolerated.
- The dose needed for pain control may be lower than doses typically used for treatment of depression.
- Tricyclic antidepressants: Anticholinergic side effects include dry mouth, sedation, and urinary hesitancy. Secondary amines such as nortriptyline or desipramine have less of these effects and are most commonly used.
- SNRIs: Duloxetine and venlafaxine are most commonly used. In a randomized cross-over trial with 231 patients with chemotherapy-induced neuropathy, duloxetine improved the Brief Pain Inventory score and quality of life as measured by Functional Assessment of Cancer Therapy (FACT)-Neurotoxicity assessment (51).

Anticonvulsants

- Start low and titrate up as tolerated. The patient may get relief from neuropathic pain at relatively low doses.
- Gabapentin: The starting dose is 100-mg TID, but there is a large dosing range and doses may be titrated up to 1,200-mg TID as needed. Sedation can be a dose-limiting toxicity.
- Pregabalin: The starting dose is 50-mg TID and may be doubled over time. Fluid retention and peripheral edema may occur.

Fatigue

Cancer-related fatigue is the most common and distressing symptom affecting patients who are undergoing chemotherapy and/or RT, or who have metastatic disease. Fatigue can disrupt functionality and affect activities of daily living for months after treatment, and for some patients indefinitely (52).

Physicians should screen patients for fatigue at each visit or this symptom may get lost in the assessment for more "pressing" problems, such as pain or nausea/vomiting.

Correctable factors that may contribute to fatigue and their primary treatments include:

- Anemia—transfusion
- Pain—analgesic medications
- Depression—psychosocial interventions and antidepressants
- Poor nutrition—consultation with nutritionist for consideration of dietary supplements, and strategies to improve nutrition in the face of altered taste or nausea
- Medications—decrease or discontinue medications that may contribute to fatigue if possible, such as opiates, antidepressants, and antiemetics

General approaches to treatment:

- Physical activity: This is a key recommendation. Although it may be counter-intuitive to think that fatigue should be treated with exercise, several studies have demonstrated benefit to this approach, including a large meta-analysis and a Cochrane analysis (53,54). After verifying that it is safe for the patient to be active, an exercise program that includes endurance activities intended to increase cardiovascular fitness, such as walking or swimming, can decrease fatigue and increase quality of life. In some cases, the patient may benefit from a referral to physical therapy or occupational therapy.
- Psychostimulants: Clinical trials have yielded mixed results on the effectiveness of methylphenidate for cancer-related fatigue, but there is some evidence that patients with very advanced disease may experience the most benefit. Dosing is 5 to 10 mg in the morning, and may be repeated, but not later than 1:00 p.m. to avoid interference with sleep.

BRAIN METASTASES

Brain metastases are a common problem in patients with NSCLC. Lung cancer accounts for approximately one-half of all brain metastases that are diagnosed and this number is rising (55). The prognosis for patients with brain metastases is poor with the median survival of untreated patients being approximately 1 month. With treatment, the overall median survival after diagnosis is typically still less than 1 year (56). Brain metastases also cause significant neurologic, cognitive, and emotional difficulties.

Diagnosis

The differential diagnosis for brain metastases includes infection, paraneoplastic disease, bleeding, and radiation necrosis. Surgical resection is considered when the diagnosis is uncertain or where large lesions are causing neurologic symptoms as a result of mass effect. Patchell et al. randomized patients with solitary brain metastases to surgical resection with whole-brain RT (WBRT) versus biopsy and WBRT and found that approximately 10% of patients had tumors other than metastases (57).

The imaging study of choice for the diagnosis of brain metastases is MRI. These lesions typically arise within the gray/white matter junction. Approximately 80% of the lesions are found in the cerebral hemispheres and 15% in the cerebellum. Most brain metastases intensely enhance with gadolinium contrast as a result of disruption of the blood–brain barrier. Symptoms can include headache, confusion, nausea, vomiting, focal neurologic deficits such as weakness or slurring of speech, and seizures. Many patients remain asymptomatic.

Treatment

Corticosteroids: Symptom management usually starts with corticosteroids since these lesions tend to cause significant vasogenic edema. Corticosteroids decrease this edema and thereby improve symptoms. The corticosteroid of choice is typically dexamethasone at 16 mg per day in two to four doses. Patients should also receive prophylaxis from ulcer development with either an H2 blocker or a proton pump inhibitor. If patients are on steroids for extended periods of time, they may also need antifungal prophylaxis for oral candidiasis. Corticosteroids can cause significant side effects including weight gain, Cushingoid appearance, proximal muscle weakness, hyperglycemia, fluid retention, and, if tapered too quickly, adrenal insufficiency. Despite this, steroids are incredibly effective in helping to alleviate symptoms of brain metastases (58).

Whole Brain Radiotherapy

Whole brain radiotherapy (WBRT) is an extremely effective way of treating intracranial metastases from NSCLC. The appropriate use of WBRT can provide rapid improvement of neurologic symptoms and quality of life, and can be beneficial in patients whose metastases are surgically inaccessible or who are poor surgical candidates. In randomized trials, the use of adjuvant WBRT following resection or stereotactic radiosurgery (SRS) has been proven to improve local control of brain metastases and decrease the likelihood of neurologic death (59). However, WBRT has come under criticism recently due to the possibility of RT-induced neurocognitive decline (60,61). WBRT is an excellent treatment of choice and can provide effective symptom relief in patients who:

- Have metastases that are too large or too numerous for SRS
- Have metastases that are too disseminated for surgery or SRS
- Have a performance status that does not allow for surgery (62)

Response rates following WBRT vary, with multiple effective dose and fractionation schemes. In multiple RTOG studies, complete or partial responses have been documented in greater than half of patients treated. However, despite these efforts, median survival remains poor, in the range of 2.4 to 7.1 months. As a result of these studies, the RTOG devised a recursive partitioning analysis, which subdivides patients into three prognostic classes:

- Class I: KPS ≥70; less than 65 years of age; controlled primary; no extracranial metastases (median survival = 7.1 months)
- Class II: not class I or class III (median survival = 4.2 months)
- Class III: KPS less than 70 (median survival = 2.3 months) (63)

A more sophisticated analysis was done by Sperduto et al. in which primary histology was included in the graded prognostic assessment (64). This was felt to be a more sensitive tool for predicting outcomes in patients with brain metastases. The median survival of patients with NSCLC and brain metastases was 7 months.

Another use of WBRT is as adjuvant therapy following surgery or SRS. MRI imaging reveals that about 80% of patients have more than one metastasis and about 50% have three or more metastases, so treating microscopic disease is of value. Furthermore, 70% of patients with brain metastases experience relapse after resection if WBRT is omitted (65).

Stereotactic Radiosurgery

SRS is now considered standard practice for patients with four or fewer brain metastases based on validation in multiple prospective trials. Doses of 15 to 24 Gy prescribed to the margin of the contrast enhancing lesion based upon MRI scan are frequently utilized (66). In RTOG 9508, 333 patients with three or fewer brain metastases were randomized to WBRT with or without a SRS boost. An interesting outcome from this trial was that patients with single brain metastases were found to have improved overall survival with the addition of a SRS boost, establishing a new standard of care for patients with single brain metastases (67). Chang et al. conducted a single-institution randomized trial of SRS with or without WBRT (68). Fifty-eight patients with one to three brain metastases and recursive partitioning analysis (RPA) class I or II were randomized and stratified by RPA class, number of lesions, and radio-resistant histologies. SRS doses were similar to those in RTOG 9508 and the WBRT dose was 30 Gy in 12 fractions. The trial was stopped early due to decreased survival on the WBRT arm. More recently, Brown et al. presented data from 213 patients with one to three brain metastases who were randomized to SRS with or without WBRT. Decline in cognitive function, specifically immediate recall, memory, and verbal fluency, was more frequent with the addition of WBRT to SRS. Adjuvant WBRT did not improve overall survival despite better disease control in the brain (61). This data suggest that WBRT may cause excess neurocognitive dysfunction and that SRS alone is a new standard of care for patients with limited brain metastases.

Another area of increased interest involves the use of adjuvant SRS after surgical resection. Patchell et al. had previously shown the benefit of adjuvant WBRT in improving local control in the brain and in the resection cavity (59). However, with the fear of WBRT toxicities, some clinicians feel that SRS to the resection cavity can replace WBRT. Soltys et al. conducted a retrospective review of 72 patients with 76 resection cavities treated with SRS from 1998 to 2006 with a median margin dose of 18.6 Gy (range 15–30 Gy) (69). Local control of the resection cavity was 88% and 79% at 6 and 12 months, respectively, which compared favorably to historic controls. Unfortunately, other investigators have not been able to duplicate these impressive results (70). This may be due to the difficulty in identifying the postoperative resection cavity and targeting it with SRS. A clinical trial, NCCTG N107C, which randomized patients to adjuvant WBRT (37.5 Gy in 15 fractions) versus SRS to the surgical resection bed (12–20 Gy in a single fraction) has recently closed to accrual. Hopefully, the results from this trial will help settle the controversy regarding the effectiveness of adjuvant SRS.

WBRT Versus SRS

The current trend in radiation oncology is to utilize SRS alone while avoiding WBRT. In this approach, patients with a limited number of brain metastases are treated with SRS without WBRT and are closely monitored. If new intracranial metastases arise, repeat SRS is performed. The intent is to eliminate WBRT or at least delay it for as long as possible in order to avoid excess neurotoxicity.

One argument for SRS is that brain metastases may be oligometastatic, so there is only a need to treat the disease seen on MRI scan. However, older autopsy data refute this notion (71). In addition, several trials to support the use of WBRT and SRS showed an improvement in survival in patients who received both modalities. Pirzkall et al. reported that for patients with brain metastases without extracranial disease, the median survival following SRS alone was 8.3 months compared to 15.4 months for patients treated with SRS plus WBRT (72). A retrospective study from the Mayo Clinic reported an overall survival benefit in patients who received adjuvant WBRT after resection compared to those who did not (5 years, 21% vs. 4%) (73). Other studies suggest a high rate of intracranial failure and reduced local control when WBRT is omitted or delayed. In a phase III study from the Japanese Radiation Oncology Study Group, 99-1, patients were randomized to SRS alone versus SRS plus WBRT (74). The 6-month freedom from new brain metastases rate was 48% on the SRS alone arm and 82% on the SRS plus WBRT arm (P = .003). The actuarial 1-year brain tumor control rate for lesions treated with SRS was also better with SRS plus WBRT compared to SRS alone (86% vs. 70%). These studies point out that the failure to control intracranial disease by omitting or delaying WBRT may negatively impact local control and survival.

While neurologic status and quality of life can be impacted negatively by WBRT, the withholding of WBRT increases the intracranial failure rate, which may then worsen neurologic deterioration due to disease progression in the brain (75). In an effort to mitigate the neurocognitive toxicity associated with WBRT, neuro-protective agents and novel RT delivery techniques are being explored. NRG-CC001 is randomizing patients to WBRT with hippocampal avoidance plus the neuroprotector, memantine, versus standard WBRT with memantine. The results of this trial may support the delivery of WBRT with lower concern for cognitive decline.

Conclusions

- The use of WBRT is declining despite evidence supporting its efficacy.
- For patients with greater than four brain metastases, whole brain remains the standard of care.
- For patients with one to four brain metastases, SRS alone is a reasonable option with close surveillance for progressive brain disease.
- After resection of a brain metastasis, the question of adjuvant SRS to the resection cavity or WBRT will hopefully be answered by a randomized trial that has recently completed accrual.
- Innovative strategies with neuroprotective medications and novel RT techniques are being explored to mitigate neurocognitive decline in patients receiving cranial radiation for brain metastases.

END-OF-LIFE CARE

Palliative care is patient- and family-centered health care that focuses on pain and other distressing symptoms, while incorporating psychosocial and spiritual care according to the patient and family needs. Palliative care begins at diagnosis and should be delivered concurrently with disease-directed, life-prolonging therapy. When these therapies are no longer effective, palliative care becomes the main focus of care (8). Palliative care can improve both quality of life and survival when introduced early to patients with advanced cancer. In a seminal study, 151 patients with metastatic NSCLC were randomized to receive early palliative care plus standard oncologic care versus standard oncologic care alone (76). The palliative care intervention consisted of a meeting with a member of the palliative care team at least monthly, during which physical and psychosocial symptoms, goals of care, and decision making were addressed. Quality of life and mood were assessed at baseline and 12 weeks later. Early palliative care led to significant improvements in both quality of life and mood. As compared to patients receiving standard care, patients receiving early palliative care had less aggressive care at the end of life, but longer survival. Another study utilizing an early palliative care intervention showed benefit at 4 months in spiritual well-being, symptom severity, and satisfaction with care for patients with multiple tumor types, including lung, gastrointestinal (GI), genitourinary (GU), breast, and gynecologic cancers (77).

The American Society of Clinical Oncology (ASCO) convened a panel to issue a provisional clinical opinion on the integration of palliative care into standard oncologic care. The panel's expert consensus was that combined standard oncologic care and palliative care should be considered early in the course of illness for any patient with metastatic cancer and/or high symptom burden, because data have shown improvement in symptoms, quality of life, and patient satisfaction, with reduced caregiver burden (78). Therefore, oncologists should be encouraged to address their patients' symptoms early and continuously throughout the course of treatment, and to have open discussions regarding goals of care, particularly at transition points in treatment.

KEY POINTS

- Cough: Cough is one of the most common symptoms associated with lung cancer, and is treated primarily with antitussives and opiates. Dexamethasone is recommended for cough resulting from radiation pneumonitis.

- Dyspnea: The mainstays of treatment of dyspnea are oxygen, opiates, benzodiazepines, and nonpharmacologic measures.
- Intrathoracic symptoms: RT is an effective local palliative treatment if symptoms are localized. It can often accomplish urgent palliation of hemoptysis, airway obstruction, or SVC syndrome.
- Pain: Pain from bone metastases is treated with NSAIDs, opiates, and bisphosphonates or RANKL inhibitors. Neuropathic pain is treated with antidepressants and anticonvulsants, and opiates in severe cases.
- Bone metastases: External beam RT can provide significant palliation of pain from bone metastases in 50% to 80% of patients. In patients with more disseminated disease, radiopharmaceuticals can provide durable pain relief.
- Fatigue: Treat any correctable causes of fatigue, such as anemia, poor nutrition, and reduction or discontinuation of medications causing sedation. Encourage light exercise daily.
- Brain metastases: For patients with greater than four lesions, whole brain radiation remains the standard of care. For four or fewer lesions, SRS alone can be considered.
- Palliative care: Early introduction of palliative care services for patients with advanced lung cancer results in improvement in symptoms, quality of life, and patient satisfaction, with reduced caregiver burden.

REFERENCES

1. Walling AM, Weeks JC, Kahn KL, et al. Symptom prevalence in lung and colorectal cancer patients. *J Pain Symptom Manage*. 2015;49(2): 192-202.
2. Molassiotis A, Smith JA, Bennett MI, et al. Clinical expert guidelines for the management of cough in lung cancer: report of a UK Task Group on Cough. *Cough*. 2010;6:9.
3. Molassiotis A, Bailey C, Caress A, et al. Interventions for cough in cancer. *Cochrane Database Syst Rev*. 2015;5:CD007881.
4. Doona M, Walsh D. Benzonatate for opioid-resistant cough in advanced cancer. *Palliat Med*. 1998;12(1):55-58.
5. Pavesi L, Subburaj S, Porter-Shaw K. Application and validation of a computerized cough acquisition system for objective monitoring of acute cough: a meta-analysis. *Chest*. 2001;120(4):1121-1128.

6. Yancy WS, Mccrory DC, Coeytaux RR, et al. Efficacy and tolerability of treatments for chronic cough: a systematic review and meta-analysis. *Chest*. 2013;144(6):1827-1838.
7. Gross NJ. Pulmonary effects of radiation therapy. *Ann Intern Med*. 1977;86(1):81-92.
8. Levy M, Smith T, Alvarez-Perez A, et al. Palliative care version 1.2016. *J Natl Compr Canc Netw*. 2016;14(1):82-113.
9. Jennings AL, Davies AN, Higgins JP, et al. A systematic review of the use of opioids in the management of dyspnoea. *Thorax*. 2002;57(11):939-944.
10. Bezjak A. Palliative therapy for lung cancer. *Semin Surg Oncol*. 2003;21(2):138-147.
11. Bleehen NM, Girling DJ, Machin D, Stephens RJ. A Medical Research Council (MRC) randomised trial of palliative radiotherapy with two fractions or a single fraction in patients with inoperable non-small-cell lung cancer (NSCLC) and poor performance status. Medical Research Council Lung Cancer Working Party. *Br J Cancer*. 1992;65(6):934-941.
12. Bleehen NM, Girling DJ, Fayers PM, Aber VR, Stephens RJ. Inoperable non-small-cell lung cancer (NSCLC): a Medical Research Council randomised trial of palliative radiotherapy with two fractions or ten fractions. Report to the Medical Research Council by its Lung Cancer Working Party. *Br J Cancer*. 1991;63(2):265-270.
13. Teo P, Tai TH, Choy D, et al. A randomized study on palliative radiation therapy for inoperable non small cell carcinoma of the lung. *Int J Radiat Oncol Biol Phys*. 1988;14(5):867-871.
14. Simpson JR, Francis ME, Perez-Tamayo R, et al. Palliative radiotherapy for inoperable carcinoma of the lung: final report of a RTOG multi-institutional trial. *Int J Radiat Oncol Biol Phys*. 1985;11(4):751-758.
15. Macbeth FR, Bolger JJ, Hopwood P, et al. Randomized trial of palliative two-fraction versus more intensive 13-fraction radiotherapy for patients with inoperable non-small cell lung cancer and good performance status. Medical research council lung cancer working party. *Clin Oncol (R Coll Radiol)*. 1996;8(3):167-175.
16. Bezjak A, Dixon P, Brundage M, et al. Randomized phase III trial of single versus fractionated thoracic radiation in the palliation of patients with lung cancer (NCIC CTG SC.15). *Int J Radiat Oncol Biol Phys*. 2002;54(3):719-728.
17. Falk SJ, Girling DJ, White RJ, et al. Immediate versus delayed palliative thoracic radiotherapy in patients with unresectable locally advanced non-small cell lung cancer and minimal thoracic symptoms: randomised controlled trial. *BMJ*. 2002;325(7362):465.
18. Barton R, Kirkbride P. Special techniques in palliative radiation oncology. *J Palliat Med*. 2000;3(1):75-83.
19. Gollins SW, Burt PA, Barber PV, et al. Long-term survival and symptom palliation in small primary bronchial carcinomas following treatment with intraluminal radiotherapy alone. *Clin Oncol (R Coll Radiol)*. 1996;8(4):239-246.

20. Stout R, Barber P, Burt P, et al. Clinical and quality of life outcomes in the first United Kingdom randomized trial of endobronchial brachytherapy (intraluminal radiotherapy) vs. external beam radiotherapy in the palliative treatment of inoperable non-small cell lung cancer. *Radiother Oncol*. 2000;56(3):323-327.
21. Nunnelee JD. Superior vena cava syndrome. *J Vasc Nurs*. 2007;25(1): 2-5; quiz 6.
22. Roberts JR, Bueno R, Sugarbaker DJ. Multimodality treatment of malignant superior vena caval syndrome. *Chest*. 1999;116(3):835-837.
23. Rowell NP, Gleeson FV. Steroids, radiotherapy, chemotherapy and stents for superior vena caval obstruction in carcinoma of the bronchus: a systematic review. *Clin Oncol (R Coll Radiol)*. 2002;14(5):338-351.
24. Flounders JA. Oncology emergency modules: superior vena cava syndrome. *Oncol Nurs Forum*. 2003;30(4):E84-E90.
25. Wilson LD, Detterbeck FC, Yahalom J. Clinical practice. Superior vena cava syndrome with malignant causes. *N Engl J Med*. 2007;356(18):1862-1869.
26. García Mónaco R, Bertoni H, Pallota G, et al. Use of self-expanding vascular endoprostheses in superior vena cava syndrome. *Eur J Cardiothorac Surg*. 2003;24(2):208-211.
27. Van Den Beuken-Van Everdingen MH, De Rijke JM, Kessels AG, et al. Prevalence of pain in patients with cancer: a systematic review of the past 40 years. *Ann Oncol*. 2007;18(9):1437-1449.
28. Decroisette C, Monnet I, Berard H, et al. Epidemiology and treatment costs of bone metastases from lung cancer: a French prospective, observational, multicenter study (GFPC 0601). *J Thorac Oncol*. 2011;6(3):576-582.
29. Chow E, Harris K, Fan G, et al. Palliative radiotherapy trials for bone metastases: a systematic review. *J Clin Oncol*. 2007;25(11):1423-1436.
30. Fairchild A, Barnes E, Ghosh S, et al. International patterns of practice in palliative radiotherapy for painful bone metastases: evidence-based practice. *Int J Radiat Oncol Biol Phys*. 2009;75(5):1501-1510.
31. Lutz S, Berk L, Chang E, et al. Palliative radiotherapy for bone metastases: an Astro evidence-based guideline. *Int J Radiat Oncol Biol Phys*. 2011;79(4):965-976.
32. Yarnold JR. 8 Gy single fraction radiotherapy for the treatment of metastatic skeletal pain: randomised comparison with a multifraction schedule over 12 months of patient follow-up. Bone pain trial working party. *Radiother Oncol*. 1999;52(2):111-121.
33. Steenland E, Leer JW, Van Houwelingen H, et al. The effect of a single fraction compared to multiple fractions on painful bone metastases: a global analysis of the Dutch Bone Metastasis Study. *Radiother Oncol*. 1999;52(2):101-109.
34. Foro P, Algara M, Reig A. Randomized prospective trial comparing three schedules of palliative radiotherapy. Preliminary results. *Oncologia*. 1998;21:55-60.

35. Hartsell WF, Scott CB, Bruner DW, et al. Randomized trial of short-versus long-course radiotherapy for palliation of painful bone metastases. *J Natl Cancer Inst.* 2005;97(11):798-804.
36. Jeremic B, Shibamoto Y, Acimovic L, et al. A randomized trial of three single-dose radiation therapy regimens in the treatment of metastatic bone pain. *Int J Radiat Oncol Biol Phys.* 1998;42(1):161-167.
37. Kaasa S, Brenne E, Lund JA, et al. Prospective randomised multicenter trial on single fraction radiotherapy (8 Gy × 1) versus multiple fractions (3 Gy × 10) in the treatment of painful bone metastases. *Radiother Oncol.* 2006;79(3):278-284.
38. Nielsen OS, Bentzen SM, Sandberg E, et al. Randomized trial of single dose versus fractionated palliative radiotherapy of bone metastases. *Radiother Oncol.* 1998;47(3):233-240.
39. Roos DE, Turner SL, O'brien PC, et al. Randomized trial of 8 Gy in 1 versus 20 Gy in 5 fractions of radiotherapy for neuropathic pain due to bone metastases (Trans-Tasman Radiation Oncology Group, Trog 96.05). *Radiother Oncol.* 2005;75(1):54-63.
40. Sande TA, Ruenes R, Lund JA, et al. Long-term follow-up of cancer patients receiving radiotherapy for bone metastases: results from a randomised multicentre trial. *Radiother Oncol.* 2009;91(2):261-266.
41. ASTRO. Choosing Wisely, 2013. https://www.astro.org/choosing wiselylist
42. Friedell HL, Storaasli JP. The use of radioactive phosphorus in the treatment of carcinoma of the breast with widespread metastases to bone. *Am J Roentgenol Radium Ther.* 1950;64(4):559-575.
43. Blake GM, Zivanovic MA, Mcewan AJ, et al. Sr-89 therapy: strontium kinetics in disseminated carcinoma of the prostate. *Eur J Nucl Med.* 1986;12(9):447-454.
44. Sciuto R, Festa A, Pasqualoni R, et al. Metastatic bone pain palliation with 89-Sr and 186-Re-HEDP in breast cancer patients. *Breast Cancer Res Treat.* 2001;66(2):101-109.
45. Eary JF, Collins C, Stabin M, et al. Samarium-153-EDTMP biodistribution and dosimetry estimation. *J Nucl Med.* 1993;34(7):1031-1036.
46. Collins C, Eary JF, Donaldson G, et al. Samarium-153-EDTMP in bone metastases of hormone refractory prostate carcinoma: a phase I/II trial. *J Nucl Med.* 1993;34(11):1839-1844.
47. Serafini AN, Houston SJ, Resche I, et al. Palliation of pain associated with metastatic bone cancer using samarium-153 lexidronam: a double-blind placebo-controlled clinical trial. *J Clin Oncol.* 1998;16(4): 1574-1581.
48. Cleeland CS, Body JJ, Stopeck A, et al. Pain outcomes in patients with advanced breast cancer and bone metastases: results from a randomized, double-blind study of denosumab and zoledronic acid. *Cancer.* 2013;119(4):832-838.
49. World Health Organization. WHO's cancer pain ladder for adults, 2014. http://www.who.int/cancer/palliative/painladder/en

50. Swarm RA, Abernethy AP, Anghelescu DL, et al. Adult cancer pain. *J Natl Compr Canc Netw*. 2013;11(8):992-1022.
51. Smith EM, Pang H, Cirrincione C, et al. Effect of duloxetine on pain, function, and quality of life among patients with chemotherapy-induced painful peripheral neuropathy: a randomized clinical trial. *JAMA*. 2013;309(13):1359-1367.
52. Berger AM, Mooney K, Alvarez-Perez A, et al. Cancer-related fatigue, version 2.2015. *J Natl Compr Canc Netw*. 2015;13(8):1012-1039.
53. Tomlinson D, Diorio C, Beyene J, et al. Effect of exercise on cancer-related fatigue: a meta-analysis. *Am J Phys Med Rehabil*. 2014;93(8):675-686.
54. Mishra SI, Scherer RW, Snyder C, et al. Exercise interventions on health-related quality of life for people with cancer during active treatment. *Cochrane Database Syst Rev*. 2012;8:CD008465.
55. Yawn BP, Wollan PC, Schroeder C, et al. Temporal and gender-related trends in brain metastases from lung and breast cancer. *Minn Med*. 2003;86(12):32-37.
56. Sundström JT, Minn H, Lertola KK, et al. Prognosis of patients treated for intracranial metastases with whole-brain irradiation. *Ann Med*. 1998;30(3):296-299.
57. Patchell RA, Tibbs PA, Walsh JW, et al. A randomized trial of surgery in the treatment of single metastases to the brain. *N Engl J Med*. 1990;322(8):494-500.
58. Borgelt B, Gelber R, Larson M, et al. Ultra-rapid high dose irradiation schedules for the palliation of brain metastases: final results of the first two studies by the radiation therapy oncology group. *Int J Radiat Oncol Biol Phys*. 1981;7(12):1633-1638.
59. Patchell RA, Regine WF. The rationale for adjuvant whole brain radiation therapy with radiosurgery in the treatment of single brain metastases. *Technol Cancer Res Treat*. 2003;2:111-115.
60. Mehta M. The dandelion effect: treat the whole lawn or weed selectively. *J Clin Oncol*. 2011;29(2):121-124.
61. Brown P, Asher A, Ballman K, et al. NCCTG N0574 (Alliance): a phase III randomized trial of whole brain radiation therapy (WBRT) in addition to radiosurgery (SRS) in patients with 1 to 3 brain metastases. (Abstract). *J Clin Oncol*. 2015;33(18 suppl):LBA4.
62. Coia LR. The role of radiation therapy in the treatment of brain metastases. *Int J Radiat Oncol Biol Phys*. 1992;23(1):229-238.
63. Gaspar L, Scott C, Rotman M, et al. Recursive partitioning analysis (RPA) of prognostic factors in three Radiation Therapy Oncology Group (RTOG) brain metastases trials. *Int J Radiat Oncol Biol Phys*. 1997;37(4):745-751.
64. Sperduto PW, Chao ST, Sneed PK, et al. Diagnosis-specific prognostic factors, indexes, and treatment outcomes for patients with newly diagnosed brain metastases: a multi-institutional analysis of 4,259 patients. *Int J Radiat Oncol Biol Phys*. 2010;77(3):655-661.

65. Patchell RA, Tibbs PA, Regine WF, et al. Postoperative radiotherapy in the treatment of single metastases to the brain: a randomized trial. *JAMA*. 1998;280(17):1485-1489.
66. Shaw E, Scott C, Souhami L, et al. Single dose radiosurgical treatment of recurrent previously irradiated primary brain tumors and brain metastases: final report of RTOG protocol 90-05. *Int J Radiat Oncol Biol Phys*. 2000;47(2):291-298.
67. Andrews DW, Scott CB, Sperduto PW, et al. Whole brain radiation therapy with or without stereotactic radiosurgery boost for patients with one to three brain metastases: phase III results of the RTOG 9508 randomised trial. *Lancet*. 2004;363(9422):1665-1672.
68. Chang EL, Wefel JS, Hess KR, et al. Neurocognition in patients with brain metastases treated with radiosurgery or radiosurgery plus whole-brain irradiation: a randomised controlled trial. *Lancet Oncol*. 2009;10(11):1037-1044.
69. Soltys SG, Adler JR, Lipani JD, et al. Stereotactic radiosurgery of the postoperative resection cavity for brain metastases. *Int J Radiat Oncol Biol Phys*. 2008;70(1):187-193.
70. Narayana A. A Phase II trial of stereotactic radiosurgery boost following surgical resection for solitary brain metastases. *J Clin Oncol*. 2006; 24(18S):1552.
71. Khuntia D, Brown P, Li J, et al. Whole-brain radiotherapy in the management of brain metastasis. *J Clin Oncol*. 2006;24(8):1295-1304.
72. Pirzkall A, Debus J, Lohr F, et al. Radiosurgery alone or in combination with whole-brain radiotherapy for brain metastases. *J Clin Oncol*. 1998;16(11):3563-3569.
73. Smalley SR, Laws ER, O'fallon JR, et al. Resection for solitary brain metastasis. Role of adjuvant radiation and prognostic variables in 229 patients. *J Neurosurg*. 1992;77(4):531-540.
74. Aoyama H, Shirato H, Tago M, et al. Stereotactic radiosurgery plus whole-brain radiation therapy vs stereotactic radiosurgery alone for treatment of brain metastases: a randomized controlled trial. *JAMA*. 2006;295(21):2483-2491.
75. Regine WF, Huhn JL, Patchell RA, et al. Risk of symptomatic brain tumor recurrence and neurologic deficit after radiosurgery alone in patients with newly diagnosed brain metastases: results and implications. *Int J Radiat Oncol Biol Phys*. 2002;52(2):333-338.
76. Temel JS, Greer JA, Muzikansky A, et al. Early palliative care for patients with metastatic non-small-cell lung cancer. *N Engl J Med*. 2010;363(8):733-742.
77. Zimmermann C, Swami N, Krzyzanowska M, et al. Early palliative care for patients with advanced cancer: a cluster-randomised controlled trial. *Lancet*. 2014;383(9930):1721-1730.
78. Smith TJ, Temin S, Alesi ER, et al. American Society of Clinical Oncology provisional clinical opinion: the integration of palliative care into standard oncology care. *J Clin Oncol*. 2012;30(8):880-887.

Appendix A: TNM Classification for Lung Cancer

Table A.1 TNM classification for lung cancer: AJCC 7th edition

TNM descriptors		
Primary tumor (T)		
Tx	Primary tumor cannot be assessed, or the tumor is proven by the presence of malignant cells in sputum or bronchial washing but is not visualized by imaging or bronchoscopy	
T0	No evidence of primary tumor	
Tis	Carcinoma in situ	
T1	Tumor ≤3 cm in greatest dimension, surrounded by lung or visceral pleura, no bronchoscopic evidence of invasion more proximal than the lobar bronchus (not in the main bronchus); superficial spreading of tumor in the central airways (confined to the bronchial wall)	
	T1a	Tumor ≤2 cm in the greatest dimension
	T1b	Tumor >2 cm but ≤3 cm in the greatest dimension
T2	Tumor >3 cm but ≤7 cm or tumor with any of the following: Invades visceral pleura Involves the main bronchus ≥2 cm distal to the carina Associated with atelectasis/obstructive pneumonitis extending to hilar region but not involving the entire lung	
	T2a	Tumor >3 cm but ≤5 cm in the greatest dimension
	T2b	Tumor >5 cm but ≤7 cm in the greatest dimension
T3	Tumor >7 cm or one that directly invades any of the following: chest wall (including superior sulcus tumors), diaphragm, phrenic nerve, mediastinal pleura, or parietal pericardium; or tumor in the main bronchus <2 cm distal to the carina but without involvement of the carina; or associated atelectasis/obstructive pneumonitis of the entire lung or separate tumor nodule(s) in the same lobe	
T4	Tumor of any size that invades any of the following: mediastinum, heart, great vessels, trachea, recurrent laryngeal nerve, esophagus, vertebral body, or carina; or separate tumor nodule(s) in a different ipsilateral lobe	

(*continued*)

Table A.1 TNM classification for lung cancer: AJCC 7th edition (*continued*)

TNM descriptors		
Regional lymph nodes (N)		
Nx	Regional lymph nodes cannot be assessed	
N0	No regional node metastasis	
N1	Metastasis in ipsilateral peribronchial and/or ipsilateral hilar lymph nodes and intrapulmonary nodes, including involvement by direct extension	
N2	Metastasis in the ipsilateral mediastinal and/or subcarinal lymph node(s)	
N3	Metastasis in the contralateral mediastinal, contralateral hilar, ipsilateral or contralateral scalene, or supraclavicular lymph nodes	
Distant metastasis (M)		
Mx	Distant metastasis cannot be assessed	
M0	No distant metastasis	
M1	Distant metastasis	
	M1a	Separate tumor nodule(s) in a contralateral lobe; tumor with pleural nodules or malignant pleural (or pericardial) effusion
	M1b	Distant metastasis

Anatomic stage grouping: AJCC 7th edition

Stage	T	N	M
IA	T1a	N0	M0
	T1b	N0	M0
IB	T2a	N0	M0
IIA	T1a	N1	M0
	T1b	N1	M0
	T2a	N1	M0
	T2b	N0	M0
IIB	T2b	N1	M0
	T3	N0	M0

(*continued*)

Anatomic stage grouping: AJCC 7th edition (*continued*)

Stage	T	N	M
IIIA	T1	N2	M0
	T2	N2	M0
	T3	N2	M0
	T3	N1	M0
	T4	N0	M0
	T4	N1	M0
IIIB	T4	N2	M0
	T1	N3	M0
	T2	N3	M0
	T3	N3	M0
	T4	N3	M0
IV	T Any	N Any	M1a or 1b

Source: Edge S, Byrd DR, Compton CC, Fritz AG, Greene FL, Trotti A (eds). *AJCC Cancer Staging Handbook*. 7th ed. New York, NY: Springer; 2010:299-323. Used with the permission of the American Joint Committee on Cancer (AJCC), Chicago, Illinois. The original source for this material is the *AJCC Cancer Staging Manual, Seventh Edition* (2010) published by Springer Science and Business Media LLC, www.springer.com.

Table A.2 Proposed TNM classification for lung cancer: AJCC 8th edition

TNM descriptors	
Primary tumor (T)	
Tx	Primary tumor cannot be assessed or tumor proven by presence of malignant cells in sputum or bronchial washings but not visualized by imaging or bronchoscopy
T0	No evidence of primary tumor
Tis	Carcinoma in situ
T1	Tumor ≤3 cm in greatest dimension surrounded by lung or visceral pleura without bronchoscopic evidence of invasion more proximal than the lobar bronchus (i.e., not in the main bronchus) **T1a(mi)—Minimally invasive adenocarcinoma** **T1a—Tumor ≤1 cm in greatest dimension** **T1b—Tumor >1 cm but ≤2 cm in greatest dimension** **T1c—Tumor >2 cm but ≤3 cm in greatest dimension**

(*continued*)

Table A.2 Proposed TNM classification for lung cancer: AJCC 8th edition (*continued*)

T2	Tumor >3 cm **but ≤5 cm** or tumor with any of the following features: **Involves main bronchus regardless of distance from the carina but without involvement of the carina;** or invades visceral pleura;or **associated with atelectasis or obstructive pneumonitis that extends to the hilar region, involving part or all of the lung** **T2a—Tumor >3 cm but ≤4 cm in greatest dimension** **T2b—Tumor >4 cm but ≤5 cm in greatest dimension**
T3	**Tumor >5 cm but ≤7 cm in greatest dimension** or associated with separate tumor nodule(s) in the same lobe as the primary tumor or directly invades any of the following structures: chest wall (including the parietal pleura and superior sulcus tumors), phrenic nerve, and parietal pericardium
T4	**Tumor >7 cm in greatest dimension** or associated with separate tumor nodule(s) in a different ipsilateral lobe than that of the primary tumor or invades any of the following structures: **diaphragm,** mediastinum, heart, great vessels, trachea, recurrent laryngeal nerve, esophagus, vertebral body, and carina
Regional lymph nodes (N)	
Nx	Regional lymph nodes cannot be assessed
N0	No regional lymph node metastasis
N1	Metastasis in ipsilateral peribronchial and/or ipsilateral hilar lymph nodes and intrapulmonary nodes, including involvement by direct extension
N2	Metastasis in ipsilateral mediastinal and/or subcarinal lymph node(s)
N3	Metastasis in contralateral mediastinal, contralateral hilar, ipsilateral or contralateral scalene, or supraclavicular lymph node(s)
Distant metastasis (M)	
M0	No distant metastasis
M1	Distant metastasis present M1a Separate tumor nodule(s) in a contralateral lobe; tumor with pleural or pericardial nodule(s) or malignant pleural or pericardial effusion **M1b Single extrathoracic metastasis** **M1c Multiple extrathoracic metastases in one or more organs**

Note: Changes to the 7th edition are highlighted in **bold**.

Proposed anatomic stage groupings: AJCC 8th edition

Stage	T	N	M
Occult carcinoma	TX	N0	M0
Stage 0	Tis	N0	M0
Stage IA1	**T1a(mi)**	**N0**	**M0**
	T1a	**N0**	**M0**
Stage IA2	**T1b**	**N0**	**M0**
Stage IA3	**T1c**	**N0**	**M0**
Stage IB	T2a	N0	M0
Stage IIA	T2b	N0	M0
Stage IIB	**T1a–c**	**N1**	**M0**
	T2a	**N1**	**M0**
	T2b	N1	M0
	T3	N0	M0
Stage IIIA	**T1a–c**	**N2**	**M0**
	T2a–b	N2	M0
	T3	N1	M0
	T4	N0	M0
	T4	N1	M0
Stage IIIB	**T1a–c**	**N3**	**M0**
	T2a–b	N3	M0
	T3	**N2**	**M0**
	T4	N2	M0
Stage IIIC	**T3**	**N3**	**M0**
	T4	**N3**	**M0**
Stage IVA	**Any T**	**Any N**	**M1a**
	Any T	**Any N**	**M1b**
Stage IVB	**Any T**	**Any N**	**M1c**

Note: Changes to the 7th edition are highlighted in **bold**.
Source: Goldstraw P, Chansky K, Crowley J, et al. The IASLC Lung Cancer Staging Project: proposal for revision of the TNM staging groupings in the forthcoming (eighth) edition of the TNM classification for lung cancer. *J Thorac Oncol.* 2016;11:39-51.

Appendix B: Regional Lymph Node for Lung Cancer Staging

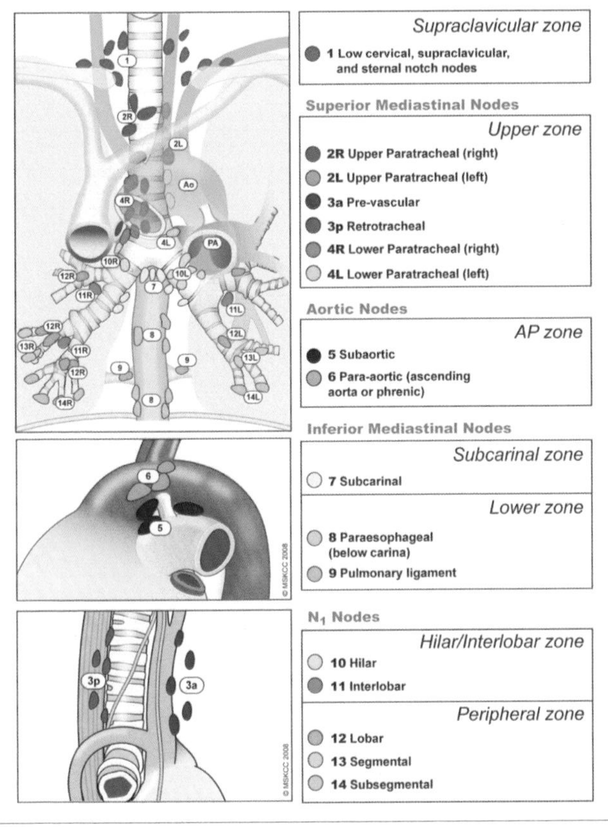

Figure B.1 Regional Lymph Node Stations for Lung Cancer Staging: The IASLC Lymph Node Map
Source: From Edge S, Byrd DR, Compton CC, Fritz AG, Greene FL, Trotti A (eds). *AJCC Cancer Staging Handbook*. New York, NY: Springer; 2010:303. Originally reprinted from *Journal of Thoracic Oncology*, 4(5), Valerie W. Rusch, et. al, The IASLC Lung Cancer Staging Project: A Proposal for a New International Lymph Node Map in the Forthcoming Seventh Edition of the TNM Classification for Lung Cancer, pp. 568–577, Copyright 2009, with permission from Elsevier.

Appendix C: Commonly Used Systemic Treatment Regimens

The following is not a comprehensive listing of all regimens that have been evaluated for patients with thoracic malignancies, but rather a list of the most commonly used regimens based on efficacy and tolerability. Some of the suggested doses and schedules differ from those in the cited references. These adjustments have been made primarily to improve tolerability and are based on clinical experience.

All drugs are administered intravenously (IV) and on day 1 of each cycle unless otherwise noted (e.g., PO = orally). Trial names and clinically relevant comments are provided in parentheses.

NON-SMALL-CELL LUNG CANCER

Adjuvant Chemotherapy—Stage IB–III

The regimens for which references are provided have been evaluated in randomized, adjuvant therapy trials. Other platinum-based regimens are acceptable based on equivalence noted in randomized trials in patients with advanced-stage disease. Cisplatin-based regimens are preferred in the curative setting, but carboplatin can be substituted if patients are ineligible for or intolerant of cisplatin.

a. Cisplatin 50 mg/m^2 days 1 and 8 + vinorelbine 25 mg/m^2 days 1, 8, 15, and 22 q 28 days × 4 cycles (JBR.10) (1)
b. Cisplatin 100 mg/m^2 day 1 + vinorelbine 30 mg/m^2 days 1, 8, 15, and 22 q 28 days × 4 cycles (ANITA; not favored due to high-dose cisplatin) (2)
c. Cisplatin 75 mg/m^2 day 1 + gemcitabine 1,000–1,200 mg/m^2 days 1 and 8 q 21 days × 4 cycles (ECOG 1505) (3)
d. Cisplatin 75 mg/m^2 + pemetrexed 500 mg/m^2 q 21 days × 4 cycles (ECOG 1505; non-squamous only) (3)
e. Cisplatin 75 mg/m^2 + docetaxel 75 mg/m^2 × 4 cycles (ECOG 1505) (3).
f. Cisplatin 80 mg/m^2 day 1 + etoposide 100 mg/m^2 days 1–3 q 21 days × 4 cycles (IALT) (4)
g. Carboplatin AUC 5 day 1 (or day 8) + gemcitabine 1,000 mg/m^2 days 1 and 8 q 21 days × 4 cycles

h. Carboplatin AUC 5 + pemetrexed 500 mg/m^2 q 21 days × 4 cycles (non-squamous only)
i. Carboplatin AUC 6 + paclitaxel 200 mg/m^2 q 21 days × 4 cycles (CALGB 9633) (5)

Combined Modality Therapy—Stage III

1. *Concurrent Chemoradiotherapy*
   a. Cisplatin 50 mg/m^2 days 1 and 8 + etoposide 50 mg/m^2 days 1–5 (or etoposide 100 mg/m^2 days 1–3) q 28 days × 2 cycles plus concurrent definitive thoracic RT 60 Gy (6)
   b. Cisplatin 75 mg/m^2 + pemetrexed 500 mg/m^2 q 21 days × 3 cycles plus concurrent definitive thoracic RT 60-66 Gy followed by consolidation pemetrexed 500 mg/m^2 q 21 days × 4 cycles (PROCLAIM; non-squamous only) (7)
   c. Carboplatin AUC 5 + pemetrexed 500 mg/m^2 q 21 days × 3 cycles plus concurrent definitive thoracic RT 64-68 Gy followed by consolidation pemetrexed 500 mg/m^2 q 21 days × 3 cycles (non-squamous only) (8)
   d. Carboplatin AUC 2 + paclitaxel 45 mg/m^2 once a week × 6 weeks plus concurrent definitive thoracic RT 63 Gy followed by consolidation carboplatin AUC 6 day 1 + paclitaxel 200 mg/m^2 day 1 q 21 days × 2 cycles (LAMP) (9)
   e. Carboplatin AUC 5 day 1 + etoposide 100 mg/m^2 days 1–3 q 28 days × 2 cycles plus concurrent definitive thoracic RT 60-66 Gy
2. *Neo-adjuvant Concurrent Chemoradiation*
   a. Cisplatin 50 mg/m^2 days 1 and 8 + etoposide 50 mg/m^2 days 1–5 (or etoposide 100 mg/m^2 days 1–3) q 28 days × 2 cycles with concurrent RT 45 Gy followed by surgical resection followed by cisplatin 50 mg/m^2 days 1 and 8 + etoposide 50 mg/m^2 days 1–5 (or etoposide 100 mg/m^2 days 1–3) q 28 days × 2 cycles (Intergroup 0139) (10)
   b. Carboplatin AUC 5 day 1 + etoposide 100 mg/m^2 days 1–3 q 28 days × 2 cycles with concurrent RT 45 Gy followed by surgical resection followed by carboplatin AUC 5 day 1 + etoposide 100 mg/m^2 days 1–3 q 28 days × 2 cycles

Advanced Disease: First-Line Therapy

1. *Driver Mutation-Negative—Squamous*

   Carboplatin-based regimens are favored in the palliative setting due to excessive nonhematologic toxicity associated with cisplatin.

   a. Carboplatin AUC 5 day 8 + gemcitabine 1,000 mg/m^2 days 1 and 8 q 21 days × 4–6 cycles (administering carboplatin on day 8 results in fewer dose reductions and treatment delays due to myelosuppression) (11)

b. Carboplatin AUC 5 day 1 + gemcitabine 1,000–1,250 mg/m^2 days 1 and 8 q 21 days × 4–6 cycles (12,13)
c. Carboplatin AUC 6 + paclitaxel 200 mg/m^2 q 21 days × 4–6 cycles (14)
d. Carboplatin AUC 6 day 1 + *nab*-paclitaxel 100 mg/m^2 days 1, 8, and 15 q 21 days × 4–6 cycles (14)
e. Cisplatin 75 mg/m^2 day 1 + gemcitabine 1,000–1,250 mg/m^2 days 1 and 8 q 21 days × 4–6 cycles (ECOG 1594) (15,16)
f. Carboplatin AUC 6 + docetaxel 75 mg/m^2 q 21 days × 4–6 cycles (TAX 326) (17)
g. Cisplatin 75 mg/m^2 day 1 + gemcitabine 1,250 mg/m^2 days 1 and 8 + necitumumab 800 mg days 1 and 8 q 21 days × 6 cycles followed by maintenance necitumumab 800 mg days 1 and 8 q 21 days (SQUIRE) (18)

2. *Driver Mutation-Negative—Non-Squamous*

   Carboplatin-based regimens are favored in the palliative setting due to excessive nonhematologic toxicity associated with cisplatin.

   a. Carboplatin AUC 5-6 + pemetrexed 500 mg/m^2 q 21 days × 4 cycles followed by maintenance pemetrexed 500 mg/m^2 q 21 days (PRONOUNCE) (19,20)
   b. Carboplatin AUC 5-6 + pemetrexed 500 mg/m^2 + bevacizumab 15 mg/kg q 21 days × 4–6 cycles followed by maintenance bevacizumab 15 mg/kg q 21 days *or* pemetrexed 500 mg/m^2 q 21 days (PointBreak; insufficient data to support the use of both bevacizumab *and* pemetrexed as maintenance therapy) (21)
   c. Carboplatin AUC 6 + paclitaxel 200 mg/m^2 + bevacizumab 15 mg/kg q 21 days × 4–6 cycles followed by maintenance bevacizumab 15 mg/kg q 21 days (ECOG 4599) (22)
   d. Cisplatin 75 mg/m^2 + pemetrexed 500 mg/m^2 q 21 days × 4 cycles followed by maintenance pemetrexed 500 mg/m^2 q 21 days (PARAMOUNT) (23)

3. *Driver Mutation-Negative—Elderly or PS 2*

   a. Gemcitabine 1,000–1,200 mg/m^2 days 1 and 8 q 21 days (MILES) (24)
   b. Pemetrexed 500 mg/m^2 q 21 days (non-squamous only) (25)
   c. Vinorelbine 25–30 mg/m^2 days 1 and 8 q 21 days (ELVIS) (26)
   d. Docetaxel 36 mg/m^2 days 1, 8, and 15 q 28 days (27)
   e. Carboplatin AUC 5 + pemetrexed 500 mg/m^2 q 21 days × 4 cycles (non-squamous only) (28)

   f. Carboplatin AUC 6 day 1 + paclitaxel 80 mg/m² days 1, 8, and 15 q 28 days × 4 cycles (IFCT-0501) (29)
   g. Carboplatin AUC 6 day 1 + *nab*-paclitaxel 100 mg/m² days 1, 8, and 15 q 21 days × 4 cycles (14)
4. *Driver Mutation-Negative — High PD-L1 Expression*
   a. Pembrolizumab 200 mg q 21 days (KEYNOTE-024; ≥50% tumor cells PD-L1-positive only) (76)
5. *EGFR Mutation-Positive*
   a. Erlotinib 150 mg PO QD (EURTAC) (30)
   b. Afatinib 40 mg PO QD (LUX-Lung 3; LUX-Lung 6) (31)
   c. Gefitinib 250 mg PO QD (IPASS) (32)
6. *ALK or ROS1 Rearrangement-Positive*
   a. Crizotinib 250 mg PO BID (33,34)

Subsequent Therapy

1. *Driver Mutation-Negative*
   a. Nivolumab 3 mg/kg q 14 days (CheckMate 017; CheckMate 057) (35,36)
   b. Pembrolizumab 2 mg/kg (or 200 mg) q 21 days (KEYNOTE-001; PDL1-positive only) (37)
   c. Docetaxel 60–75 mg/m² q 21 days (38,39)
   d. Docetaxel 30–36 mg/m² days 1, 8, and 15 q 28 days (40)
   e. Docetaxel 75 mg/m² + ramucirumab 10 mg/kg q 21 days (REVEL) (41)
   f. Pemetrexed 500 mg/m² q 21 days (non-squamous only) (42)
   g. Gemcitabine 1,000 mg/m² days 1 and 8 q 21 days (43)
   h. Erlotinib 150 mg PO QD (BR.21; patients not selected by EGFR mutation status) (44)
2. *EGFR Mutation-Positive*
   a. Osimertinib 80 mg PO QD (for EGFR T790M-positive progressive disease) (45)
3. *ALK Rearrangement-Positive*
   a. Alectinib 600 mg PO BID (46)
   b. Ceritinib 600–750 mg PO QD (750 mg QD frequently causes significant GI toxicity and fatigue, so reasonable to start at 600 mg QD) (47)

SMALL CELL LUNG CANCER

1. Limited-Stage Disease
   a. Cisplatin 75 mg/m² day 1 + etoposide 100 mg/m² days 1–3 q 21 days (q 28 days during RT) × 4 cycles with concurrent

RT 60–70 Gy with once-daily fractionation or 45 Gy with twice-daily fractionation (48)

b. Cisplatin 60 mg/m^2 day 1 + etoposide 120 mg/m^2 days 1–3 q 21 days (q 28 days during RT) × 4 cycles with concurrent RT 45 Gy with twice-daily fractionation or 60–70 Gy with once-daily fractionation (49)

c. Carboplatin AUC 5-6 day 1 + etoposide 100 mg/m^2 days 1–3 q 21 days (q 28 days during RT) × 4 cycles with concurrent definitive thoracic RT (50)

2. Extensive-Stage Disease
   a. Carboplatin AUC 5 day 1 + etoposide 100 mg/m^2 days 1–3 q 21 days × 4 cycles (51)
   b. Cisplatin 75 mg/m^2 day 1 + etoposide 100 mg/m^2 days 1–3 q 21 days × 4 cycles (52)
   c. Cisplatin 60 mg/m^2 day 1 + etoposide 120 mg/m^2 days 1–3 q 21 days × 4 cycles (53)
   d. Cisplatin 60 mg/m^2 day 1 + irinotecan 60 mg/m^2 days 1, 8, and 15 q 28 days × 4 cycles (54)
   e. Carboplatin AUC 4 + irinotecan 175 mg/m^2 q 21 days × 4 cycles (55)
   f. Carboplatin AUC 5 day 1 + irinotecan 50 mg/m^2 days 1, 8, and 15 q 28 days × 4 cycles (56)
3. Subsequent Therapy
   a. Topotecan 1.0–1.5 mg/m^2 IV days 1–5 q 21 days (1.5 mg/ m^2 is difficult to give due to excessive myelotoxicity and fatigue; 1.0–1.2 mg/m^2 days 1–4 or days 1–5 is more practical) (57,58)
   b. Topotecan 2.3 mg/m^2 PO days 1–5 q 21 days (59)
   c. Topotecan 3–4 mg/m^2 IV days 1, 8, and 15 q 28 days (60)
   d. Paclitaxel 200 mg/m^2 q 21 days or 80 mg/m^2 days 1, 8, and 15 q 28 days (61,62)
   e. Etoposide 50 mg/m^2 PO days 1–14 q 21 days (published as 50 mg/m^2 PO days 1–21 q 28 days with significant myelotoxicity and neutropenic fever) (63)
   f. Temozolomide 200 mg/m^2 PO days 1–5 q 28 days (64)
   g. Nivolumab 3 mg/m^2 q 14 days (CheckMate 032) (65)
   h. Cyclophosphamide 1,000 mg/m^2 + doxorubicin 45 mg/m^2 + vincristine 2 mg q 21 days (57)

MESOTHELIOMA

1. First-Line Therapy
   a. Cisplatin 75 mg/m^2 + pemetrexed 500 mg/m^2 q 21 days × 4–6 cycles (66)

   b. Cisplatin 75 mg/m^2 + pemetrexed 500 mg/m^2 + bevacizumab 15 mg/kg q 21 days × 4–6 cycles followed by maintenance bevacizumab 15 mg/kg q 21 days (67)
   c. Carboplatin AUC 5 + pemetrexed 500 mg/m^2 q 21 days × 4–6 cycles (68)
   d. Pemetrexed 500 mg/m^2 q 21 days (69)
2. Subsequent Therapy
   a. Gemcitabine 1,000–1,250 mg/m^2 days 1 and 8 q 21 days (70)
   b. Vinorelbine 30 mg/m^2 days 1, 8, and 15 q 28 days (71)

THYMOMA

1. First-Line Therapy
   a. Cyclophosphamide 500 mg/m^2 + doxorubicin 50 mg/m^2 + cisplatin 50 mg/m^2 q 21 days × 4–6 cycles (72)
   b. Cisplatin 60 mg/m^2 day 1 + etoposide 120 mg/m^2 days 1–3 q 21 days × 4–6 cycles (alternatively, cisplatin 75 mg/m^2 day 1 [or carboplatin AUC 5] + etoposide 100 mg/m^2 days 1–3 q 21 days × 4–6 cycles) (73)
2. Subsequent Therapy
   a. Pemetrexed 500 mg/m^2 q 21 days (74)
   b. Paclitaxel 200 mg/m^2 q 21 days or 80 mg/m^2 days 1, 8, and 15 q 28 days (75)

REFERENCES

1. Winton T, Livingston R, Johnson D, et al. Vinorelbine plus cisplatin vs. observation in resected non-small-cell lung cancer. *N Engl J Med.* 2005;352:2589-2597.
2. Douillard JY, Rosell R, De Lena M, et al. Adjuvant vinorelbine plus cisplatin versus observation in patients with completely resected stage IB-IIIA non-small-cell lung cancer (Adjuvant Navelbine International Trialist Association [ANITA]): a randomised controlled trial. *Lancet Oncol.* 2006;7:719-727.
3. Wakelee HA, Dahlberg SE, Keller SM, et al. E1505: adjuvant chemotherapy +/- bevacizumab for early stage NSCLC—outcomes based on chemotherapy subsets. *J Clin Oncol.* 2016;34:15S:436s.
4. Arriagada R, Bergman B, Dunant A, et al. Cisplatin-based adjuvant chemotherapy in patients with completely resected non-small-cell lung cancer. *N Engl J Med.* 2004;350:351-360.
5. Strauss GM, Herndon JE, Maddaus MA, et al. Adjuvant paclitaxel plus carboplatin compared with observation in stage IB non-small-cell lung cancer: CALGB 9633 with the Cancer and Leukemia Group B, Radiation Therapy Oncology Group, and North Central Cancer Treatment Group Study Groups. *J Clin Oncol.* 2008;26:5043-5051.

6. Hanna N, Neubauer M, Yiannoutos C, et al. Phase III study of cisplatin, etoposide, and concurrent chest radiation with or without consolidation docetaxel in patients with inoperable stage III non-small cell lung cancer: the Hoosier Oncology Group and U.S. Oncology. *J Clin Oncol.* 2008;26:5755-5760.
7. Senan S, Brade A, Wang L, et al. PROCLAIM: randomized phase III trial of pemetrexed-cisplatin or etoposide-cisplatin plus thoracic radiation therapy followed by consolidation chemotherapy in locally advanced non-small cell lung cancer. *J Clin Oncol.* 2016;34:953-962.
8. Choy H, Schwartzberg LS, Dakhil SR, et al. Phase 2 study of pemetrexed plus carboplatin or pemetrexed plus cisplatin with concurrent radiation therapy followed by pemetrexed consolidation in patients with favorable prognosis inoperable stage IIIA/B non-small cell lung cancer. *J Thorac Oncol.* 2013;8:1308-1316.
9. Belani CP, Choy H, Bonomi P, et al. Combined chemotherapy regimens of paclitaxel and carboplatin for locally advanced non-small cell lung cancer: a randomized phase II locally advanced multi-modality protocol. *J Clin Oncol.* 2005;23:5883-5891.
10. Albain KS, Swann RS, Rusch VW, et al. Radiotherapy plus chemotherapy with or without surgical resection for stage III non-small cell lung cancer: a phase III randomized controlled trial. *Lancet.* 2009;374:379-386.
11. Yoshimura M, Imamura F, Ueno K, et al. Gemcitabine/carboplatin in a modified 21-day administration schedule for advanced-stage non-small-cell lung cancer. *Clin Lung Cancer.* 2006;8:208-213.
12. Rudd RM, Gower NH, Spiro SG, et al. Gemcitabine plus carboplatin versus mitomycin, ifosfamide, and cisplatin in patients with stage IIIB or IV non-small-cell lung cancer: a phase III randomized study of the London Lung Cancer Group. *J Clin Oncol.* 2005;23:142-153.
13. Sederholm C, Hillerdal G, Lamberg K, et al. Phase III trial of gemcitabine plus carboplatin versus single-agent gemcitabine in the treatment of locally advanced or metastatic non-small-cell lung cancer: the Swedish Lung Cancer Study Group. *J Clin Oncol.* 2005;23:8380-8388.
14. Socinski MA, Bondarenko I, Karaseva NA, et al. Weekly nab-paclitaxel in combination with carboplatin versus solvent-based paclitaxel plus carboplatin as first-line therapy in patients with advanced non-small-cell lung cancer: final results of a phase III trial. *J Clin Oncol.* 2012;30:2055-2062.
15. Schiller JH, Harrington D, Belani CP, et al. Comparison of four chemotherapy regimens for advanced non-small-cell lung cancer. *N Engl J Med.* 2002;346:92-98.
16. Scagliotti GV, Parikh P, von Pawel J, et al. Phase III study comparing cisplatin plus gemcitabine with cisplatin plus pemetrexed in chemotherapy-naïve patients with advanced-stage non-small-cell lung cancer. *J Clin Oncol.* 2008;26:3543-3551.

17. Fossella F, Pereira JR, von Pawel J, et al. Randomized, multinational, phase III study of docetaxel plus platinum combinations versus vinorelbine plus cisplatin for advanced non-small-cell lung cancer: the TAX 326 Study Group. *J Clin Oncol.* 2003;21:3016-3024.
18. Thatcher N, Hirsch FR, Luft AV, et al. Necitumumab plus gemcitabine and cisplatin versus gemcitabine and cisplatin alone as first-line therapy in patients with stage IV squamous non-small-cell lung cancer (SQUIRE): an open-label, randomized, controlled phase 3 trial. *Lancet Oncol.* 2015;16:763-774.
19. Zinner RG, Obasaju CK, Spigel DR, et al. Randomized, open-label, phase III study of first-line pemetrexed + carboplatin followed by maintenance pemetrexed versus paclitaxel + carboplatin + bevacizumab followed by maintenance bevacizumab in patients with advanced non-squamous non-small-cell lung cancer. *J Thorc Oncol.* 2015;10:134-142.
20. Gronberg BH, Bremnes RM, Flotten O, et al. Phase III study by the Norwegian Lung Cancer Study Group: pemetrexed plus carboplatin compared to gemcitabine plus carboplatin as first-line chemotherapy in advanced non-small-cell lung cancer. *J Clin Oncol.* 2009;27:3217-3224.
21. Patel JD, Socinski MA, Garon EB, et al. PointBreak: a randomized phase III study of pemetrexed plus carboplatin and bevacizumab followed by maintenance pemetrexed and bevacizumab versus paclitaxel plus carboplatin and bevacizumab followed by maintenance bevacizumab in patients with stage IIIB or IV non-squamous non-small-cell lung cancer. *J Clin Oncol.* 2013;31:4349-4357.
22. Sandler A, Gray R, Perry MC, et al. Paclitaxel-carboplatin alone or with bevacizumab for non-small-cell lung cancer. *N Engl J Med.* 2006; 355:2542-2550.
23. Paz-Ares L, de Marinis F, Dediu M, et al. Maintenance therapy with pemetrexed plus best supportive care versus placebo plus best supportive care after induction therapy with pemetrexed plus cisplatin for advanced non-squamous non-small-cell lung cancer (PARAMOUNT): a double-blind, phase 3, randomised controlled trial. *Lancet Oncol.* 2012;13:247-255.
24. Gridelli C, Perrone F, Gallo C, et al. Chemotherapy for elderly patients with advanced non-small-cell lung cancer: the Multicenter Italian Lung Cancer in the Elderly Study (MILES) phase III randomized trial. *J Natl Cancer Inst.* 2003;95:362-372.
25. Weiss GJ, Langer C, Rosell R, et al. Elderly patients benefit from second-line cytotoxic chemotherapy: a subset analysis of a randomized phase III trial of pemetrexed compared with docetaxel in patients with previously treated advanced non-small-cell lung cancer. *J Clin Oncol.* 2006;24:4405-4411.
26. Effects of vinorelbine on quality of life and survival of elderly patients with advanced non-small-cell lung cancer. The Elderly Lung Cancer Vinorelbine Italian Study Group. *J Natl Cancer Inst.* 1999;91:66-72.
27. Lilenbaum R, Rubin M, Samuel J, et al. A randomized phase II trial of two schedules of docetaxel in elderly or poor performance status

patients with advanced non-small cell lung cancer. *J Thorac Oncol.* 2007;2:306-311.

28. Zukin M, Barrios CH, Pereira JR, et al. Randomized phase III trial of single-agent pemetrexed versus carboplatin and pemetrexed in patients with advanced non-small-cell lung cancer and Eastern Cooperative Oncology Group performance status of 2. *J Clin Oncol.* 2013;31:2849-2853.
29. Quoix E, Zalcman G, Oster JP, et al. Carboplatin and weekly paclitaxel doublet chemotherapy compared with monotherapy in elderly patients with advanced non-small-cell lung cancer: IFCT-0501 randomised phase 3 trial. *Lancet.* 2011;378:1079-1088.
30. Rosell R, Carcereny E, Gervais R, et al. Erlotinib versus standard chemotherapy as first-line treatment for European patients with advanced EGFR mutation-positive non-small-cell lung cancer (EURTAC): a multicentre, open-label, randomised phase 3 trial. *Lancet Oncol.* 2012;13:239-246.
31. Yang JC, Wu YL, Schuler M, et al. Afatinib versus cisplatin-based chemotherapy for EGFR mutation-positive lung adenocarcinoma (LUX-Lung 3 and LUX-Lung 6): analysis of overall survival data from two randomised, phase 3 trials. *Lancet Oncol.* 2015;16:141-151.
32. Mok TS, Wu YL, Thongprasert S, et al. Gefitinib or carboplatin-paclitaxel in pulmonary adenocarcinoma. *N Engl J Med.* 2009;361:947-957.
33. Solomon BJ, Mok T, Kim DW, et al. First-line crizotinib versus chemotherapy in ALK-positive lung cancer. *N Engl J Med.* 2014;371:2167-2177.
34. Shaw AT, Ou SHI, Bang YJ, et al. Crizotinib in ROS1-rearranged non-small-cell lung cancer. *N Engl J Med.* 2014;371:1963-1971.
35. Brahmer J, Reckamp KL, Baas P, et al. Nivolumab versus docetaxel in advanced squamous-cell non-small-cell lung cancer. *N Engl J Med.* 2015;373:123-135.
36. Borghaei H, Paz-Ares L, Horn L, et al. Nivolumab versus docetaxel in advanced non-squamous non-small-cell lung cancer. *N Engl J Med.* 2015;373:1627-1639.
37. Garon EB, Rizvi NA, Hui R, et al. Pembrolizumab for the treatment of non-small-cell lung cancer. *N Engl J Med.* 2015;372:2018-2028.
38. Shepherd FA, Dancey J, Ramlau R, et al. Prospective randomized trial of docetaxel versus best supportive care in patients with non-small cell lung cancer previously treated with platinum-based chemotherapy. *J Clin Oncol.* 2000;18:2095-2103.
39. Fossella FV, DeVore R, Kerr RN, et al. Randomized phase III trial of docetaxel versus vinorelbine or ifosfamide in patients with advanced non-small cell lung cancer previously treated with platinum-containing chemotherapy regimens. *J Clin Oncol.* 2000;18:2354-2362.
40. Di Maio M, Perrone F, Chiodini P, et al. Individual patient data meta-analysis of docetaxel administered once every 3 weeks compared with once every week second-line treatment of advanced non-small-cell lung cancer. *J Clin Oncol.* 2007;25:1377-1382.

41. Garon EB, Ciuleanu TE, Arrieta O, et al. Ramucirumab plus docetaxel versus placebo plus docetaxel for second-line treatment of stage IV non-small-cell lung cancer after disease progression on platinum-based therapy (REVEL): a multicenter, double-blind, randomized phase 3 trial. *Lancet.* 2014;384:665-673.
42. Hanna N, Shepherd FA, Fossella FV, et al. Randomized phase III trial of pemetrexed versus docetaxel in patients with non-small-cell lung cancer previously treated with chemotherapy. *J Clin Oncol.* 2004;22:1589-1597.
43. Crino L, Mosconi AM, Scagliotti G, et al. Gemcitabine as second-line treatment for advanced non-small cell lung cancer: a phase II trial. *J Clin Oncol.* 1999;17:2081-2085.
44. Shepherd FA, Pereira JR, Ciuleanu T, et al. Erlotinib in previously treated non-small-cell lung cancer. *N Engl J Med.* 2005;353:123-132.
45. Janne PA, Yang JC, Kim DW, et al. AZD9291 in EGFR inhibitor-resistant non-small-cell lung cancer. *N Engl J Med.* 2015;372:1689-1699.
46. Shaw AT, Gandhi L, Gadgeel S, et al. Alectinib in ALK-positive, crizotinib-resistant, non-small-cell lung cancer: a single-group, multicenter, phase 2 trial. *Lancet Oncol.* 2016;17:234-242.
47. Shaw AT, Kim DW, Mehra R, et al. Ceritinib in ALK-rearranged non-small-cell lung cancer. *N Engl J Med.* 2014;370:1189-1197.
48. Saito H, Takada Y, Ichinose Y, et al. Phase II study of etoposide and cisplatin with concurrent twice-daily thoracic radiotherapy followed by irinotecan and cisplatin in patients with limited-disease small-cell lung cancer: West Japan Thoracic Oncology Group 9902. *J Clin Oncol.* 2006;24:5247-5252.
49. Turrisi AT, Kim K, Blum R, et al. Twice-daily compared with once-daily thoracic radiotherapy in limited small-cell lung cancer treated concurrently with cisplatin and etoposide. *N Engl J Med.* 1999;340:265-271.
50. Bogart JA, Herndon JE, Lyss AP, et al. 70 Gy thoracic radiotherapy is feasible concurrent with chemotherapy for limited-stage small-cell lung cancer: analysis of Cancer and Leukemia Group B study 39808. *Int J Radiat Oncol Biol Phys.* 2004;59:460-468.
51. Socinski MA, Smit EF, Lorigan P, et al. Phase III study of pemetrexed plus carboplatin compared with etoposide plus carboplatin in chemotherapy-naïve patients with extensive-stage small-cell lung cancer. *J Clin Oncol.* 2009;27:4787-4792.
52. Fink TH, Huber RM, Heigener, et al. Topotecan/cisplatin compared with cisplatin/etoposide as first-line treatment for patients with extensive disease small-cell lung cancer: final results of a randomized phase III trial. *J Thorac Oncol.* 2012;7:1432-1439.
53. Hanna N, Bunn PA, Langer C, et al. Randomized phase III trial comparing irinotecan/cisplatin with etoposide/cisplatin in patients with previously untreated extensive-stage small-cell lung cancer. *J Clin Oncol.* 2006;24:2038-2043.

54. Noda K, Nishiwaki Y, Kawahara M, et al. Irinotecan plus cisplatin compared with etoposide plus cisplatin for extensive small-cell lung cancer. *N Engl J Med.* 2002;346:85-91.

55. Hermes A, Bergman B, Bremmes R, et al. Irinotecan plus carboplatin versus oral etoposide plus carboplatin in extensive small-cell lung cancer: a randomized phase III trial. *J Clin Oncol.* 2008;26:4261-4267.

56. Schmittel A, Fischer von Weikersthal L, Sebastian M, et al. A randomized phase II trial of irinotecan plus carboplatin versus etoposide plus carboplatin treatment in patients with extended disease small-cell lung cancer. *Ann Oncol.* 2006;17:663-667.

57. Von Pawel J, Schiller JH, Shepherd FA, et al. Topotecan versus cyclophosphamide, doxorubicin, and vincristine for the treatment of recurrent small-cell lung cancer. *J Clin Oncol.* 1999;17:658-667.

58. Huber RM, Reck M, Gosse H, et al. Efficacy of a toxicity-adjusted topotecan therapy in recurrent small cell lung cancer. *Eur Respir J.* 2006;27:1183-1189.

59. O'Brien MER, Ciuleanu TE, Tsekov H, et al. Phase III trial comparing supportive care alone with supportive care with oral topotecan in patients with relapsed small-cell lung cancer. *J Clin Oncol.* 2006;24:5441-5447.

60. Shipley DL, Hainsworth JD, Spigel DR, et al. Topotecan: weekly intravenous schedule similar to standard 5-day IV schedule as second-line therapy for relapsed small cell lung cancer—a Minnie Pearl Cancer Research Network phase II trial. *J Clin Oncol.* 2006;24(18S):384s.

61. Smit EF, Fokkema E, Biesma B, et al. A phase II study of paclitaxel in heavily pretreated patients with small-cell lung cancer. *Br J Cancer.* 1998;77:347-351.

62. Yamamoto N, Tsurutani J, Yoshimura N, et al. Phase II study of weekly paclitaxel for relapsed and refractory small cell lung cancer. *Anticancer Res.* 2006;26:777-781.

63. Johnson DH, Greco FA, Strupp J, et al. Prolonged administration of oral etoposide in patients with relapsed or refractory small-cell lung cancer: a phase II trial. *J Clin Oncol.* 1990;8:1613-1617.

64. Zauderer MG, Drilon A, Kadota K, et al. Trial of a 5-day dosing regimen of temozolomide in patients with relapsed small cell lung cancers with assessment of methylguanine-DNA methyltransferase. *Lung Cancer.* 2014;86:237-240.

65. Antonia SJ, Lopez-Martin JA, Bendell J, et al. Nivolumab alone and nivolumab plus ipilumumab in recurrent small-cell lung cancer (CheckMate 032): a multicenter, open-label, phase 1/2 trial. *Lancet Oncol.* 2016;17:883-895.

66. Vogelzang NJ, Rusthoven JJ, Symanowski J, et al. Phase III study of pemetrexed in combination with cisplatin versus cisplatin alone in patients with malignant pleural mesothelioma. *J Clin Oncol.* 2003;21:2636-2644.

67. Zalcman G, Mazieres J, Margery J, et al. Bevacizumab for newly diagnosed pleural mesothelioma in the Mesothelioma Avastin Cisplatin Pemetrexed Study (MAPS): a randomised, controlled, open-label, phase 3 trial. *Lancet*. 2015;387:1405-1414.

68. Ceresoli GL, Zucali PA, Favaretto AG, et al. Phase II study of pemetrexed plus carboplatin in malignant pleural mesotherlioma. *J Clin Oncol*. 2002;24:1443-1448.

69. Taylor P, Castagneto B, Dark G, et al. Single-agent pemetrexed for chemonaive and pretreated patients with malignant pleural mesothelioma. *J Thorac Oncol*. 2008;3:764-771.

70. van Meerbeeke JP, Baas P, Debruyne C, et al. Phase II study of gemcitabine in patients with malignant pleural mesothelioma. *Cancer*. 1999;85:2577-2582.

71. Steele JPC, Shamash J, Evans MT, et al. Phase II study of vinorelbine in patients with malignant pleural mesothelioma. *J Clin Oncol*. 2000;18:3912-3917.

72. Loehrer PJ Sr., Kim K, Aisner SC, et al. Cisplatin plus doxorubicin plus cyclophosphamide in metastatic or recurrent thymoma: final results of an intergroup trial. The Eastern Cooperative Oncology Group, Southwest Oncology Group, and Southeastern Cancer Study Group. *J Clin Oncol*. 1994;12:1164-1168.

73. Giaccone G, Ardizzoni A, Kirkpatrick A, et al. Cisplatin and etoposide combination chemotherapy for locally advanced or metastatic thymoma. A phase II study of the European Organization for Research and Treatment of Cancer Lung Cancer Cooperative Group. *J Clin Oncol*. 1996;14:814-820.

74. Loehrer PJ, Yiannoutsos CT, Dropcho S, et al. A phase II trial of pemetrexed in patients with recurrent thymoma or thymic carcinoma. *J Clin Oncol*. 2006;24(18S):383s.

75. Lemma GL, Lee JW, Aisner SC, et al. Phase II study of carboplatin and paclitaxel in advanced thymoma and thymic carcinoma. *J Clin Oncol*. 2011;29:2060-2065.

76. Reck M, Rodriguez-Abreu D, Robinson AG, et al. Pembrolizumab versus chemotherapy for PD-L1-positive non-small-cell lung cancer. *N Engl J Med*. Published online ahead of print on October 8, 2016. doi: 10.1056/NEJMoa1606774

Index

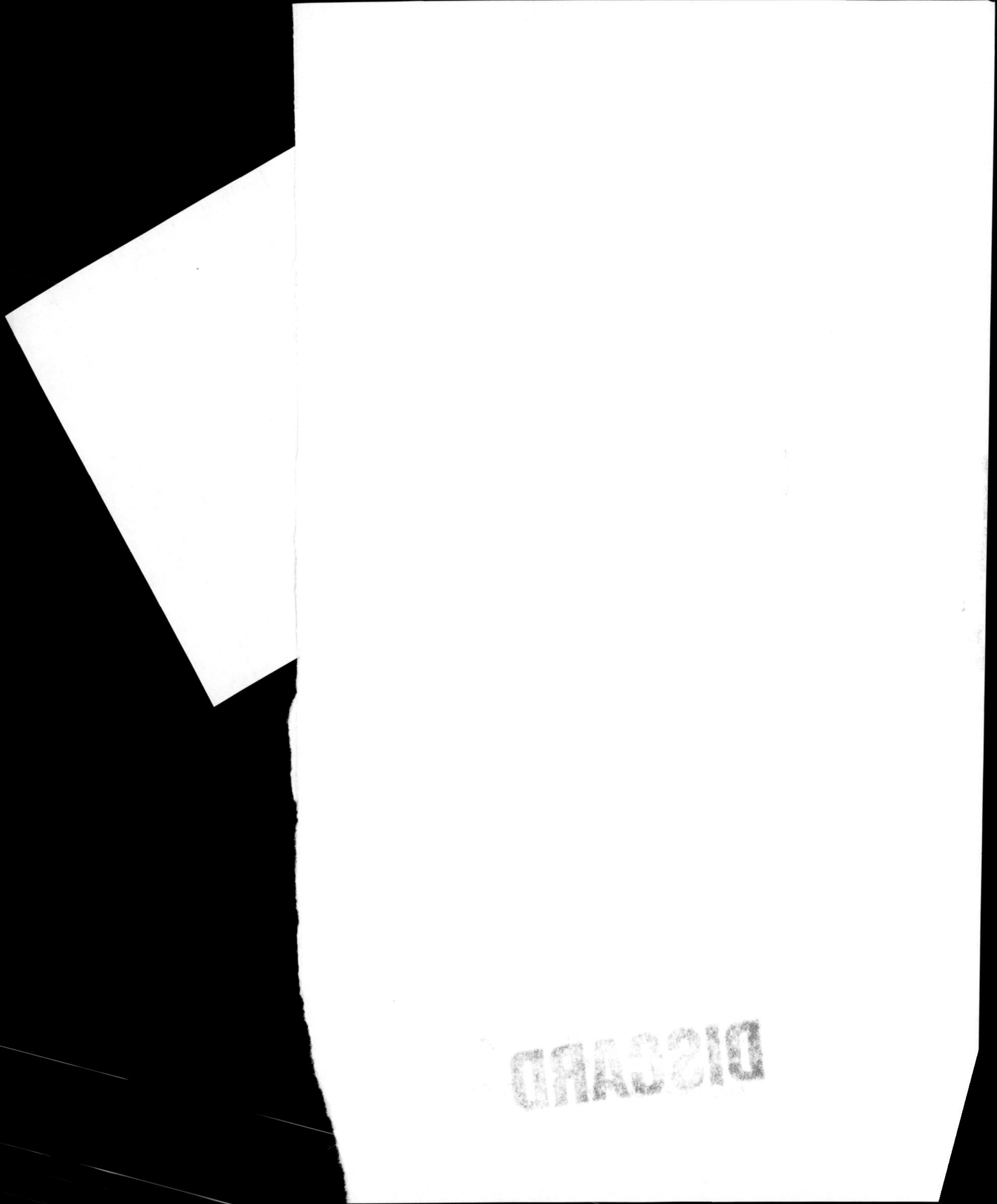

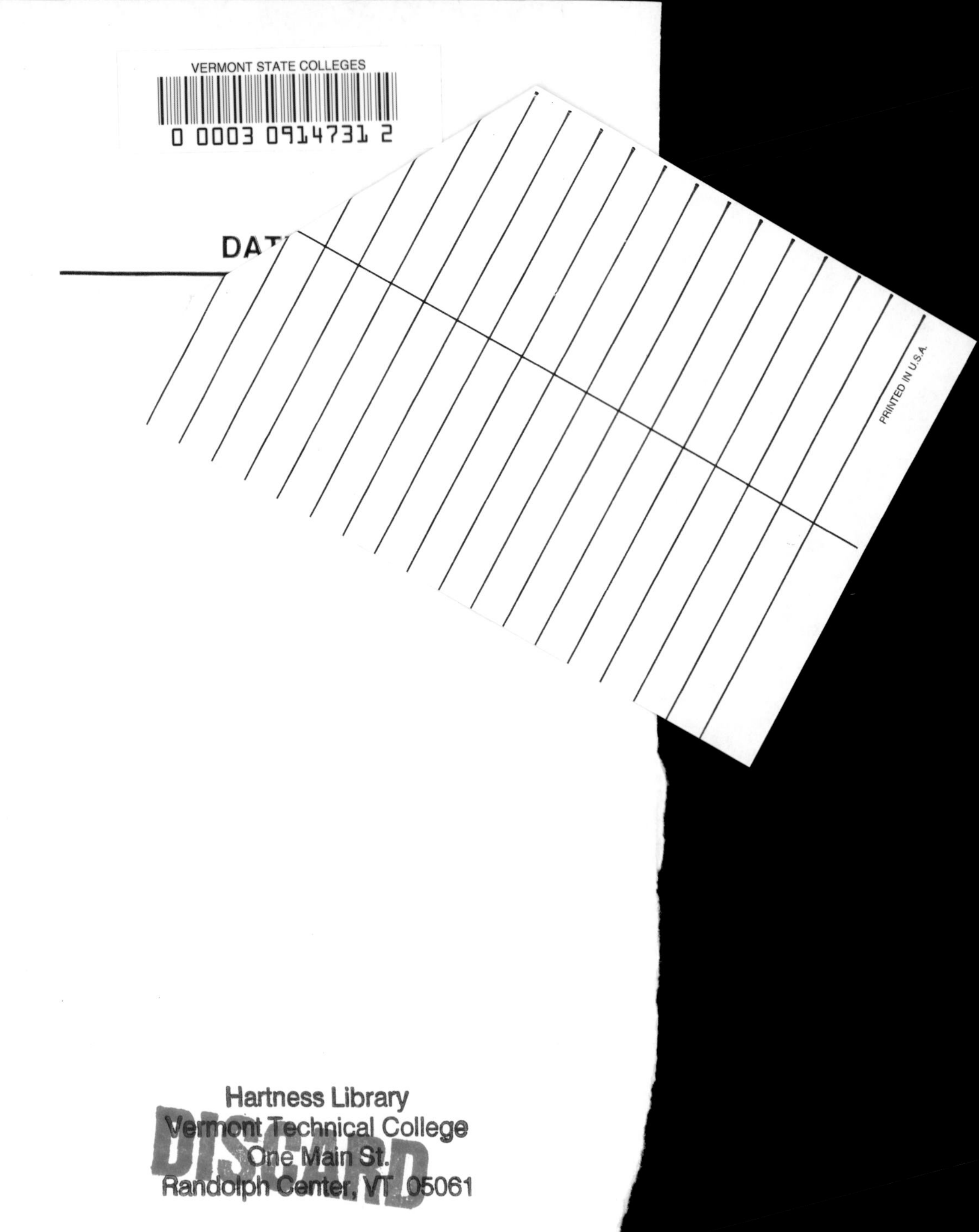
VERMONT STATE COLLEGES
0 0003 0914731 2
DAT
PRINTED IN U.S.A.